# Pain:

## Its anatomy, physiology and treatment

### Second Edition

## Aage R. Møller, PhD (DMedSci)

*The University of Texas at Dallas*

*Richardson, TX*

AAGE R MØLLER PUBLISHING 2014

PAIN: Its Anatomy, Physiology, and Treatment
By Aage R. Møller, Ph.D. (D. Med. Sci.) The University of Texas at Dallas
School of Behavioral and Brain Sciences,
800 W. Campbell Road
Richardson, TX 75080

Front cover by Monica Javidnia.
The anatomy picture is from Price, D.D., *Psychological and neural mechanisms of the affective dimension of pain*. Science, 2000. 288: p. 1769-1772, reprinted with the permission from AAAS. The insert picture is from Bingel, U. and I. Tracey, *Imaging CNS Modulation of Pain in Humans*, Physiology, 2008. 23: p. 371-380, reprinted by the permission of the American Physiological Society.

Dr. AAGE R. MØLLER is a Distinguished Lecturer in Behavioral and Brain Sciences and he is the Founders Professor of The University of Texas at Dallas.

Dr. Møller has a PhD, (DMedSci.) from the Karolinska Institut, (School of Medicine), Stockholm, Sweden. He was on the faculty of the Karolinska Institut for 10 years, on the faculty of the University of Pittsburgh School of Medicine for 19 years, first as Associate Professor of Otolaryngology, and later as Tenured Professor of Neurological Surgery. Since 16 years he is Professor of Cognition and Neuroscience at The University of Texas School of Behavioral and Brain Sciences.

He teaches courses on "Biology of Pain", "Human Functional Neuroanatomy", "Sensory Physiology", "Neural Plasticity and Disorders of the Nervous System" and "Intraoperative Neurophysiologic Monitoring, Part I and II" in the Neuroscience Program of The University of Texas at Dallas School of Behavioral and Brain Sciences.

ISBN-13: 978-1499206470
ISBN-10: 149920647X
© Aage R. Møller, Publishing, 2014

# Acknowledgements

The material in this book is based on my teaching of both undergraduate and graduate courses in the "Biology of Pain". I thank my students for their contributions to this book, for their comments and questions, My students' comments have improved many aspects of the book. I thank especially Jan Steinbrecher for valuable suggestions regarding the book. I specifically thank Paige Wahl for editing the manuscript of the first edition. I am grateful to Monica Javidnia and Irene Cunha for their work on many of the illustrations in the book. Monica Javidnia designed the front cover. Michael Wiseman copyedited the second edition of this book. It would not have been possible to write this book without the continuing support from The University of Texas at Dallas School of behavioral and Brain Sciences.

# List of abbreviations

5-HT: 5- Hydroxytryptophan (Serotonin)

**A**
ABL: Basolateral nucleus (of the amygdala)
ACC: Anterior cingulate cortex
ACE: Central nucleus (of the amygdala)
ACR: American College of Rheumatology
ACTH: Adenocorticotropic hormone
AD: Adenosine
ADP: Adenosine diphosphate
ADR: Adverse drug reactions
AL: Lateral nucleus (of the amygdala)
ALC: Acetyl-l-carnitine
ALS: Amyotropic lateral sclerosis
ALXR: Lipoxin A4 receptor
AMB: Nucleus ambiguous
AMPA: 2-amino-3-(5-methyl-3-oxo-1,2-oxazol-4-yl) propanoic acid
Amyg: Amygdala
ANS: Autonomic nervous system
AP: Anterior pituitary
ATP: Adenosine triphosphate

**B**
BA: Brodmann's area
BDNF: Brain derived neurotrophic factor
BG: Basal ganglia
BMI: Body mass index
BNST: Brainstem

**C**
CBD: cannabidiol
CCD: Chronic compression of the dorsal root ganglion
CCK: Cholecystokinin
CDG: Compression of the dorsal root ganglion
CG: Coeliac ganglion
CGRP: Calcitonin gene-related peptide
CI: Confidence interval
CN: Cardiac nerves
CNIV: Cranial nerve IV (trochlear nerve)
CNIX: Cranial nerve IX (glossopharyngeal nerve)
CNS: Central nervous system
CNV: Cranial nerve V (trigeminal nerve)
CNVII: Cranial nerve VII (facial nerve)
CNX: Cranial nerve X (vagus nerve)
CNXI: Cranial nerve XI (spinal accessory nerve)
COX-1: Cyclooxygenase 1
COX-2: Cyclooxygenase 2
CP: Central pain
CPSN: Central pain signaling neurons
CPSP: Central post stroke pain
CRPS-1: Complex regional pain syndrome - Type 1
CRPS-2: Complex regional pain syndrome - Type 2
CT: Computerized tomography
CTS: Carpal tunnel syndrome
CVLM: Caudal ventrolateral medulla
CWP: Chronic widespread pain

**D**
DBS: Deep brain stimulation
DH: Disc herniation
DLPFC: Dorsolateral prefrontal cortex
DLPT: Dorsolateral pontine tegmentum
DQ: Disability questionnaire
DRN: Dorsal reticular nucleus
DRG: Dorsal root ganglia
DRN: Dorsal raphae nucleus
DSM-IV: Diagnostic and Statistical Manual of Mental Disorders

**E**
EA: Electrical acupuncture
EAA: Excitatory amino acids
EMG: Electromyographic
ENK: Enkephalin
EPSP: Excitatory postsynaptic potential
ES: Effect of exercise
ESI: Epidural steroid injection

**F**
FDA: Food and Drug Administration (USA)
FM: Fibromyalgia
fMRI: Functional magnetic resonance imaging

**G**
GABA$_A$: Gamma amino butyric acid receptor - Type A
GABA$_B$: Gamma amino butyric acid receptor - Type B
GAD: Glutamic acid decarboxylase
GLT-1: Glutamate transporter-1
GPCR: G protein-coupled receptor
GPN: Glossopharyngeal neuralgia

**H**
HFS: Hemifacial spasm
HGN: Hypogastric nerve
HIV: Human immunodeficiency virus
HPA: Hypothalamus-pituitary-adrenal axis
HT: Hypothalamus
HTM: High threshold mechanoreceptors
HYP: Hypothalamus
HZ: Herpes zoster

**I**
IASP: International Association for the Study of Pain
IL-6: Interleukin-6
IL: Interleukin
ILC: Infralimbic cortex
IML: Intermediolateral cell column
INS: Insular cortex
IONM: Intraoperative neurophysiological monitoring
IR: Immunoreactivity
IS: Inflammatory soup

**K**
KA: Kainate A (glutamate receptor)

**L**
LC: Locus coeruleus
LEB: Lumbar epidural blockade
LOX: Lipooxygenase
LPb: Lateral parabrachial area
LTD: Long-term depression
LTM: Low threshold mechanoreceptors
LTP: Long-term potentiation
LTR: Local twitch response

**M**
M/SP: Myenteric or submucosal plexus
M1: Primary motor cortex
MA: Manual acupuncture
MARK: Mitogen-activated protein kinase
MCG: Middle cervical ganglia
MCP-1: Monocyte chemotactic protein-1
MDvc: Medial dorsal
MEG: Magnetoencephalography
MMP-2: Matrix metalloproteinase-2
MMPI: Minnesota Multiphasic Personality Inventory
mPFC: Medial prefrontal cortex
MRI: Magnetic resonance imaging
MSH: Melanocyte stimulating hormone
MVD: Microvascular decompression

**N**
NA: Norepinephrine
nAChRs: Nicotinic acetylcholine receptors
NG: Nodose ganglion
NGF-IR: NGF immunoreactivity
NGF: Nerve growth factor
NIDA: National Institute of Drug Abuse
NKA: Neurokinase A
NMDA: N-methyl-D-aspartate
NNT: Number needed to treat
NO; nitric oxide
NOR: Norepinephrine
NRM: Nucleus raphe magnus
NRS: Numeric Rating Scale
NSAID: Non-steroid anti-inflammatory drugs
NTS: Nucleus tractus solitarius

**O**
OR: Odds ratio

## P
PAF: Platelet activating factor
PAG: Periaqueductal gray
PBN: Parabrachial nucleus
PCC: Posterior cingulate cortex
PD: Parkinson's disease
PDN: Painful diabetic neuropathy
PET: Positron emission tomography
PG: Prostaglandins
$PGE_2$: Prostaglandins $E_2$
PHN: Post-herpetic neuralgia
PLP: Phantom limp pain
PMA: Premotor areas
PMv: Ventral premotor area
PN: Pelvic nerve
PND: Painful diabetes neuropathy
PNS: Peripheral nerve stimulation
PPC: Posterior parietal complex
PPS: Pulses per second
PTSD: Posttraumatic stress disorders

## Q
QSART: Quantitative sudomotor axon reflex test
QST: Quantitative sensory testing

## R
RA: Rheumatoid arthritis
RCT: Randomized controlled trials
RDA: Recommended daily allowance
RR: Risk ration
RSD: Reflex sympathetic dystrophy
rTMS: Repetitive transcranial magnetic stimulation
RVM: Rostral ventromedial medulla

## S
S: Stellate ganglion
S2: Secondary somatosensory cortex SA: Spontaneous activity
SCG: Superior cervical ganglia
SCS: Spinal cord stimulation
SG: Sympathetic ganglion
SI: Primary somatosensory cortex
SII: Secondary somatosensory cortex

SMA: Supplementary motor area
SMP: Sympathetic maintained pain
SNRI: Serotonin noradrenalin reuptake inhibitors
SP: Substance P
SPB: Spinoparabrachial
SPM: Pro-resolving lipid mediators
SSRI: Selective serotonin reuptake inhibitors
STT: Spinothalamic tract

## T
TAK1: Transforming growth factor-activated kinase 1
TCA: Tricyclic antidepressants
TENS: Transderm electrical nerve stimulation
TGN: Trigeminal neuralgia
THC: tetrahydrocanabidiol
TMD: Temporomandibular diseases
TMJ: Temporo-mandibular joint
TMS: Transcranial magnetic stimulation
TNF-alpha: Tumor necrosis factor alpha
TPA: Tissue type plasminogen activator
TRT: Tinnitus retraining therapy
TSN: Thoracic splanchic nerves
TTT: Trigothalamic tract
TX: Thromboxane

## U
UPR: Unfolded protein response

## V
VAS: Visual analog scale
VLM: Ventrolateral medulla
VMC: Vasomotor centers
VMpo: Ventromedial posterior (nucleus of thalamus)
VNS: Vagus nerve stimulation nerve stimulation
VPI: Ventral posterior inferior (nucleus of thalamus)
VPL: Ventral posterolateral (nucleus of thalamus)
VZV: Varicella zoster virus

## W

WDR: Wide dynamic range (nuclei)
WHO: World Health Organization

# Preface

Pain is complex; it can be regarded as an adverse phenomenon that deserves treatment to become eliminated, but at the same time, some forms of pain are absolutely necessary for a normal life. Pain often signals the need for changing behavior and it warns of dangers from trauma and diseases. Many people are afraid of pain; some are afraid of dying because they believe it will be painful. Some forms of pain may give pleasure to some individuals; it may have a role in sexual behavior. Some individuals with some diseases, such as autism, have an abnormal perception of pain.

The appearance of pain is complex. It may be regarded as a perception, but pain is not a sense like hearing and vision. Pain is often regarded to be a symptom of a physical disease. Pain in itself is not life threatening (except when it cases a person to commit suicide), but it decreases the quality of life.

Pain is a fascinating yet frightening subject, from wherever and however it is viewed. It has emotional features and medical features. Understanding its neuroanatomy and neurophysiology is interesting and challenging. Pain is often a symptom of trauma or a physical disease, but the cause of many forms of pain is unknown. Pain is common in various kinds of trauma, but the appearance of pain can be complex. Pain can last a short time (acute pain) or it can last a long time (chronic pain). While there are ample treatments available for acute pain, treatment of chronic pain and idiopathic pain, especially, is challenging, but rewarding.

Some forms of pain can be described as a physical stimulus that creates a mental perception. Other forms of pain are caused by pathologies or plastic changes in the spinal cord or brain. Some forms of pain are complex and are accompanied by other symptoms. For example, complex regional pain syndromes are disorders where abnormal activation of the autonomic nervous system plays an important role.

Neuropathic pain is often accompanied by an abnormal response to touch (allodynia) and to light to moderate painful stimulations (hyperpathia). Chronic inflammation and arthritis are common causes of chronic pain.

Pain may be purposeful and beneficial to an individual, it may be purposeful, but not beneficial to an individual, or it may not be purposeful nor beneficial to an individual person. Some forms of pain are life-saving bodily functions with a clear purpose. Other forms of pain have no benefit. Some forms of pain are just a nuisance. Chronic pain can cause severe suffering and it has a risk of being accompanied by affective disorders such as depression.

Treatment and management of pain is discussed in the book. Old treatments and their side effects are discussed together with treatments that have been developed only recently. The risks associated with commonly used painkillers; especially severe side effects such as lever damage are discussed in detail. The book describes recent studies of alternatives to common pain medication such as cannabis, which has been shown to be effective in relieving some forms of chronic pain that has been difficult to control using traditional medical treatments. The concept of a placebo and its role in the treatment and testing of treatments, especially of medications, is discussed. Coping with pain and how to learn to cope is an important aspect of pain management that will be discussed. The evolution of pain, the purposefulness, and the benefit to an individual of different kinds of pain will be discussed.

All that should induce interest from many branches of science, humanity, and medicine. Yet, pain is mostly disregarded in medical education despite about half of those who seek medical assistance do so for pain or have pain as a cause of the disease for which they seek help. The treatment of chronic pain is generally second-rate and often unsatisfactory. Pain occupies very small parts of textbooks of neuroscience, neurology, and psychology. Its anatomy and physiology are taught sparsely in our universities.

The book is an attempt to provide basic information about pain. It is focused on neuroscience, but it also discusses other aspects of pain including treatment. The reason is that I teach both an undergraduate and a graduate course on the biology of pain in our neuroscience program. This book will discuss pain as seen from many different angles. The book provides a comprehensive description of the anatomy and physiology of the different forms of pain. It will describe what we know about the anatomical, physiological, and chemical basis for pain. It discusses what can cause pain and how to reduce the risk of pain. It will also discuss the emotions of pain, suffering, and affective components, and how chronic pain may affect an individual person. The role of activation of neural plasticity in many forms of pain will be discussed. Finally, it will discuss how to treat pain and why so many people have untreated or poorly treated pain.

This book has three sections. The first section discusses general aspects of pain and the second section discusses pain caused by stimulation of specific receptors, nociceptors. The third section concerns pain that is not caused by stimulation of pain receptors, but instead caused by changes in the function of the spinal cord and the brain, induced by activation of neural plasticity. The third section discusses similarities between pain and other diseases that are caused by activation of neural plasticity.

There are pain conditions where the pathology is mixed with components of receptor induced pain and pain caused by functional changes in the spinal cord and the brain. An example is low back pain and it will be discussed in both sections.

This book
- Discusses pain as seen from many different angles
- Provides an understanding of what we know about the anatomical, physiological, and chemical basis for pain
- Discuses the emotions of pain, suffering, and affective components
- Discusses how chronic pain may affect an individual person
- Discusses coping with pain
- Discusses what can cause pain
- Discusses how to reduce the risk of pain
- Discusses treatment of pain

In summary, the book provides a multidisciplinary, comprehensive, and broad coverage of up-to-date knowledge about pain, including the anatomy and physiology of many forms of pain, and it explains the basis for many forms of treatment and management of pain including recently discovered treatments. The material is in a form that is suitable as a text for medical education and for those who do research in pain. The book is also written to make it useful for the informed patient.

The book is derived from my teaching of both undergraduate and graduate courses on the "Biology of Pain" in the Neuroscience Program in the School of Behavioral and Brain Sciences at The University of Texas at Dallas since 2008.

Dallas, April 2014
Aage R. Møller

# TABLE OF CONTENTS

# SECTION I
# BASICS ABOUT PAIN

## CHAPTER 1

*Introduction* ................................................................................................................. 11
*Why is it essential to understand pain?* ....................................................................... 12
*Why does the medical profession pay so little attention to pain?* ............................... 14
*How does this book address the subject of pain?* ....................................................... 16

## CHAPTER 2
## What is Pain

*Abstract* ....................................................................................................................... 19
*Introduction* ................................................................................................................. 20
*Pain is subjective* ........................................................................................................ 22
*Perception and interpretation of pain* ......................................................................... 24
    Pain has two different components .......................................................................... 24
*Classification of pain* .................................................................................................. 25
*Is pain a sense?* ........................................................................................................... 32
*Pain and cognition* ...................................................................................................... 32
    Personality profiles of chronic pain ......................................................................... 33
    Sensitivity to pain varies .......................................................................................... 33
    Catastrophizing ........................................................................................................ 34
*What can affect pain?* ................................................................................................. 35
    Pain may elicit body reactions ................................................................................. 37
*Benefit and purposefulness of pain* ............................................................................ 38
*Evolution of pain* ........................................................................................................ 39
*Pain as a diagnostic tool* ............................................................................................. 41
    Patients use different words to describe their pain .................................................. 42
    Amputation pain ....................................................................................................... 44
    Self-inflicted pain ..................................................................................................... 44
    Pain inflicted by other individuals ........................................................................... 45

*Neuroscience of pain* ........................................................................................................... *45*
    Is pain a disease? ............................................................................................................ 48
    Ways to reduce pain ....................................................................................................... 48
*Treatment of pain* ................................................................................................................ *48*
*What can cause pain and what can pain cause?* ............................................................... *50*
    What can cause pain? ..................................................................................................... 50
    What can pain cause? ..................................................................................................... 52
*Epidemiology of pain* ........................................................................................................... *54*
    Prevalence of pain .......................................................................................................... 55
    Chronic widespread pain (CWP) ................................................................................. 59
    How reliable are epidemiological data? ..................................................................... 60
*Pain and affective disorders* ................................................................................................ *60*

# SECTION II
# PHYSIOLOGICAL PAIN

## CHAPTER 3
## Somatic Pain

*Abstract* ................................................................................................................................. *65*
*Introduction* .......................................................................................................................... *67*
*Nature of somatic pain* ........................................................................................................ *68*
    Painful stimuli have a local effect ................................................................................ 70
    Tissue damage ................................................................................................................. 71
*Receptors for pain, heat, and cold and their innervation* ................................................ *72*
    Innervation of pain receptors ........................................................................................ 73
    Aδ and C-fibers carry different kinds of pain sensations ......................................... 74
    Bottom-up and top-down communication of pain signals ..................................... 75
    Neuroanatomy of somatic pain .................................................................................... 75
*The dorsal horn* .................................................................................................................... *75*
*The trigeminal nucleus* ....................................................................................................... *78*
*Pain pathways* ...................................................................................................................... *79*
*Ascending pain pathways* ................................................................................................... *80*
    Spinothalamic tract ........................................................................................................ 80
    Lateral spinothalamic tract ............................................................................................ 81
    Anterior spinothalamic tract ......................................................................................... 83
    Projections of C-fibers .................................................................................................... 84
*The spinomesencephalic and spinoreticular tracts* ......................................................... *86*
*The role of the vagus nerve* ................................................................................................ *87*

*Central projections of pain* ......................................................................................................... *89*
    The role of the thalamus ........................................................................................... 92
    The role of the dorsomedial thalamus ..................................................................... 92
    The amygdala ............................................................................................................. 94
*Anatomical basis for central modulation of physiological pain* ............................................. *96*
    Descending systems ................................................................................................... 97
    Periaqueductal grey (PAG) ........................................................................................ 99
    The rostral ventromedial medulla (RVM).............................................................. 100
    The dorsolateral pontomesencephalic tegmentum pathway (DLPT) ................. 102
*Other descending pathways* ..................................................................................................... *103*
*Itch* ............................................................................................................................................. *104*
    Itch receptors ............................................................................................................ 105
    Neural pathways ...................................................................................................... 106
    Central representation of itching ............................................................................ 106
    Discrimination between pain and itching ............................................................. 108
    Itching as a side effects of administration of opioid ............................................ 109

# CHAPTER 4
# Visceral Pain

*Abstract*...................................................................................................................................... *111*
*Introduction* ............................................................................................................................... *112*
*Anatomy* ..................................................................................................................................... *113*
    Receptors .................................................................................................................. 113
    Afferent nerve fibers ............................................................................................... 114
    Cardiac pain ............................................................................................................. 122
*Central pathways for visceral pain* .......................................................................................... *123*
    The vagus nerve and visceral pain ........................................................................ 123
    The vagus nerve and the illness response ............................................................. 125
    Visceral organ cross-sensitization .......................................................................... 127
*Referred pain* ............................................................................................................................. *127*
    An odd manifestation of referred pain ................................................................. 130
*The role of the sympathetic nervous system in visceral pain* ................................................ *130*
*Involvement of the dorsal column in deep pain* ..................................................................... *131*
*The role of the insula lobe in visceral pain* ............................................................................. *131*
    Deep sensations ....................................................................................................... 134

# CHAPTER 5
# Pain from Peripheral and Cranial Nerves
## The Role of Inflammation

*Abstract* ............................................................................................................................. 135
*Introduction* ..................................................................................................................... 136
*Different kinds of disorders of nerves* ............................................................................ 137
    Neuralgias ................................................................................................................... 137
    Painful neuropathies .................................................................................................. 139
    Mononeuropathies ..................................................................................................... 140
    Polyneuropathies ........................................................................................................ 145
    Neuritis (inflammation of nerves) ........................................................................... 146
    Trauma to peripheral nerves .................................................................................... 148
*How do nerves cause pain?* ............................................................................................ 149
    Slightly injured nerves ............................................................................................... 149

# CHAPTER 6
# Modulation of Physiological Pain

*Abstract* ............................................................................................................................. 153
*Introduction* ..................................................................................................................... 154
*Basis for modulation of physiological pain* ................................................................... 154
    Peripheral sensitization ............................................................................................. 155
    The role of the sympathetic nervous system in modulation receptor sensitivity ...... 157
    The role of inflammation .......................................................................................... 157
    Neural transmitters involved in peripheral sensitization ..................................... 157
    Development of mechanical hyperalgesia after injury ......................................... 160
    The gate control hypothesis ..................................................................................... 161
    Endogenous opioids modulate acute pain ............................................................. 163
    The role of the vagus nerve in control of pain ...................................................... 164

# CHAPTER 7
# Treatment of Physiological Pain

*Abstract* ............................................................................................................................. *165*
*Introduction* ...................................................................................................................... *166*
*Diagnosis of pain and its cause* ....................................................................................... *168*

*Pain medication (analgesics)* ........................................................................................... *168*
    Non-steroidal anti-inflammatory drugs (NSAID) ..................................................... 169
    Action of non-steroidal anti-inflammatory drugs (NSAID) ...................................... 175
*Opioids* ............................................................................................................................. *177*
    Action of opioids ........................................................................................................ 177
    Other side effects of administration of opioids ......................................................... 179
*Other analgesics* .............................................................................................................. *179*
    Non-analgesics that can relieve pain ......................................................................... 180
*Administration of pain medication* ................................................................................. *182*
*Tolerance and addiction* .................................................................................................. *184*
    Tolerance to opioids ................................................................................................... 184
    Addiction to opioids ................................................................................................... 184
    Sensitization from opioids ......................................................................................... 186
    Misconceptions of side effects of pain medications ................................................. 187
    The placebo effect ..................................................................................................... 187
*Treatment of the cause of pain* ....................................................................................... *188*
    Peripheral nerve neuropathy ...................................................................................... 188
*Electrical stimulation   (Neuromodulation)* .................................................................... *191*
    Surgical treatment of pain .......................................................................................... 191
    Reducing the risk of pain ........................................................................................... 192
*New avenues for treatment of physiological pain* .......................................................... *194*

# SECTION III
# PATHOLOGICAL PAIN

# CHAPTER 8
# Chronic Neuropathic Pain

| | |
|---|---|
| *Abstract* | 201 |
| *Introduction* | 203 |
| *What is chronic neuropathic pain?* | 204 |
| *Symptoms and signs of pathological pain* | 205 |
|     Perception of pain | 206 |
|     Coping | 206 |
|     Phantom sensations | 208 |
|     Hyperpathia | 209 |
|     "Wind-up" phenomenon | 209 |
|     Temporal integration at threshold | 210 |
|     Emotional components of pain | 212 |
|     Depression | 213 |
| *Causes of chronic neuropathic pain* | 214 |
| *Pathology of chronic neuropathic pain* | 216 |
|     Reorganization of central pain pathways | 218 |
|     The role of the dorsal horn (and the trigeminal nucleus) in causing chronic neuropathic pain | 219 |
|     Cortical representation of the body is dynamic | 222 |
|     Phantom limb syndrome | 224 |
| *Deafferentation pain* | 226 |
|     Cortico-thalamic loop abnormalities in deafferentation pain | 227 |
|     Perception of "self" and amputations | 229 |
|     Can pain influence body perception of "self"? | 230 |
| *Pain in connection with specific disorders* | 232 |
|     Pain after strokes | 233 |
|     Spinal cord injuries | 233 |
|     Parkinson's disease | 235 |
|     Alzheimer's disease | 235 |
|     Pain and motor disorders | 236 |
| *Neural structures especially involved in creating pathological pain* | 236 |
|     The role of changes in the dorsal horn of the spinal cord | 237 |
|     Wide dynamic range (WDR) neurons | 239 |

*Role of other parts of the brain* .................................................................................................. 241
    Motor cortical areas ................................................................................................... 241
    Limbic structures ....................................................................................................... 242
    The insula lobe ........................................................................................................... 242
    The role of the sympathetic nervous system on pain .............................................. 243
    Complex regional pain syndrome, CRPS I and II ................................................... 244
    Other complex pain conditions ................................................................................ 248
*Causes of low back pain* ..................................................................................................... 252
    Other forms of back pain ........................................................................................... 254
    Carpal tunnel syndrome ............................................................................................ 254
    Entrapment of other nerves ...................................................................................... 256
*Microvascular decompression disorders* ........................................................................... 256
*Transformations from acute pain into chronic pain* ........................................................ 258
    Cancer pain ................................................................................................................. 260

# CHAPTER 9
# Muscle Pain

*Abstract* ................................................................................................................................ 261
*Introduction* ........................................................................................................................ 262

*Pain from striate muscles* ................................................................................................... 262
    Muscle tone ................................................................................................................. 263
    Nature of muscle pain ................................................................................................ 264
    Anatomical and physiological basis for muscle pain ............................................. 264
    Cause of muscle pain ................................................................................................. 265
    Muscle spasm .............................................................................................................. 266
    How muscle contractions can cause pain ................................................................ 267
    Muscle pain that occurs together with other disorders ......................................... 269
    Fibromyalgia ............................................................................................................... 270
    Myofascial pain .......................................................................................................... 273
    Chronic fatigue syndrome ......................................................................................... 275
    Other diseases that have pain as one of their symptoms ....................................... 276

# CHAPTER 10
# Inflammatory Pain and the Immune System

*Abstract* ................................................................................................................................. 277
*Introduction* ........................................................................................................................... 278
*Mechanisms of inflammatory pain* ........................................................................................ 280
    Peripheral nerves ............................................................................................................ 282
    The role of the immune system in pain ......................................................................... 282
    Evolution of the immune system .................................................................................. 284
    The role of the immune system in strokes and other insults ....................................... 287
    The role of glial activation in pathological pain............................................................ 288
    The role of the immune system in opioid tolerance .................................................... 290

# CHAPTER 11
# Modulation of Pathological Pain

*Abstract* ................................................................................................................................. 293
*Introduction* ........................................................................................................................... 294
*Peripheral control of central pain* ......................................................................................... 295
    Central sensitization...................................................................................................... 295
*Central action of the sympathetic nervous system* ................................................................ 297
    Hyperactivity via the adrenal medulla ......................................................................... 298
*Central control of pain* .......................................................................................................... 298
    Central sensitization from prostaglandins and other prostanoids ............................... 300
    The role of activation of microglia in central sensitization ......................................... 302

*Role of descending pathways* ................................................................................................. 305
    Influence on LTP and LTD from glia activation ............................................................ 305
    Mental activity can modulate pathological pain........................................................... 306
    The reward system of the brain and pain ..................................................................... 309

# CHAPTER 12
# Treatment of Pathological Pain

*Abstract* .......................................................................................................................................... 311
*Introduction* ................................................................................................................................... 313
*Diagnosis* ....................................................................................................................................... 314
    Incorrect diagnosis ................................................................................................................... 315
    Which body part has the abnormal function that can cause pain? ....................................... 316
    Which components of pain should be aimed at treatment? ................................................... 318
*Methods used for treatment of pain in general* .......................................................................... 319
    Drug treatments ....................................................................................................................... 320
    Non-pharmacologic treatments .............................................................................................. 321
*Neuromodulation* .......................................................................................................................... 323
    Transdermal electrical nerve stimulation (TENS) ................................................................. 324
    Dorsal column stimulations .................................................................................................... 325
    Electrical Stimulation of the prefrontal and motor cortices .................................................. 326
    Use of repetitive transcranial magnetic stimulation .............................................................. 327
*The role of the vagus nerve in pain* ............................................................................................. 328
    Electrical stimulation of the vagus nerve ............................................................................... 329
*Acupuncture for relieving pain* .................................................................................................... 331
    Hypnosis ................................................................................................................................... 333
    Physical exercise ...................................................................................................................... 335
    Administration of treatments .................................................................................................. 335
*Surgical treatment of pain* ........................................................................................................... 336
*Treatment of specific pain disorders* .......................................................................................... 337
*Treatment of neuralgia* ................................................................................................................. 338
    Treatment of trigeminal neuralgia ......................................................................................... 338
    Treatment of virus induced neuralgias .................................................................................. 339
    Metabolic related peripheral nerve neuropathies ................................................................. 340
*Low back pain* ............................................................................................................................... 341
    Surgical treatment of low back pain ...................................................................................... 342
    Sciatica ...................................................................................................................................... 344
    Carpal tunnel syndrome .......................................................................................................... 344
*Deafferentation pain* ..................................................................................................................... 344
    Treatment of amputation pain ................................................................................................ 345
    Correcting distorted body image ............................................................................................ 346
    Treatment of pain from muscle spasms ................................................................................ 349
    Cancer pain ............................................................................................................................... 349
    Treatment of pain related to autonomic nervous system disorders ..................................... 350
*Stress and pain* .............................................................................................................................. 352
*Placebo effect* ................................................................................................................................ 352

*Examples of attempts to develop new methods for pain control* .................................................................. 353
   NMDA receptors ........................................................................................................................... 353
   Vitamins .......................................................................................................................................... 354
   Omega-3 ......................................................................................................................................... 355
*Immune reactions and pain* .................................................................................................................... 358
   Minocycline ................................................................................................................................... 360
*Reducing the risk of pain* ....................................................................................................................... 361
   Reducing the risk of amputation pain ......................................................................................... 362
   Importance of a person's life style .............................................................................................. 363

# APPENDIX A
# Neuroplasticity

*Appendix A* ............................................................................................................................................. 365
*Neuroplasticity* ....................................................................................................................................... 365
*Introduction* ........................................................................................................................................... 365
*What is neuroplasticity?* ........................................................................................................................ 366
   Implications of plastic changes .................................................................................................... 367
   Nature of plastic changes ............................................................................................................. 368
   What can activate neuroplasticity? .............................................................................................. 370

# APPENDIX B
# Brodmann's areas of the cerebral cortex

   Lateral surface of the brain .......................................................................................................... 371
   Medial surface ............................................................................................................................... 372

*References* .............................................................................................................................................. 375
*Subject index* .......................................................................................................................................... 397

# SECTION I
# BASICS ABOUT PAIN

## CHAPTER 1
## Introduction

Pain, however one views it, is a fascinating, yet frightening, subject. Understanding the neuroanatomy and neurophysiology of pain is interesting and challenging, and relatively simple compared to its subjective aspects. Pain is common; it is often a symptom of a single trauma or of a single physical disease. Pain is complex; it is often a symptom of many diseases and plays an important role in the diagnoses of those diseases. Pain is mysterious; it has many forms where its cause is unknown. Pain is complicated; it can be viewed as an adverse phenomenon that deserves treatment to become eliminated. Pain is beneficial; it protects the body from harm by signaling the need to change behavior and it serves as a warning signal of the dangers from trauma and disease, which is essential to leading a normal life. Pain is evolutionary; it has several forms that have evolved over time into life-saving bodily functions with a clear purpose.

Pain is temporal; it can last a short time (acute pain) or it can last a long time (chronic pain). Pain is emotional; it causes anger, frustration, depression, and even suicide. Pain is intense; it can cause people such immense fear that they are afraid to die because they believe it will be painful. Alternatively, pain can be pleasurable; some forms of pain may give pleasure to some individuals and it may have a role in sexual behavior. Ultimately, pain is subjective; it varies with each individual and their individual mental and physical health. For instance, some individuals with diseases, such as autism, can have an abnormal perception of pain. However, most forms of pain have no benefit to an individual.

The International Association for the Study of Pain (IASP) (2008) defines pain as: "an unpleasant sensory and emotional experience associated with actual or potential tissue damage or described in terms of such damage". As we will see later in this book, this is too narrow a definition of pain.

# Why is it essential to understand pain?

Pain is a major symptom in many medical conditions, and can significantly interfere with a person's life and general functioning [46]. Many forms of pain cause a reduction in the quality of life and the effect on a person may best be described as suffering. Chronic pain has been estimated to cost $ 50 Billion ($50,000 million) (annually in the USA with lower-back pain alone being the most common complaint affecting between 70 and 85 percent of adults at some time. Of these, it has been estimated that 7 million are partly or severely disabled according to Mehmet Oz, Time, March 2011. Other forms of pain also affect many people. Arthritis pain has been estimated to affect 5 million people and headaches affect an estimated 45 million people in the USA. The National Center for Health Statistics has estimated that 45 million people suffer from arthritis and back pain.

Pain caused by a primary lesion (physiological pain) or by a dysfunction in the nervous system (pathological pain) has been estimated to affect approximately 4 million people in the United States each year [75]. Often, pain is not associated with any condition of disease and no cause can be found, thus idiopathic pain.

In the United States, pain is the most common reason for seeking medical consultation or assistance and nearly half of those who seek treatment by a physician report that their primary symptom is pain [447]. The fact that about half of those who seek medical help either from their personal physician or from emergency services have pain as their primary complaint underlines the importance of pain both as a sign of disease and as a disease in itself that may or may not benefit from medical intervention.

The purpose of seeking medical attention for pain is twofold: the person with pain wants to know if the pain is a sign of a disease or, if that is not the case, the person want to have relief of her/his pain. There are many reasons why treatment of pain is challenging. The subjective nature of pain and the absence of objective tests that can determine the kind of pain and its intensity is one reason. Insufficient understanding of the pathophysiology of many of the different forms of pain is another reason for inadequate treatment of many forms of pain.

Albert Schweitzer (1953) recognized the seriousness of pain and made this following statement about pain:

"To the millions of people in every country who live and die in needless pain: We must all die. But if I can save him from days of torture, that is what I feel is my great and ever new privilege".

Pain is a challenge to the medical profession, which finds limited resources for alleviating the pain. Pain is often not given the attention it deserves from medical professions or from lay people. For instance, a person with pain is not viewed with the same degree of seriousness by his/her relatives and friends as a person with physical signs of disease. There are several reasons for this. One reason is that coverage of pain occupies very small parts of textbooks on sensory systems, neuroscience, neurology, and psychology, and pain is mostly disregarded in medical education. Teaching of the fundamentals of pain in medical schools in the United States is nearly non-existent. While the research literature about pain is abundant, readings that are suitable for teaching of medical students is limited.

# Why does the medical profession pay so little attention to pain?

This lack of attention from the medical profession may have several causes. Pain is rarely life threatening, it has no visible signs, and there are no imaging, chemical or electrophysiological tests that can tell how much or which kind of pain a patient has and if the patient has pain at all. Diagnosis of pain must be based on what the patient tells the medical professional. Patients use many different words to describe their pain.

The fact that pain itself has no physical signs sometimes results in suspicions of malingering (making up the symptoms) or making it more serious than it is. This can have the result of inadequate treatment and in legal matters; it has made jurors and judges to be suspicious regarding the seriousness of a person's pain.

Some of the disorders that have pain as a symptom have no effective treatment and the treatment must then focus on relieving the pain. While there are ample treatments available for acute pain, treatment of chronic pain and idiopathic pain, especially, is challenging, but rewarding. Some disorders that have pain as a symptom are treated surgically. Surgical treatment, in general, can cause trauma that can cause pain that persists for a long time (years) after the surgery. Often, pain cannot be eliminated, but reduced. This means management instead of curing.

Why is the medical profession unable to treat pain correctly? There are several obstacles to effective treatment of pain and many individuals with pain suffer unnecessarily because of the lack of available treatments or, more commonly, because of treatment that is not optimal or sometimes not beneficial to the patient at all. Most medical treatments have side effects of various forms. Treatment of pain is no exception. Some treatments even have a high risk of making the pain worse or causing a different from of pain. In most Western countries, including the USA, the use of the most effective pain medication (opioids) is restricted because of an often-misunderstood risk of addiction.

One important reason for failure in treatments is misdiagnosis and insufficient understanding of the pathophysiology of an individual patient's pain. Another reason is the lack of suitable treatments. The patient's general condition, such as lack of coping ability and pain-related affective disorders, is another reason for poor results of treatment distress. Poor understanding of instructions about treatment resulting in poor compliance with the administration of prescribed treatment is another factor that contributes to poor outcomes.

A considerable obstacle to effective control of pain is the way in which pain medications are administrated. Patients themselves almost always do it and that often involves errors that reduce the efficacy of the treatment and increase the risks of the treatment.

Our medical system and the sentiment of people in general is directed to treatment although it has been documented that prevention is often far more efficient and, in particular, has far less side effects. Pain is not an exception, and attempts to reduce the risk of severe pain are rarely used. This book discusses ways in which the risks of some forms of postoperative pain can be reduced.

Pain is an important diagnostic sign, but subject to many uncertainties and errors. The purpose of diagnosing pain is first and foremost to find out if the pain is a sign of a disease. If it is, the disease should be treated and, if successful, the pain will disappear. If the disease cannot be treated successfully or if no disease can be found, the pain should be the target of treatment attempts. Misdiagnosis of pain causes many treatments that are not beneficial to the patients, but harmful because of the side effects along with the economic harm that unnecessary treatment may cause to individuals and/or society.

The reasons listed above should induce interest from many branches of science, humanity, and medicine. Indeed, pain has attracted interest from people of diverse backgrounds. René Descartes (1596 – 1650), or Cartesius, a mathematician, philosopher of nature, and writer, was one of the first thinkers who devoted interest in pain. He regarded the reaction to pain as an example of an automatic function of the human body that could be emulated by mechanical devices in contrast to what he described as actions of the soul.

This dual function (dichotomy) of the human body has one part that is automatic and which may be emulated by man-made machines ("automat") and another part that is complex. Descartes referred to the complex functions as the soul and described it as a mind-body dichotomy. The dualism proposed by Descartes is still very much a part of modern science.

Despite great progress in understanding pain, there are many unknowns regarding the pathophysiology of pain. There are many misconceptions regarding the pathology and cause of many forms of pain along with several reasons why treatment of chronic pain is often unsatisfactory.

# How does this book address the subject of pain?

The purpose of this book is not only to understand the neuroanatomy and neurophysiology of pain, but also to understand its diverse symptoms. In this book, we will use the term physiological pain for the pain that is caused by activation of pain receptors (nociceptors) and the term pathological pain for the bad pain that is not caused by stimulation of nociceptors. Since these two groups of pain are different in their cause, in their nature, and, to a great extent, in their treatment, we will cover these two kinds of pain in separate sections.

The fact that neuroplasticity plays an important role in many forms of pain and that it is the main cause of a large group of chronic pain is emphasized in the book and thoroughly discussed.

Other classifications that are commonly used when describing and diagnosing pain are acute pain and chronic pain. Pain is also often classified according to the length of time it has lasted. These terms are used to discriminate between pain that lasts a short time (acute pain) from pain that lasts a long time (chronic pain). However, these terms are arbitrary and their classification is not related to the pathology. These two terms are poorly defined and the terms are often used in unscientific ways.

This book discusses physiological pain and pathological pain in two separate sections. It describes in detail our present understanding of the anatomy and physiology of physiological pain in Chapter 3 and pathological pain in Chapter 8. Chapter 8 discusses in detail the role of neuroplasticity and more recent additions to our understanding of the bases for some forms of pain, such as the role of the parts of the brain that only recently have been associated with pain.

This book provides a comprehensive description of the anatomy and physiology of different forms of both physiological and pathological pain. It describes the anatomical and physiological bases for important forms of pain such as acute and chronic pain, pain caused by bodily trauma, diseases causing pain from internal organs, and pain caused by functional changes in the spinal cord and the brain. Neuroplasticity that is activated in many forms of pain causing functional changes in the spinal cord and the brain is discussed. This book also discusses the results of many recent studies that show extensive functional connections between many regions of the brain that are involved in various forms of pain.

The close relationship between neuropathic pain and affective disorders is supported by studies that show evidence of the functional interactions between limbic structures, reward, distress, and memory structures. This book discusses what can cause pain and how to reduce the risk of pain.

Pain signals can be affected (modulated) by many systems in the spinal cord and the brain. Endogenous opiates are just one such means of modulating the neural activity of pain and thus, the intensity of pain. The autonomic nervous system plays an important role in both increasing and decreasing the strength of pain.

The autonomic nervous system, especially the sympathetic system, influences the receptors and the transmission of neural activity in the spinal cord and the brain, where higher central nervous system centers exert influence as well.

The emotional aspects of pain and suffering and coping with pain are discussed. How to learn to cope is an important aspect of pain management that will be discussed. Some of the emotional components, such as depression, fear, and other affective disorders that may accompany pain, are discussed. The book also discusses the anatomical and physiological bases for the treatment of different forms of pain. The concept of a placebo and its role in treatment and testing of treatments, especially of medications, is also discussed. The book also describes some new aspects on pain including some experimental treatments. Pain that occurs in connection with strokes and diseases, such as Parkinson's disease, fibromyalgia, and myofascial pain, will also be discussed.

The book describes which brain regions are involved in different forms of pain and what it means regarding understanding the development of different forms of pain, the prospect of intervention (management), and the effect of pain on an individual person.

The evolution of pain and the purposefulness and benefit to an individual of different kinds of pain are discussed.

More abstract matters, such as the purposefulness of pain and the negative effects of pain in relation to Darwinian developmental aspects, are also topics of this book. How neuroplasticity can contribute to "purposefulness" regarding pain and the difference between being purposeful and beneficial to an individual for different kinds of pain are discussed. In addition to the Darwinian "selection of the fittest", the brain has the ability to change its function to meet certain demands. How neuroplasticity at the same time can cause many of the negative effects of pain will also be discussed.

# CHAPTER 2
# What is Pain?

# Abstract

1. Pain can be caused by stimulation of pain receptors (nociceptors) or it can be caused by changes in the function of the spinal cord and the brain.

2. Pain caused by stimulation of pain receptors is known as physiological pain. Pain that is not caused by stimulation of pain receptors is known as pathological pain.

3. Physiological pain has a protective function and it can be a sign of disease.

4. Most forms of pathological pain have no benefit to the individual.

5. People's reaction to pain varies: it can be just a nuisance or it can affect a person's entire life negatively.

6. Pain has two different expressions, the perception or awareness of the pain and its negative effects that may be in the form of suffering.

7. Pain is often accompanied by allodynia (pain from normally innocuous stimuli such as a light touch) and hyperpathia (prolonged and exaggerated reactions to moderate pain stimulations such as a needle prick).

8. Pain itself is subjective and it has no physical signs in itself, but it may activate the autonomic system and cause muscle contractions and arouse fear.

9. The term central neuropathic pain is used for pain caused by changes in the function of the spinal cord and the brain created by activation of neuroplasticity.

10. Some diseases have pain as a part of their symptom complex, such as fibromyalgia, chronic widespread pain, and chronic fatigue syndrome.

11. Amputations of limbs cause specific forms of pain.

12. Pain may occur together with disorders such as stroke and Parkinson's disease.

13. The main complaint by people with excessive and prolonged muscle contractions, such as spasmodic torticollis, is pain (from the strong muscle contractions).

14. Different people react differently to pain and there is a relation to ethnic origin.

15. Pain is an important diagnostic tool, but its use is hampered by the fact that different people use different words to describe their pain, and that the patient's testimony cannot be verified by objective tests. Distraction affects perception of pain and there is a strong placebo effect.

16. Since approximately half of those who seek medical help have pain, treatment of pain is an important part of clinical medicine. While many forms of pain can be treated effectively by readily available pain medication, there are also forms of pain that are difficult to treat effectively.

17. Pain can affect many body functions, such as the autonomic nervous system, and it can increase blood pressure, which in turn, increases the risk of strokes and heart attacks.

# Introduction

Pain has important protective functions in warning about dangers from the environment and from inside of the body (diseases). This is good pain serving an important function for survival. Pain is often a sign of disease and plays an important role in the diagnosis of many diseases. However, most forms of pain provide no benefit to people and have only negative effects, reducing the quality of life. This form of pain, that we will call bad pain, may be regarded as a disease that should be treated to alleviate the pain. The best way of treating pain is naturally to treat the disease that causes the pain. In many situations, this is not possible and often no cause of a person's pain can be found (idiopathic pain). (Treatments of pain will be discussed in Chapters 7 and 12.) In this chapter, we will first discuss the biology of pain, which is important for the treatment or for the management of pain that cannot be totally alleviated by treatment.

Pain that only has negative effects on a person (bad pain) has many forms and causes many different reactions that can be different for different individuals. Severe pain can affect a person's entire life in major ways. It can prevent or disturb sleep and it can interfere with or prevent intellectual work. In any form, pain reduces the quality of life.

Pain itself is rarely associated with any physical signs. A person with pain has no visible signs of disease. Therefore, pain is often not given the attention it deserves from medical professions, and a person with pain is not viewed with the same degree of seriousness by his/her relatives and friends as a person with physical signs of disease.

That pain itself has no physical signs sometimes results in suspicions of malingering (making up the symptoms) or making it more serious than it is. This can have the result of inadequate treatment and in legal matters; it has made jurors and judges suspicious about the validity and the seriousness of a person's pain.

Pain is a challenge to the medical profession, which finds limited resources for alleviating the pain. Treatment of pain is also hampered by the fact that there is no objective method that can verify a person's testimony about the severity of his/her pain and which can monitor the effect of treatment.

The lack of physical signs of pain affects the way a person with pain is viewed by relatives and sometimes also with health care professionals, as has been recognized many years ago:

"The only tolerable pain is someone else's pain"
René Leriche, French surgeon (1879–1955)

The International Association for the Study of Pain (IASP) (2008) described pain as: "an unpleasant sensory and emotional experience associated with actual or potential tissue damage or described in terms of such damage". This is too narrow a definition; it includes only the experience of pain, and it especially does not include the effect of pain on the body and does not cover such forms of pathological pain that are caused by changes in the function of the central nervous system (spinal cord and brain) without stimulation of pain receptors.

Other similar kinds of pain are myofascial pain, the pain in fibromyalgia, and pain that occurs together with other disorders such as strokes and Parkinson's disease. We will discuss these disorders in Section II.

There are two main kinds of pain: pain that is caused by activation of pain receptors and pain that is not caused by activation of pain receptors, but instead is caused by changes in the function of the central nervous system (spinal cord and brain). These two kinds of pain are known as physiological pain and pathological pain, respectively. In this book, separate sections are devoted to these two kinds of pain (Sections II and III).

# Pain is subjective

Pain is a self-experience that depends on the circumstances under which it appears. Pain has no physical signs and there are no objective tests that can determine the degree of pain that a person has. In fact, no tests can tell if a person has pain at all. Both physiological pain and pathological pain occur with widely different intensities and their effect on an individual person varies widely. Only the person who has the pain can evaluate the severity of his/her pain. There are no objective methods that can determine the intensity of pain. The lack of outside signs on the person who has pain can lead to underestimation of the severity of a person's pain.

Some forms of pain may be regarded as just a nuisance; however, other forms can severely reduce the quality of life. Some forms of severe pain are best described as causing suffering and may lead to suicide. Thus, pain occurs with a wide range of severity, may cause a large degree of suffering, and may affect the entire life of a person.

Pain is not a single sensation, but a complete package that cannot be separated from other feelings such as that of fear or misery. Perceived intensity of pain often depends on the circumstances. Pain has been defined as "an unpleasant sensory and emotional experience associated with actual and potential tissue damage, or described in terms of such damage" according to Turk and Okifuji [448]. However, this definition does not cover such forms of pathological pain that are caused by changes in the function of the central nervous system (spinal cord and brain) without stimulation of pain receptors. Other similar kinds of pain are myofascial pain, the pain in fibromyalgia, and pain that occurs together with other disorders such as strokes and Parkinson's disease. We will discuss these disorders in Section II.

The lack of visible signs of pain can lead to underestimation of the severity of pain by a person's relatives and friends and even by his/her physicians. The lack of physical signs has lead judges to reduce the compensation awarded in malpractice suits involving a patient who was caused severe pain because the judge could not see any signs of pain and, therefore, was not really sure that the person did have pain.

Pain activates many different circuits in the brain including circuits such as those of the reward system. Severe pain involves the emotional part of the brain such as the amygdala and anterior cingulate cortex. This can explain why the effect of pain on a person is complex and subject to variations that can be elicited by many factors.

Pain can cause fear because of the suspicion that it is a sign of a serious disease. It can cause fear in general because it activates centers in the brain that are associated with fear. Affective disorders, such as depression, occur more often in individuals with severe pain than in individuals who do not have pain.

Pain is more related to suffering than to any other descriptions, but the degree of suffering varies between individuals and within a given individual. Factors, such as helplessness and expectation, are important for the perception of the degree of pain. What matters for an individual person, as well as for the physician who treats the person, is the person's perception of the severity of the pain.

Pain is a highly subjective matter that is related to the individual's expectation and evaluation of the cause of the pain. It very much depends on the individual's control over the situations related to whether the pain is escapable or inescapable. A person in who the suffering is under good control, but who still has pain may say, "I have pain, but pain does not have me." Catastrophizing [125, 167, 449] is the opposite, namely making the suffering worse. Catastrophizing and coping with pain are two extreme reactions to pain. Coping is a learned skill that can avoid the decrease in quality of life that is often associated with pain. Catastrophizing involves increased worrying and irrational thoughts.

A person can tolerate much more pain if it is known that it is limited in time or that the individual can control the pain such as pain experienced during dental work. The perception of pain depends on whether it is under the control of the individual (escapable) or not (inescapable) [240]. If it is possible to request a local anesthesia, many patients can endure more pain than they were prepared to if no relief was available.

This means that there is a difference in the reaction to escapable and inescapable pain. This difference is even reflected in the involvement of different anatomical parts of the periaqueductal gray (PAG) [203, 240], especially with pain of deep origin (muscles, joints, and viscera).

A person's ability to cope with pain is important. Coping is a learned skill and teaching how to cope with pain would be helpful and would alleviate much suffering.

# Perception and interpretation of pain

Perception of pain is created in a similar way as the perception of sensory signals where ambiguous images or sounds are interpreted with the help of memory and the final interpretation is assumed to be achieved by comparing the sensory input to models that reside in memory. In the same way as sensory perceptions of the same stimulus can vary considerably, there is now considerable evidence that the perception of pain is not uniquely related to the stimulus. An individual's perception of pain depends on a combination of factors such as the individual's attention to the pain and emotional state, the circumstances under which the pain was acquired, and whether it is perceived as a threatening signal.

For example, visceral pain is often perceived to be more severe than pain that originates from the surface of the body.

The perception of pain is affected by factors such as arousal, attention, distraction, and/or expectation. This means that expectations, prior experiences, and mood shape our perception of pain. In that way, pain is similar to other senses, which are also affected by these factors although to a lesser extent than for pain.

Many forms of pain are phantom perceptions and memory plays an important role regarding how a person perceives the pain [99, 189]. It has been suggested [10] that learning and memory can reformulate the coding in the cerebral cortex and thus, has relevance for the design of drug therapies [10]. This is based on evidence from different studies that shows that the cerebral cortex plays an active role in chronic pain. There is evidence that the human cortex reorganizes during times of chronic pain [10]. Distinct chronic pain conditions impact the cortex in unique ways [10].

# Pain has two different components

Most forms of pain have two components: one component is the perception of pain that is similar to the perception of sensory stimuli and the other component is an emotional and negative influence that may be best described as suffering. There are similarities between pain and tinnitus where these matters are taken into account in treating individuals with severe tinnitus [189].

According to Turk and Okifuji (2001), suffering implies a threat to the wholeness of an individual's self-concept, self-identity, and integrity. Suffering is defined as a "reaction to the physical or emotional components of pain with a feeling of uncontrollability, helplessness, intolerability, and interminableness" [448].

In attempts to treat pain, the two components of pain can often be manipulated independently. For example, treatment with opioids can take the unpleasant components away without greatly affecting the perception of pain. There are other treatments that also affect the unpleasant components without noticeably decreasing the perception of the pain (see Chapter 12).

The lowering of a person's quality of life caused by pain is another measure of the negative effects of pain. The quality of life has been described as "a person's general well-being, including mental status, stress level, sexual function, and self-perceived health status" according to Stedman's Electronic Medical Dictionary. The effect of pain on a person's quality of life depends more on the distress it causes and less on how a person perceives his or her pain. In 1931, the French medical missionary Dr. Albert Schweitzer wrote, "pain is a more terrible lord of mankind than even death itself".

The emotional effects of pain are often related to earlier experiences and it may have to do with the understanding of pain as a sign of diseases of various kinds. That most people are afraid of pain may have to do with the emotional reaction that pain causes. The emotional reactions to pain may also be explained by the extensive connections between pain circuits in the brain and the amygdala, which can be reached by pain signals and not amendable to reasoning.

Pain is often feared because the person knows so little about pain. Better knowledge about pain for the person with pain may have a beneficial effect on the pain. This has been experienced through treatment of tinnitus where teaching the patients about the auditory system is a part of a treatment known as tinnitus retraining therapy (TRT) [190].

# Classification of pain

There are many kinds of pain and different terms are used to describe each one of these different forms of pain. Many different classifications of pain have been suggested. Generally, pain has been divided into two large groups regarding whether the pain is caused by activation (stimulation) of specific receptors (pain receptors, nociceptors) or whether it is caused by changes in the function of the central nervous system (spinal cord and brain).

We will use the term physiological pain for pain caused by stimulation of receptors, and the term pathological pain for pain that is not caused by stimulation of receptors, but which is caused by changes in the function of the central nervous system (spinal cord or brain).

Woolf[485] has proposed a classification with three classes of pain: nociceptive pain, inflammatory pain, and pathological pain. Nociceptive pain is pain caused by stimulation of nociceptors activating peripheral nerve fibers that respond only to painful stimuli. Inflammatory pain is also caused by stimulation of pain receptors but the pain is associated with tissue damage and the infiltration of immune cells. Pathological pain is a disease state caused by damage to the nervous system or by abnormal function (dysfunctional pain, like in fibromyalgia, irritable bowel syndrome, tension type headache, etc.).

Pathological pain has many forms and different investigators may describe it differently. Terms such as central neuropathic pain, or central pain or chronic neuropathic pain are terms used to describe different forms of pathological pain. These different terms are often used to describe pain that involves plastic changes of neural circuits in the spinal cord, the trigeminal nucleus, and many other parts of the brain. These forms of pain may involve re-routing of information to different parts of the brain. Now it is common to use the term chronic neuropathic pain for the form of pathological pain because what Woolf has named pathological pain is often chronic. The term central neuropathic pain is used in this book to describe pain that is caused by functional changes in the spinal cord and the brain that causes pain without activation of nociceptors.

Physiological pain includes somatic pain, visceral pain, and inflammatory pain. Pathological pain includes central neuropathic pain and several disorders that have pain as one of their symptoms, such as fibromyalgia, strokes, Parkinson's disease, etc.

Pain may be classified according to which parts of the body are involved (Figure 2.1) or according to what causes the pain. Some classifications are related to the cause of the pain; often no cause to a person's pain can be found (idiopathic pain).

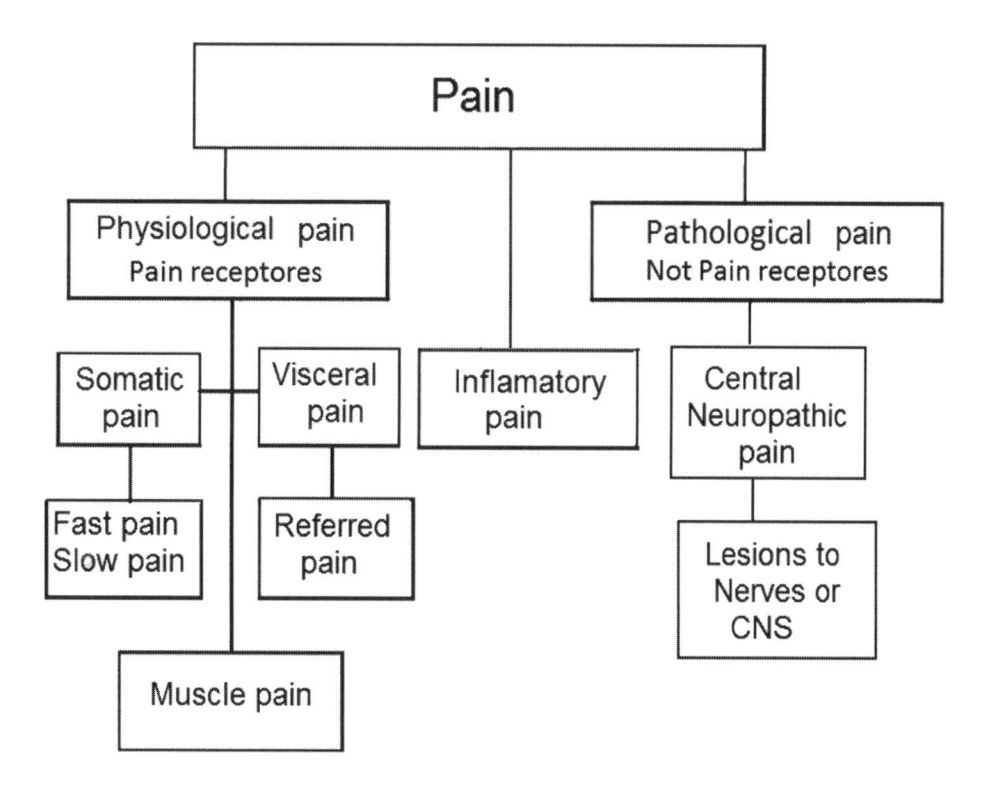

Figure 2.1 An example of the classification of different forms of pain. Data from Woolf, C.J. and M.W. Salter, Neuroplasticity: Increasing the gain in pain. Science, 2000. 288: p. 1765-1768 [489] (Artwork by Irene Cunha.)

Central neuropathic pain belongs to the group of pathological pain that is caused by changes in the function of the nervous system without any stimulation of pain receptors. It is often felt as coming from a specific location on the body while it is caused by functional changes in the spinal cord or the brain. The changes are usually caused by activation of neuroplasticity. This is a reminder that the anatomical location of the pain is not always the same as the location where the pain is felt. Not recognizing this is a common mistake that can lead to the misdiagnosis of pain disorders with subsequent treatment that is not beneficial to the patient. Pain caused by disorders of the central nervous system or by changes in the function of some parts of the central nervous system is often caused by activation of neuroplasticity.

Other classifications are based on the amount of time the pain has lasted. Acute pain and chronic pain are the terms used, but the definitions vary. Different authors have used different definitions for these two terms. Some authors have defined chronic pain as pain that lasts longer than the anticipated healing period, but this definition can only be used for pain that has a clear cause such as trauma. Other authors have used an arbitrarily defined length of time for chronic pain, such as three months or six months. Some have defined acute pain as pain that lasts less than 30 days.

Turk and Okifuji [448] defined acute pain as: "pain elicited by the injury of body tissues and activation of nociceptive transducers at the site of local tissue damage".

It is interesting that the authoritative Stedman's Medical Dictionary does not list any definition for acute or chronic pain.

Pain related to nerves is known as neuropathic pain, but that is too broad a range of disorders to be described with one term. Neurologists, therefore, often use the term only for disorders of peripheral and cranial nerves.

Pathological pain has many forms with names such as central neuropathic pain. Central neuropathic pain involves plastic changes of neural circuits in the spinal cord, the trigeminal nucleus, and many other parts of the brain. It may involve re-routing of information to many different parts of the brain.

The American Medical Association (AMA Council on Science and Public Heath has suggested two different terms to describe these two different kinds of pain, namely eudynia for pain caused by activation of pain receptors (receptor pain), which is Greek for "good pain," and the term maldynia for pain that is not caused by activation of pain receptors (maladaptive pain). Maldynia is Greek for "bad pain." Pain that is not caused by activation of pain receptors has been viewed as maladaptive because it may occur in the absence of ongoing harmful (pain receptor) stimuli and does not promote healing and repair. The Committee concluded: "as defined, maldynia is a multidimensional process that may warrant consideration as a chronic disease not only affecting sensory and emotional processing, but also producing an altered brain state based on both functional imaging and macroscopic measurements. However, the absolute clinical value of this definition is not established" [106].

Pain has been classified according to its severity. One such classification uses three groups: mild, moderate, and severe.

- Mild pain:

Does not interfere noticeably with everyday life.
- Moderate pain:

May cause some annoyance and perceived as unpleasant.
- Severe chronic pain:

Pain can affect a person's entire life in major ways.

Since the perceived severity of pain depends on many different factors, one being a person's personality, the classification of a person's pain may change over time. The perception of pain is also influenced by external circumstances.

Another classification of pain condition relates to different body systems being affected. In this classification, pain has been classified as somatic pain or visceral pain. Somatic pain is pain caused by stimulation of pain receptors (nociceptors) in the skin, joints, tendons, and muscles. Visceral pain is a form of pain that is caused by activating pain receptors in internal organs. It involves the same nervous system as that which communicates pain from the body, but processing of pain signals from internal organs is different from that of pain from superficial structures, such as the skin, skeletal muscles, tendons, joints, etc. It is also different in that the pain caused by internal organs is felt as coming from various locations on the body (referred pain), which may be different for different individuals. This may cause confusion that can lead to an incorrect diagnosis and subsequently, incorrect treatment (that is to no benefit, but which may have side effects). There is also evidence that visceral pain may, in addition, use pathways, such as the dorsal column pathway, that have earlier been regarded to be a part of the somatosensory system exclusively, carrying information from sensory receptors in the skin, joints, etc.

While somatic and visceral pain are mainly processed in the spinal cord and the trigeminal nucleus, there is some evidence that some forms of pain may be mediated by the vagus nerve and carried directly through that nerve to the brain, bypassing the spinal cord. An example is ischemia of the heart muscle (heart attack) that can present with pain that is referred to several places on the body and it may not give pain at all, but instead, give other sensations such as feeling ill. Thus, typically for sensations mediated by the vagus nerve, as we will discuss later in this book.

Muscle pain is yet another group of pain conditions. There are two main kinds of muscle pain: one that is caused by muscle contractions elicited by neural activity from $\alpha$ motoneurons and the other is caused by muscle contractions that are not caused by neural activity.

In the real world, pain is complicated. In some pain disorders, it is not known whether the pain is physiological or pathological pain. Many individuals' pain falls outside these simple classifications. Thus, many forms of pain have contributions from both physiological and pathological pain. For example, pain caused by trauma or inflammation often has a component of central neuropathic pain, indicating that neuroplasticity has been activated. There are also disorders, which earlier were assumed to be caused by mechanical insult to nerve roots (such as trigeminal neuralgia), and now, evidence points to a cause of hyperactivity in the respective nucleus. Similar pathologies may explain other pain disorders, such as low back pain, carpal tunnel syndrome, and other nerve entrapment disorders.

Low back pain is an example of a kind of pain that does not have a clear classification. It often, at least in the beginning, has a component of physiological pain, while later, pathological pain (central neuropathic pain) probably dominates. Low back pain has been assumed to be caused by entrapment of spinal nerves. This is, however, disputed and there is evidence that typical low back pain, to a great extent, is pathological pain at least after some time.

Against the theory that the pain is caused by entrapment of spinal nerves speaks the finding that people who do not have pain also have equally abnormal MRI findings without giving any symptoms [168]. This means that nerve entrapment may not be the cause of low back pain. Attempts to correct such nerve entrapments may cause pain in itself [238]. These disorders are discussed in detail in Section III on pathological pain.

Neuropathic pain is pain that is related to disorders of the central nervous system. The term neuropathic pain theoretically covers all pain that originates in the peripheral and central nervous system. However, neurologists use the term in a narrower manner to describe pain related to peripheral nerves and cranial nerves. Pain from peripheral and cranial nerves include neuralgias of various kinds. Causes of such pain are many, such as, for example, diabetes neuropathy and viral infections, but again, often no cause can be found.

Central neuropathic pain belongs to the group of pathological pain that is caused by changes in the function of the nervous system without any stimulation of pain receptors. It is often felt as coming from a specific location on the body while it is caused by functional changes in the spinal cord or the brain. The changes are usually caused by activation of neuroplasticity. This is a reminder that the anatomical location of the pain is not always the same as the location where the pain is felt. Not recognizing this is a common mistake that can lead to the misdiagnosis of pain disorders with subsequent treatment that is not beneficial to the patient.

Pain caused by disorders of the central nervous system or by changes in the function of some parts of the central nervous system is often caused by activation of neuroplasticity.

Other forms of pain from the nervous system are stroke pain, especially thalamic pain. There is recent evidence that immune reactions may be involved in the generation of pain, possibly through the action of microglia [278] (discussed in Chapters 8 and 11).

Fibromyalgia, myofascial, and chronic fatigue syndrome, also known as chronic widespread pain (CWP), are other forms of pathological pain. These disorders have pain as just one of their symptoms (discussed in Chapter 9). Fibromyalgia is a complex pain disorder that has many different forms, all of which are difficult to diagnose. Attempts to reduce some of the ambiguities in the classification of such forms of pain have been made by The American College of Rheumatology that has published attempts to arrive at a standard definition of fibromyalgia and they have coined the term chronic widespread pain (CWP), which covers fibromyalgia.

However, fibromyalgia (FM) is currently defined as the presence of both chronic widespread pain (CWP) and tender points, which must be present at an examination of 11 of 18, tested body points. Only approximately 20% of individuals with CWP have a sufficient number of tender points to be regarded as having fibromyalgia. The other 80% of individuals with fewer tender points have no clear clinical diagnosis, but their pain is most certainly not due to inflammation or damage of structures, nor is it likely to be peripheral in nature.

Pain conditions that are related to the autonomic nervous systems, such as complex regional pain syndromes (CRPS) type I and II, are in a class of their own. These disorders are complex conditions that are forms of pathological pain disorders. (CRPS type I was earlier known as reflex sympathetic dystrophy, RSD, and CRPS type II was known as causalgia.) CRPS type I is a chronic nerve disorder with pain and other signs that occur most often in the arms or legs. The symptoms often begin after a minor injury. CRPS type II is caused by an injury to a nerve. The exact diagnosis of these conditions is still controversial (we will discuss these diseases in more detail later in this book).

Individuals with Parkinson's disease (PD) often have pain. Pain may, in fact, be the first symptom of PD as shown in a recent study [155]. Pain may also occur secondary to other forms of dystonia. (Dystonia: a syndrome of abnormal muscle contraction that produces repetitive involuntary twisting movements and abnormal posturing of the neck, trunk, face, and extremities. Stedman's Electronic Medical Dictionary)

# Is pain a sense?

Pain is not regarded to be a sense, but there are many similarities and differences between pain and senses. Pain definitely reaches conscious awareness, very much like senses, and like senses, awareness of some forms of pain depends on a physical stimulus, neural transmission, and a certain degree of sensory arousal. Other forms of pain are phantom sensations similar to tinnitus that occur without any physical stimulus reaching a receptor.

Unlike sensory stimuli that are associated with evoked potentials of various kinds, there are no objective measures of the intensity of pain and not even the presence of pain except, perhaps, for some accompanying signs such as increased activation of the sympathetic nervous system that can cause sweating, increased blood pressure, and increased heart rate. It also affects the digestive system by causing increased production of hydrochloric acid in the stomach and it may cause symptoms from the intestines such as diarrhea or constipation.

The emotional brain is engaged in pain to a greater extent than sensory input. Unlike senses, pain can be affected by medical treatment. The complexity of pain and its difference from sensory activation is indicated by the fact that areas of the brain other than sensory areas, such as the premotor and the supplementary motor cortex, as well as many other regions, are active during pain.

# Pain and cognition

Pain can affect intellectual abilities. Published studies show that individuals with chronic pain complain of cognitive impairment including problems with memory and attention [265]. Melzack and Wall also noticed that many patients with pain mentioned that they experienced difficulties in completing intellectual tasks. A few studies using objective testing have found that some people with chronic pain experience impairment in attention, memory, mental flexibility, verbal ability, speed of response in a cognitive task, and speed in executing structured tasks [265]. Pain related reduced cognitive functions mostly occur in connection with chronic pain in the elderly [164].

On the basis of such findings, some authors advised clinicians to assess cognitive function in individuals with chronic pain and direct their treatment to this aspect. Tests of cognitive functions would also be valuable for monitoring the results of treatment. This is closely related to the effect of pain on the quality of life in general [318]. Many elderly individuals have several diseases for which they take different kinds of medications. Some common medications, such as β-adrenergic blockers, are known to impair memory (except one, atenolol, because it does not pass the blood-brain barrier).

# Personality profiles of chronic pain

Two of the most frequent personality profiles of individuals with chronic pain described by the Minnesota Multiphasic Personality Inventory (MMPI) are the conversion V and the neurotic triad.

The conversion V personality, so called because the higher scores on MMPI scales 1 and 3, relative to scale 2, form a "V" shape on a graph, expresses exaggerated concern over body feelings, develops bodily symptoms in response to stress, and often fails to recognize their own emotional state, including depression. The neurotic triad personality, scoring high on scales 1, 2, and 3, also expresses exaggerated concern over body feelings and develops bodily symptoms in response to stress, but is demanding and complaining as described in Raphael and Leo (2007) in the "Clinical manual of pain management in psychiatry", Washington, DC: American Psychiatric Publishing (page 58).

Some investigators have argued that it is this neuroticism that causes acute pain to turn chronic, but clinical evidence points the other way, to chronic pain causing neuroticism. When long-term pain is relieved by therapeutic intervention, scores on the neurotic triad and anxiety often fall to normal levels. Self-esteem, often low in individuals with chronic pain, also shows striking improvement once pain has resolved.

# Sensitivity to pain varies

Sensitivity to painful stimulation varies from person to person although it is naturally difficult to determine the strength of pain. Therefore, it is difficult to accurately compare pain caused in different ways.

The effect of pain on an individual person shows large variations, and there are large differences between different individuals in sensitivity to pain. The perceived severity of chronic pain depends on many different factors, one being a person's personality.

A person's perception of pain is affected by the person's attention to other matters (distraction). It also varies as a function of the time of the day. Suggestions (expectations) about treatment can affect pain perception. Just suggestions of beneficial treatment can reduce the intensity of pain in many individuals (placebo effect). Circumstances, such as accidents with injury or severe fear, can affect how pain is perceived. There may b a period after an accident where the person is totally pain free. The suppression of pain is caused by the action of the sympathetic nervous system.

# Catastrophizing

Catastrophizing may be regarded as the opposite of coping [422] (Figure 2.2). It is irrational thoughts that a bad situation will turn worse. It has to do with increased worrying, fearing the worst. Catastrophizing causes a decrease in quality of life without actual causes. Studies have shown that catastrophizing painful stimulation contributes to a more intense pain experience and increased emotional distress. Studies of the effect of catastrophizing painful experiences are few, but the findings have been consistent in showing a relation between catastrophizing and pain.

A review of the literature on the relation between catastrophizing and pain discusses different theoretical models and suggests that catastrophizing might best be viewed from the perspective of hierarchical levels of analysis, where social factors and social goals may play a role in the development and maintenance of catastrophizing [422].

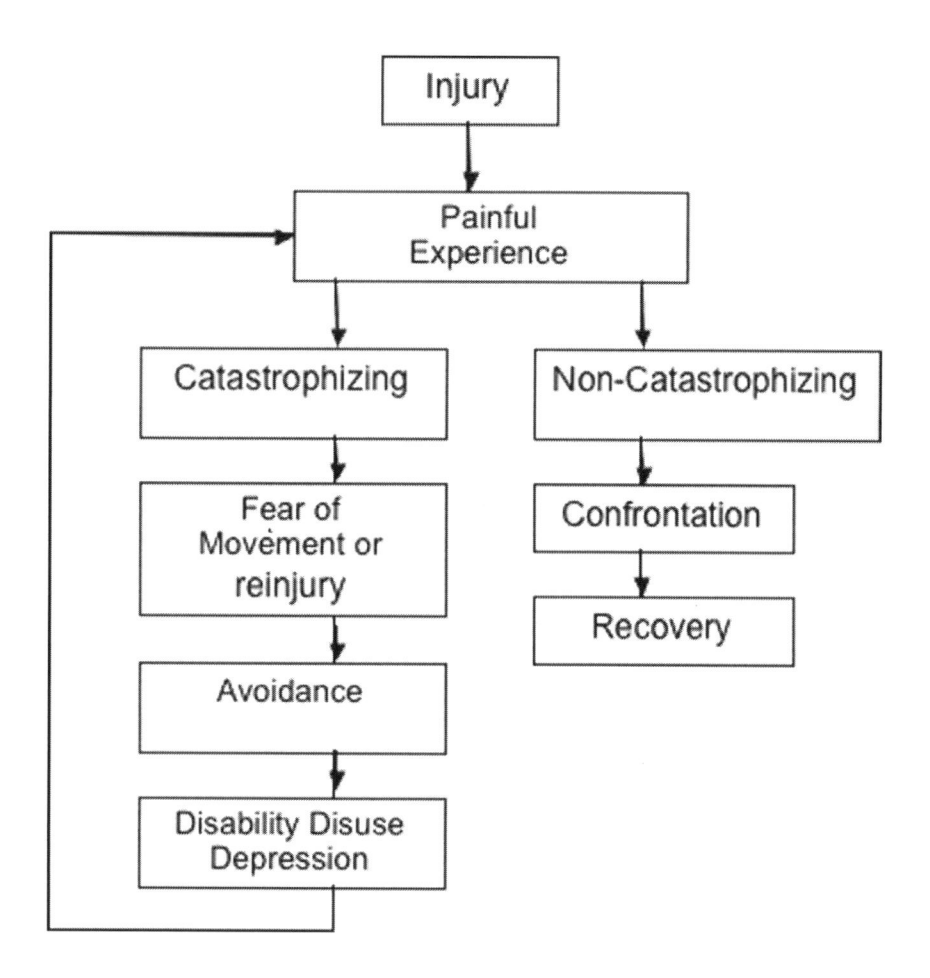

Figure 2.2 Cognitive-behavioral model of fear of movement and injury (fear-avoidance belief). (Data from "Fear of movement/(re) injury in chronic low back pain and its relation to behavioral performance". Vlaeyen JW, Kole-Snijders AM, Boeren RG, van Eek H. Pain. 1995 Sep; 62(3): 363-72 [455]). (Artwork by Irene Cunha.)

# What can affect pain?

In general, all forms of pain are affected by many high central nervous system activities. Distraction and attention to the pain affects its intensity. Also, the time of the day affects how pain is perceived and to what extent it affects a person.

The "fight and flight" reaction can abolish pain sensations during a brief period after an accident and wounds do not cause pain sensations immediately after trauma such as from being shot or subject to explosions. Anxiety and stress can both increase and decrease the perceived strength of pain sensations. Relaxation decreases the perceived strength of pain sensations.

Hypnosis has been shown to be effective in treating many pain conditions (see Chapter 12) and may be regarded as an extreme form of relaxation. This and the placebo effect indicate considerable influence from high central nervous system structures on the perception of many forms of pain.

There are objective signs that somatic pain can be affected by central influence of various kinds. For example, a study where PET scans were used to indicate brain activation from painful stimuli presented together with a sound (tones) has shown signs of activation of an area of the somatosensory cortex (left hand PET scans in Figure 2.3) when the participant paid attention to the painful stimuli (heat). However, when the participant was asked to pay attention to the tone, this activation was smaller and an area of the auditory cortex showed signs of activation (right hand PET scans).

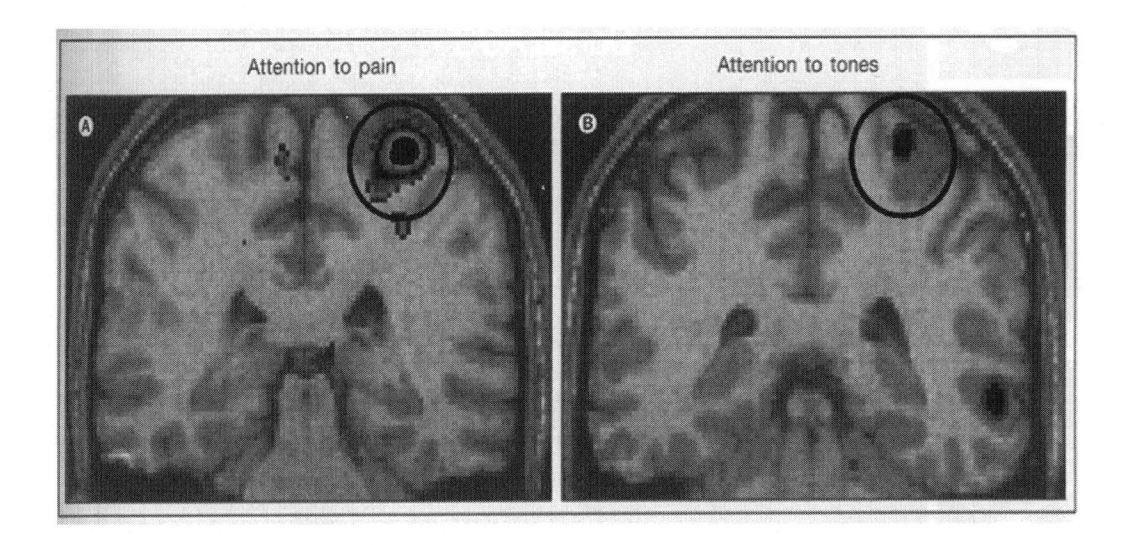

Figure 2.3 Averaged PET scans centered over the primary somatosensory cortex (red circle). A painful (heat) stimulus presented together with a tone while the participants were asked to pay attention to either the pain stimulus (left hand MRI) or the tone (right hand MRI). (From Bushnell, M.C. and A.V. Apkarian, Representation of pain in the brain, in Wall and Melzack's Textbook of Pain, S.B. McMahon and M. Koltzenburg, Editors. 2006, Elsevier: Amsterdam. p. 107-124 [59], adapted from Bushnell, M.C., et al., Pain perception: is there a role for primary somatosensory cortex? Proc Natl Acad Sci U S A, 1999. 96(14): p. 7705-9. Reprinted with the permission of the National Academy of Sciences [60].)

Increased sensitivity to pain, hyperalgesia, often occurs when a person has had pain for a long time and some medications, such as opioids, promote the development of hyperalgesia. The efficacy of medical treatment such as using opioids decreases when used over long periods. This phenomenon that is known as tolerance is discussed in Chapter 7.

There are more fundamental abnormalities in pain perception. Absence or largely reduced pain perception (congenital analgesia) is a serious congenital anomaly that increases the risks of fatal injuries and such individuals rarely reach a high age. Episodic analgesia is another abnormality.

Some disorders are associated with abnormal pain perception and reactions to painful stimuli. The clearest one is seen in autistic individuals who often have reduced sensitivity to painful stimuli and sometimes seem to enjoy painful simulations. Some individuals may enjoy pain during sexual activities.

Finally, it must be mentioned that opioids are produced in the body (endogenous opioids) and can suppress or reduce pain.

# Pain may elicit body reactions

Pain often increases muscle tonus. Acute pain, such as that of the hands and feet, can elicit a reflex known as the withdrawal reflex. Pain can activate the autonomic nervous system; mainly increasing the activity of the sympathetic nervous system, which can cause changes in body functions, including elevation of blood pressure, increased heart rate, and increased sweating. Increased sympathetic activity also affects the digestive apparatus.

The sympathetic nervous system can affect the sensation of pain, thus acting as a negative or a positive feedback that can either increase or decrease the pain. Pain can activate the sympathetic nervous system, which in turn can increase the pain (see sympathetic maintained pain, SMP). The suppression of pain that may occur after serious trauma is probably also caused by activation of the sympathetic nervous system.

The sympathetic nervous system can weaken the immune system, but that is less visual. Less is known about how pain can activate the parasympathetic nervous system. Both afferent and efferent parasympathetic activity is thought to play a role in the modulation of immunoreactions [433], which is important regarding pain (see Chapters 10 and 14). The vagus nerve plays an important role in this respect [32].

# Benefit and purposefulness of pain

Pain can be purposeful or not and it can be beneficial or not to an individual person. That pain is purposeful means that it accurately signals and identifies a problem and its anatomical localization. Some forms of pain are beneficial to an individual because the pain serves as a warning of danger from external sources, which can be avoided by appropriate action.

Pain can serve to protect wounds during healing by discoursing manipulation of the wound. Pain from trauma is both purposeful and beneficial to an individual by signaling the location on the body of the trauma and encouraging that the trauma be terminated.

Pain from disorders of muscles, joints, and tendons can be both purposeful and beneficial by identifying the body location of the disorder and promoting rest to avoid damage or remedies for treating the disorder in question. If it is possible to reduce tissue damage by appropriate intervention, these kinds of warnings are beneficial to a person. Pain from trauma may, therefore, be both purposeful and beneficial to an individual. For example, pain from damaged joints may be purposeful and beneficial because pain would identify the problem and discourage use of the joints, thus reducing the risk that further damage would develop.

Pain from headaches caused by trauma, tumors, etc. may be purposeful by accurately signaling the problem and its (gross) anatomical localization, but it may not be beneficial because little could be done to cure the disease before the beginning of modern medicine and surgery. Common idiopathic headaches are neither purposeful nor beneficial. While the common headache can be regarded as a message, it is unclear what it means and it is unclear what the benefits are of receiving this message.

Most forms of pathological pain are not even purposeful and do not serve any beneficial function for an individual person. The common kind of low back pain may be regarded as beneficial at least in its initial part because it promotes rest, which is beneficial for healing injuries. Pain from neuralgias from viral infections may be purposeful in that the pain accurately signals the disease and its anatomical location, but it was not beneficial before adequate medications became available.

Pain caused by disorders of internal organs may be purposeful when it correctly signals problems and their anatomical location, but may not be beneficial if nothing can be done to improve the situation. Often, the pain is not localized to the organ that is diseased, but in a different place (referred pain). This can eliminate the purposefulness of the pain. An example where pain serves a purpose without being beneficial to an individual person is the pain felt from appendicitis.

Pain properly signals a severe and life threatening problem, but before the advent of modern medicine and surgery, there was nothing that a person could do in reaction to such a warning. This means that pain from appendicitis is purposeful, but it was not beneficial before surgery or antibiotics were available.

Thus, there are many situations where pain is purposeful, such as warning about diseases and risks of trauma to the body. However, from an evolutionary point of view, pain as a warning about disorders is only beneficial if the warning makes it possible to avoid or reverse the situation that pain warned about. Most forms of central neuropathic pain do not seem to be purposeful because such pain does not accurately indicate the anatomical location of the disease and it is not beneficial to a person. This form of pain seems to be entirely harmful, decreasing the quality of life for many people.

Pain can also be a side effect of treatment, especially surgical treatment. Such pain may be purposeful because it correctly tells that some harm has been done, but it may not be beneficial to the person who had surgery because what caused the harm cannot be reversed.

# Evolution of pain

The ability to feel pain is absolutely essential and people who are born without the sensation of pain have a shorter life expectancy. This is because of the absence of warning in connection with diseases and accidents indicating that the general benefit from physiological pain comes from the experience that individuals who are born without pain sensation (congenital analgesia) have a shorter lifespan than people with normal pain functions. This is a clear indication that pain is important for survival.

Many different protective mechanisms of the body have evolved during the millions of years of evolution. Pain is one of these and it still fulfills an important function as a warning of various kinds of dangers to the body. The forms of pain that signal danger to the body are important for survival and may, therefore, have evolved in accordance with the Darwinian hypothesis of survival of the fittest and reproduction. This kind of pain is known as the good pain because it is beneficial to an individual person.

While some forms of pain can be one of the most important protective functions of the body, pain can also be harmful and occur without any beneficial function. This is known as the bad pain.

Pain from trauma is a warning that aims at stopping the trauma or a warning about diseases and disorders. The classical withdrawal reflex, automatically pulling a hand or foot away from touching a hot object, for example, is a very clear automatic action from pain, even before the pain has reached consciousness. Descartes, who used it as an example of how some functions of the body can be an "automata", extensively discussed the withdrawal reflex and he described the other side of body functions that were not automatic as that of the soul. We still use this dual description, but more commonly use the terms body and mind.

Dualism describes mental phenomena as different from physical phenomena. This concept of dualism that Cartesius suggested is still, to some extent, valid for describing mental phenomena as being different from physical phenomena; the functions of which can be replicated by machines (including computers). Monoideism regards all functions of the human body and depends on physical phenomena.

How pathological pain has evolved is difficult to understand since it does not seem to promote survival nor does it favor the fittest. It is surprising that pathological pain, such as central neuropathic pain, has survived so many years of evolution. Pathological pain, such as common headaches and central neuropathic pain, in general, does not promote survival, but seems to be entirely harmful. In that way, pain may be similar to the immune system, which also is important for survival, but which can be harmful when it attacks important structures of the body. One would expect that evolution would have eliminated infectious diseases and cancer by improving the efficacy of the immune system.

A strong immune system also has disadvantages such as causing autoimmune disorders. It has recently been hypothesized that there is an optimal level of efficacy of the immune system, where more efficient actions would also increase the harmful effects of the immune system such as increasing the number of autoimmune disorders.

Perhaps, similar questions can be asked regarding pain; where eliminating pain that is not purposeful would also reduce the beneficial effects of other forms of pain and, therefore, not serve the purpose of survival of the fittest as is assumed to be the goal of Darwinian evolution. The existence of pathological pain may be the price paid for having sufficient sensitivity and activation of pain to provide appropriate warnings, thus contributing to protection.

Pain is only one of the body's many protective functions. Other protective functions are the immune system and the ability to adapt to changing environmental interactions with body functions (summarized in Figure 2.4).

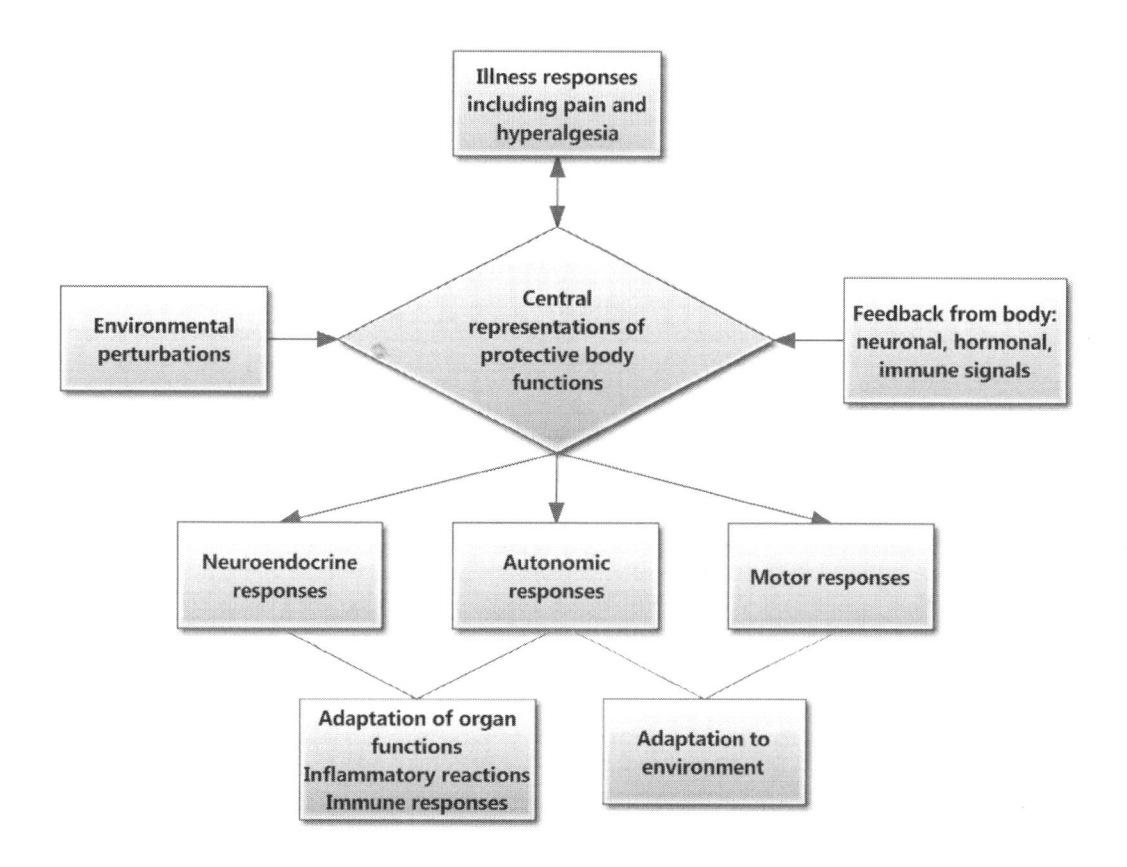

Figure 2.4 Protective mechanisms: inputs, central representation, and outputs (After Jänig, W. and J.D. Levine, Autonomic-endocrine-immune interactions in acute and chronic pain, S.B. McMahon and M. Koltzenburg, Editors. 2006, Elsevier: Amsterdam. p. 205-218 and Jänig, W. and H.J. Häbler, Sympathetic nervous system: contribution to chronic pain. Prog. Brain Res., 2000. 129: p. 451-68 [180].) (Artwork by Monica Javidnia.)

# Pain as a diagnostic tool

Pain is an important diagnostic sign of disease and used extensively as a diagnostic means. The use of a patient's description of his/her pain is an important diagnostic sign, but subject to many uncertainties and errors.

# Patients use different words to describe their pain

Different patients may use the same words to describe different forms of pain or different patients may use different words to describe the same pain. Many people who seek medical help want to have their pain treated, but a physician must always have in mind that the pain a patient describes may be a sign of a disease. The physician must, therefore, rely on the patient's description of his/her pain for diagnosing the cause and for suggesting what tests would be appropriate in addition to the patient's description of the pain. It is a major problem that different people can describe the same pain differently. That people use very different words to describe their pain has been documented by Dr. Melzack who reported the different words and terms used by patients who visited his pain clinic (Table 2.1).

## TABLE 2.1

### SENSORY

| Temporal | Spatial | Punctate Pressure | Incisive Pressure | Constrictive Pressure | Traction Pressure | Thermal | Brightness | |
|---|---|---|---|---|---|---|---|---|
| FLIKERING | | | | | | | TINGLING ITCHY | 1 |
| QUIVERING PULSING THROBBING BEATING POUNDING | JUMPING FLASHING SHOOTING | PRICKING BORING | SHARP CUTTING LACERATING | PINCHING PRESSING GNAWING CRAMPING | TUGGING PULLING | HOT | SMARTING STINGING | 2 |
| | | DRILLING STABBING LANCINATING | | CRUSHING | WRENCHING | BURNING SCALDING SEARING | | 3 4 5 |

### SENSORY / AFFECTIVE / EVALUATIVE

| Dullness | Sensory: Misc. | Tension | Autonomic | Fear | Punishment | Affective: Misc. | Anchor words | | |
|---|---|---|---|---|---|---|---|---|---|
| | | | | | | | MILD | | 1 |
| DULL SORE | TENDER | | | | | | DISCOMFORTING | ANNOYING | 2 |
| HURTING ACHING HEAVY | TAUT RASPING SPLITTING | TIRING EXHAUSTING | SICKENING SUFFOCATING | FEARFUL FRIGHTFUL TERRIFYING | PUNISHING GRUELLING CRUEL VICIOUS KILLING | WRETCHED BLINDING | DISTRESSING HORRIBLE EXCRUTIATING | TROUBLESOME MISERABLE INTENSE UNBEARABLE | 3 4 5 |

Table 2.1 What patients use to describe their pain in the emergency room as recorded by Dr. Melzack. The scales on the right hand side of the graphs show the frequency of the use of the different words given in the table. This study has later been the basis for the McGill pain questionnaire. From Wall, P., "Pain: The Science of suffering". Maps of the Mind, ed. S. Rose. 2000, New York: Columbia University Press [459].

Diagnosing diseases based on pain is hampered by ambiguities in the patients' descriptions of their pain. An incorrect diagnosis of pain causes many treatments that are not beneficial to the patients, and may be harmful because of the side effects of worthless treatment and economic harm that such treatment may cause to individuals and/or society. Many incidents of chronic pain especially have no known cause (idiopathic), but may anyhow get a diagnosis, which then will most likely be incorrect, which may be worse than not having a diagnosis at all.

The fact that pain is not a constant perception and its effect on a person depends on the circumstances further complicates communication between patients with pain and their health professionals. A patient's description of his/her pain depends on many factors including the emotional value the patient places on the pain, whether the person perceives the pain as a sign of a serious disorder, or whether the person has control over his/her pain or not.

If the pain is regarded as being inescapable, its negative emotional effect is greater than when it is regarded to be escapable. We will discuss this aspect of pain later in this book.

Where is the pain, when did it start, is it constant, what is the character (burning, stinging, etc.) are common questions asked to patients who appear in the emergency room, a hospital, or a physician or surgeon's office.

The answers to these questions should direct the attention to the structure that is pathological and the answer to the question about when it started should tell something about what caused the pain. It certainly does so in many cases, but not in all. Pain from internal organs is felt to come from the surface of the body, but the location from where it comes is not directly related to the anatomical location of the structure that is pathologic. Referred pain is the term that describes this phenomenon and, to make things worse, there are considerable individual variations in where pain is felt from pathologies in a specific structure and pathologies that are expected to cause pain, such as ischemia of the heart muscle, do not always cause pain. Pathological pain is pain that is caused by functional changes in the central nervous system and the pain is often referred to specific locations of the body, thus giving erroneous impressions of the anatomical location of the pathology.

The use of the time when pain first occurred to identify the events that caused the pathology is also subject to errors. Many biological systems have a large degree of reserves and pathologies, such as pain from peripheral nerves (neuropathy) which normally progress slowly and at first, it just uses the reserves; therefore, not producing any symptoms. Symptoms first appear when the reserves are used up which may take some time after the event that caused the beginning of the pathology. Therefore, the start of the pain is not a valid indicator of when the pathology began.

Diagnosis of pain is discussed in more detail in the chapter on treatment of pain (Chapters 7 and 12).

# Amputation pain

Amputations are often associated with phantom sensations, including pain (phantom pain). More surprising, perhaps, is that similar phantom perceptions occur in rheumatology in connection with diseases such as rheumatoid arthritis, fibromyalgia, and complex regional pain syndrome (CRPS) because of a motor/sensory conflict [258].

Central neuropathic pain is a form of a phantom sensation, i.e. a sensation that is caused by a change in function without any detectable change in morphology. We will discuss these forms of pathologies in detail in other chapters in this book.

Clinical findings support the assumption of cortical sensory reorganization as a cause of phantom sensations [258] including pain and altered body image in rheumatology patients in the same manner as has previously been hypothesized for amputees with phantom limb pain (PLP). These pathologies can be explained as a motor/sensory conflict. It has been shown that this conflict can be corrected by the use of appropriate visual sensory input, such as using a mirror [71, 347]. Studies support the hypothesis that a mismatch between motor output and sensory input creates sensory disturbances, including pain, in rheumatology patients and healthy volunteers [258].

# Self-inflicted pain

There are many forms of self-inflicted pain. Athletes who often expect pain from their training say: no pain, no gain. There are psychiatric causes of enjoying pain (masochistic behavior). Some individuals enjoy pain in connection with sexual activity. Many autistic individuals seem to enjoy pain and have other abnormalities in sensations of stimulation of the somatosensory system [289, 456]. These forms of perception of pain may be related to the involvement of the reward system of the brain.

# Pain inflicted by other individuals

Torture and punishment are examples of the use of the negative effects of pain either as a punishment or in threatening of people. Different kinds of warfare involve inflicting body harm and thereby, pain. Many societies use pain as punishment. Some parents use pain as punishment of their children and some adults use pain to solve personal conflicts.

# Neuroscience of pain

The neuroscience of pain is complex and the function of the neural structures involved in pain is plastic, which means their function can change. The physiological and anatomical basis for pain is complex and poorly understood. For these reasons, large parts of this book are devoted to the neuroscience of pain.

Neural activity elicited by stimulation of pain receptors (nociceptors) causes physiological pain. The neural signals are first processed extensively in the spinal cord or in the trigeminal nucleus and from there; it can reach many different parts of the brain for further processing. For example, pain can be modulated by stimulation of receptors that respond to innocuous stimulation and from the spinal cord and the brain. The basis for the well-known gating hypothesis concerns processes in the dorsal horn of the spinal cord (or the caudal trigeminal nucleus). Pain engages many parts of the brain, including emotional parts. The immune system [121], autonomic nervous system, and the reward network including the basal ganglia [165] are also involved. This may explain why pain can cause so many different reactions.

Pain signals from the body may reach primary and secondary somatosensory cortices, the prefrontal cortex, the anterior cingulate cortex, limbic structures, such as the amygdala and hippocampus, and the insular lobe. There is evidence of involvement of the insular lobe in pathological pain, but so far, no treatment methods have been developed that target the insula.

Pain that is caused by activation of pain receptors (physiological pain) can be modulated (increased or decreased) as the information travels through the spinal cord (or in the trigeminal nucleus) to the brain.

Cartesius understood that the brain was the receiver of the information and caused the flexor muscles in the leg to contract (in fact, the withdrawal reflex does not involve the brain; it is solely a matter of the spinal cord). He, however, did not realize that the central nervous system sends information back to the pain receptors where it can modify their response (Figure 2.5).

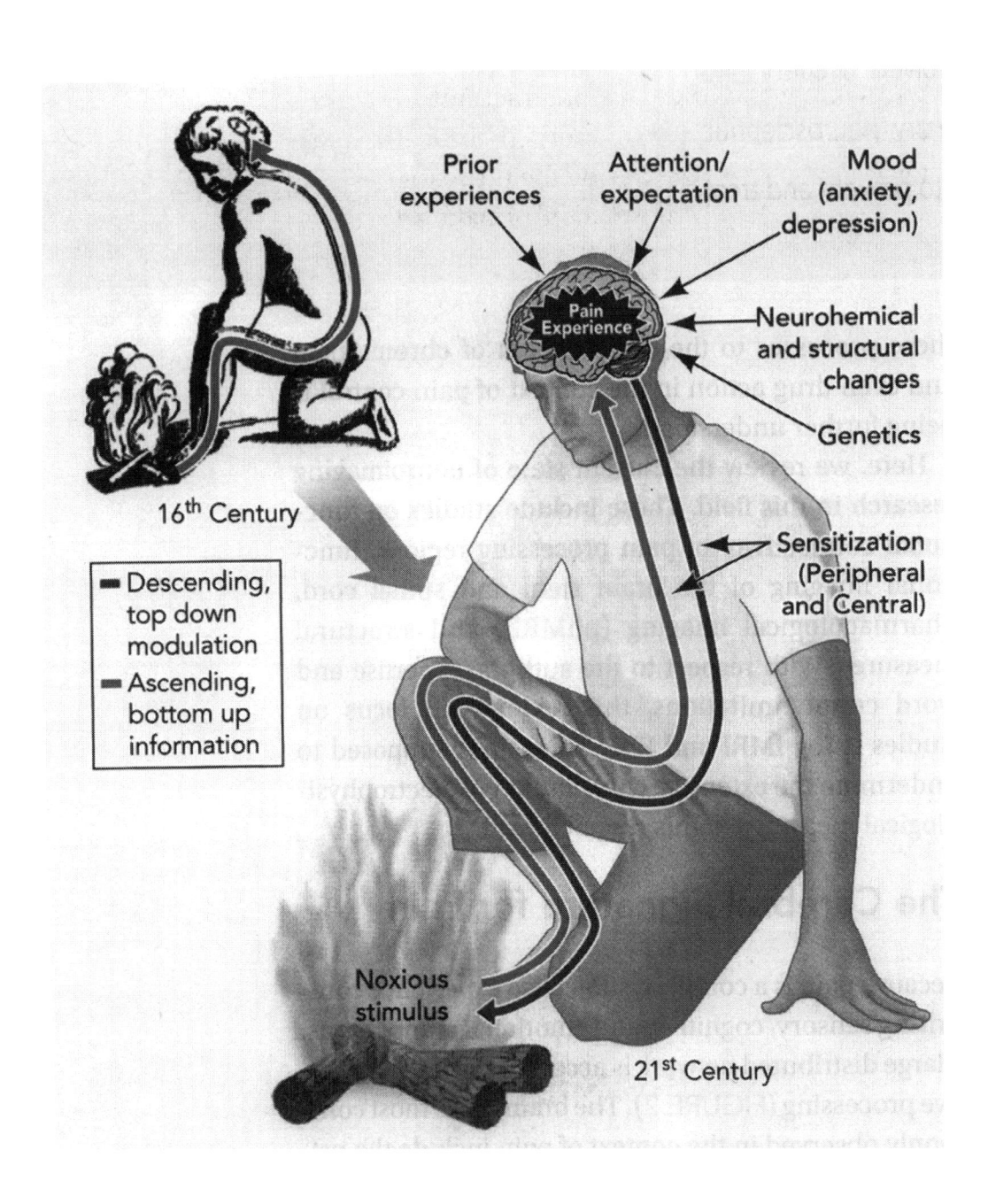

Figure 2.5 Left: Cartesian view of pain. According to the classical Cartesian view, pain was considered to be a hard-wired system in which pain receptor input was passively transmitted along sensory channels to the brain. Right: 21st century view of pain. Pain is acknowledged to represent a multidimensional experience that is influenced by both bottom-up and top-down modulatory influences. From René Descartes. L'homme de Rene Descartes. Paris: Charles Angot (1664); from Bingel, U. and I. Tracey, Imaging CNS Modulation of Pain in Humans. Physiology 2008. 23: p. 371-380. Reprinted with the permission of The American Physiological Society [35].

Descartes believed in a connection from sensory (pain) receptors to the brain and no more. He thought pain signals traveled straight to the brain. We now have a different view and there is considerable evidence that the perception of pain is much more complex and that the experience of pain is not all caused by the physical characteristics of a pain receptor stimulus. We know that there are extensive descending neural pathways that can modify (modulate) the neural activity elicited by activation of pain receptors before it reaches the brain (discussed in detail in Chapter 6).

Some forms of pain may be caused by neural activity that is generated in the spinal cord and the brain without stimulation of pain receptors (pathological pain). Examples are central neuropathic pain, differentiation pain, sympathetically maintained pain (SMP), and disorders such as migraine, myofascial pain, fibromyalgia, and many other rare forms of pain disorders. Common headaches may also be a form of pathological pain.

Pathological pain, the bad pain, has many forms, but a common feature is that it is generated without any pain receptors (nociceptors) being stimulated. It may activate similar structures as are activated in the spinal cord and the brain by stimulating pain receptors or perhaps it activates yet other brain structures. Activation of neuroplasticity plays an important role in creating many forms of pathological pain. One form of pathological pain is central neuropathic pain caused by changes in the function of the spinal cord and the brain through activation of neuroplasticity and which may occur alone or together with pain caused by stimulation of pain receptors. Physiological (receptor) pain may promote development of central neuropathic pain (pathological pain).

This book describes our present understanding of the anatomy and physiology in detail of physiological pain in Chapter 3 and pathological pain in Chapter 8. Chapter 8 discusses the role of neuroplasticity in detail and describes more recent additions to our understanding of the bases for some forms of pain, such as the role of parts of the brain that only recently have been associated with pain. (Neuroplasticity is discussed in Appendix A.)

# Is pain a disease?

Approximately 50% of people who seek medical help either by a physician or at the emergency room do so for pain. Pain in itself is rarely life threatening. Modern medicine often seems to have as its first goal to preserve and extend life while paying less attention to the quality of life. Pain has no visible signs and there are no medical tests, such as imaging of various kinds, chemical tests, or electrophysiology tests that can detect and quantify a person's pain. Many different forms of pain that occur without any known cause (idiopathic pain) belong to the group of pathological pain that is caused by maladaptive (bad) plastic changes in the spinal cord or the brain. Pain that is not caused by a disease or trauma may be regarded as a disease in itself.

# Ways to reduce pain

There are many ways that the sensation of pain and its adverse effects can be reduced. Administration of medications of various kinds is the best known, but there are many other forms of treatment, which will be discussed in detail in Chapter 7 and 12. There are also several systems in the spinal cord and the brain that can reduce or suppress the sensation of pain. There are naturally produced painkillers, endogenous opioids that normally suppress pain. There are also mechanisms in the body that can increase the perception of pain either by sensitizing pain receptors or by sensitizing central nervous system circuits. How circuits in the spinal cord and the brain can modulate pain will be discussed in detail in Chapter 6. Also, pathological pain can be modulated (discussed in Chapter 11).

# Treatment of pain

Pain where the cause is known is naturally best treated by treating the underlying disorder. However, often the underlying disorder does not have any effective treatment or the cause of the pain is not known (idiopathic pain). Idiopathic pain must be treated as a disease, but there are several obstacles to effective treatment of pain (when there is no known cause, when the cause cannot be found, or when the cause cannot be treated successfully).

The complexity of the spinal cord, the brain, and the human body, in general, together with the fact that body functions have developed and been optimized through millions of years, have made many attempted interventions unsuccessful, such as has been experienced from the development of ever more active medical treatments for many diseases including pain. Treatment of physiological pain is discussed in Chapter 7 and treatment of pathological pain is discussed in Chapter 12.

Little is taught in medical school about pain and its treatment and the available treatments are often unsatisfactory and known treatments may be applied inadequately. While there is extensive literature about pain and its treatment, some of it is not in the most accessible form. It is also not always obvious which medical specialty is best suited to manage an individual person's pain.

Many times irrelevant factors determine the choice of treatment. Now, medications are popular because it (seemingly) requires the least involvement of the person with pain. The other often preferred treatment is surgery of some kind. That is often preferred because it is portrayed as a way to "get it over with".

Unfortunately, surgery does not always fulfill its promises and it can have serious side effects. Some surgical operations make the pain for which the operation was done just worse, causing disappointment for the patient and for the surgeon. Most forms of operations cause pain that may last a long time after the operation.

Many people suffer unnecessarily from pain. The specific reasons for this are incorrect diagnosis and incorrect treatment. Many physicians and surgeons have insufficient knowledge about pain and its treatment causing use of incorrect treatment or inadequate use of existing, effective treatments. A further obstacle in achieving good pain control is the fact that in most Western countries, including the USA, the use of the most effective pain medication is restricted by laws, often because of misunderstood risks of addiction.

Patients' failure to follow adequate rules for administrations is not unique to the treatment of pain, but it is often one of the causes of poor results of treatment. Side effects of paracetamol are a typical example of a drug that has good pain relieving effects when administered correctly, but very severe side effects when not administered correctly. This is similar to the situation with antibiotics where incorrect administration (stopping treatment too early) is one of the more important reasons for the development of resistive strains.

The medical profession's suggested solution is to restrict the use of antibiotics, ignoring the fact that it is failure to follow the correct rules for administration of the drugs, not the drugs themselves.

Again to cite Albert Schweitzer (1953) who recognized the seriousness of pain and made the following statement about pain:

*"To the millions of people in every country who live and die in needless pain: We must all die. But if I can save him from days of torture, that is what I feel is my great and ever new privilege."*

The belief that a person is being treated with an active treatment (medication or surgical treatment) while instead an inactive treatment is used, reduces the perception of pain and its effects on many people. This is known as the placebo effect; it is present in many individuals with pain. The placebo effect is real and not just psychological, but the effect lasts only a very short time. We will discuss this in more detail in Chapters 7 and 12.

# What can cause pain and what can pain cause?

The "cause of pain" may mean what has initiated the pain or it may mean what has activated pain circuits in the nervous system, stimulated pain receptors, or changed the function of the nervous system.

While the questions we discussed above about what can cause pain are common, what pain can cause is rarely considered. The question about how pain can affect the body is in fact equal to, or more important than, the question about what causes pain.

## What can cause pain?

Causes of pain in the meaning of what has initiated the pain are many. Tissue damage from trauma or inflammation of various forms is common causes of pain, but many forms of pain occur from other reasons and pain often occurs without any known cause.

Surgery is a form of trauma and pain occurs after most forms of surgery. Peripheral and cranial nerve neuropathies are frequent causes of pain.

Virus infections or metabolic causes, such as diabetes neuropathy, are frequent causes of pain. Life style can cause pain, such as painful alcohol neuropathy or joint pain from being overweight or obese (which increases the risk of getting diabetes type 2, which is often accompanied by painful neuropathy). Functional changes in the spinal cord and the brain are common causes of pain, often brought about by plastic changes.

Somatic pain can be caused by directly stimulating pain receptors such as from burning (temperature) and exposure to chemicals of various kinds. Compression of peripheral nerves and spinal nerve roots is often assumed to be the cause of a person's pain such as common back pain. However, similar root compression also is found in individuals who do not have pain [168].

Compression of nerves and nerve roots mainly affect fibers of large diameter having little effect on the small fibers that mediate pain such as C-fibers and Aδ fibers. This means that mechanical compression of a normal mixed nerve or nerve root such as spinal nerves are unlikely to cause pain, but may affect Aβ and Aα fibers, causing sensory and motor deficits rather than pain. Small diameter (pain fibers) is only sensitive to compression when damaged or inflamed. This means that remedying the inflammation or waiting for a damaged nerve to heal would be a gentler and more effective (and less expensive) treatment than surgical decompression that is now a common treatment.

There are pain receptors in the nerve sheets of peripheral nerves (nervi nervorum), which may cause pain when a nerve is compressed. Dorsal root ganglia (DRG) are sensitive to compression and that has also been hypothesized as a cause of some forms of back pain. This means that it is uncertain how the changes in spinal nerve roots that are so clear from MRI imaging really are the causes of common back pain.

Nerve root compression is common and seems to be harmless in most instances. However, blaming spinal root compression for causing pain is also common, but is often an example of mistaking coincidence for causality. This is a common cause of incorrect diagnosis of common pain conditions such as low back pain and carpal tunnel syndrome. Carpal tunnel syndrome has similarities with low back pain in that it is believed that the cause is mechanical compression (entrapment) of a peripheral nerve (in this case, the nerves at the wrist).

This has caused many surgical operations for pain to be made on the indication of root compression. Anyhow, it seems that the surgeons who do not operate on indications of pain, and only do surgery on the indication of motor weakness, are correct in their choice of patients.

Trauma is a frequent cause of receptor (physiological) pain and such pain is expected to disappear when the wound is healed. If that does not occur, the reason for the prolonged pain may be that the acute physiological pain has activated neuroplasticity and caused changes in the function of the central nervous system; thus, causing pathological pain through activation of neuroplasticity.

Activation of neuroplasticity causing changes in the function of the spinal cord and the brain is a common cause of chronic pain. Plastic changes are often ignored as a cause and instead, structural abnormalities that are present may be assumed to cause the pain although there is evidence that similar changes occur frequently in individuals without pain. It is also often experienced that the correction of the anatomical abnormalities, such as entrapment of spinal nerves, does not relieve pain.

There is evidence that pain can signal disorders before other signs or tests. A somewhat unexpected disorder that presents with facial pain is lung cancer before tests are able to detect such malignancy [373].

# What can pain cause?

Pain can have many effects on many different body functions. Pain activates the sympathetic nervous system and this occurs normally in connection with both physiological and pathological pain, and both in acute and chronic pain. Increased activation of the sympathetic nervous system has many immediate, as well as long-term, consequences. On the short tern, the most visible effects are increased blood pressure and heart rate and perhaps sweating.

Pain definitely affects the digestive system; most obvious perhaps, is the effect of increased secretion of hydrochloric acid in the stomach. Pain also affects the motility of the intestines and secretions in the intestines, causing either diarrhea or constipation.

Increased sympathetic activation in itself increases pain. This means that pain begets pain, thus a form of positive feedback that is uncommon in a biological system. All of these effects of pain should be a sufficient incentive to take appropriate actions regarding keeping pain down. The fact that pain can make pain worse (through activation of the sympathetic nervous system) has consequences for the treatment of pain in general. It is yet another reason that pain must be treated aggressively, with the aim of reducing the pain as much as possible.

It also means that medication or other treatments of chronic pain should be administered on a regular basis and in amounts that are sufficient to eliminate or reduce the pain as much as possible. It also means that pain medication should be taken when having no or very little pain. This is difficult to get people to do. People are used to taking pain medication only when it hurts and are afraid of taking too much pain medication.

In fact, taking pain medication before the pain recurs will result in having to take less pain medication than what is the case when only taking the medication when the pain is apparent.

If the short-term effects of pain on body functions are bad, the long-term effects are even worse. Elevated blood pressure (hypertension) increases the risk for cardiovascular diseases, such as myocardial infarction, and it increases the risk of strokes.

Its effect on the digestive system, such as increasing the production of acids in the stomach, increases the risks for stomach ulcers and bleeding, erosion of the esophagus, and it probably increases the risk of stomach cancer. Increased sympathetic activation also affects the immune system, which can have wide and mostly unknown effects. It means that pain is not only unpleasant, but it is definitely a risk to general health because it causes both transient and permanent damage to vital body systems and promotes and causes diseases.

The argument that people often use is that they will take as little pain medication as possible and, therefore, only take medication when the pain is strong is as equally flawed as the argument that it is not beneficial to do physical exercise because it causes increased heart rates and that a person only has a certain number of heart beats.

In fact, physical exercise causes fewer heartbeats because the long-term decrease in heart rate after physical exercise is much greater than the increase during the actual exercise. The same is the case for pain medication for chronic pain; taking medication regularly before the pain occurs requires less total medication than taking it when the pain has recurred at full strength. It is naturally unfortunate that opioids, which are the most effective pain medication that have the fewest side effects, are surrounded with suspicions of causing addictions. The associated restrictions in the use of opioids are an obstacle in achieving effective pain control (see Chapter 7).

# Epidemiology of pain

Epidemiology is the science of the distribution of diseases in a given population at a given time. Basic epidemiological studies of diseases employ two different measures, namely the incidence and the prevalence. The incidence rate is the number of new occurrences of the disease within a certain period, usually one year.

The other measure, prevalence, is the number of people who have the disease at a given time in a specified population such as, for example, women or men in a certain region, men and women in certain age groups, or people of certain ethnicity. The incidence rate and the duration of the disease determine the prevalence.

Understanding the incidence and prevalence of a disease in a defined population is important for the improvement of health and the design of programs for prevention of diseases. Accurate determination of the prevalence of a condition, such as pain (or tinnitus), that does not have objective signs depends on the ability to define the symptoms of the disease in the questionnaire that is given to the participants in studies of the epidemiology of pain. Thereby, the use of different inclusion criteria in the different studies can explain some of the differences in the results obtained in different studies. For studies on the prevalence of pain, the greatest challenge lies in defining the pain. Epidemiological data regarding diseases, such as pain and tinnitus that only have subjective characteristics, relies on self-reported measures. Many investigators have proposed classification schemes for pain and different studies may use different definitions of the symptoms.

Pain varies widely among individuals, not only in strength, but also in the way the pain appears, and an individual's pain can vary widely from time to time. Many forms of chronic pain change from day to day and even change over the course of one day. The lack of objective signs of pain is another source of uncertainty in studies of this disorder, and only self-reported evaluations of a person's tinnitus are available. The perception of pain is also influenced by external circumstances. These factors all make it difficult to obtain an accurate estimate of the prevalence of pain that affects a person's life and this is one of the reasons that the results reported by different epidemiologic studies differ considerably. Similar reasons make reports on the prevalence of tinnitus vary from study to study.

Only a few epidemiologic studies have attempted to distinguish between the different kinds of pain or the different causes of the pain they are studying. In that way, pain has many similarities with tinnitus [296].

# Prevalence of pain

The prevalence of pain reported in the literature varies widely. Pain affects different groups of people differently, such as different age groups. It is known that different groups of people seem to feel pain differently and, in particular, are affected to different degrees by pain. People of Finnish ethnicity seem to be less sensitive to pain than other groups of people and people from southern Europe are more sensitive to pain than people from northern Europe. It is, therefore, important to define the part of the population that is studied.

One study shows that some pain was reported by 86 of individuals above the age of 65 (Iowa study, 1994). Another study shows prevalence of severe pain of 33 for people at age 77 and above (Swedish study, 1996). The results of a telephone survey of 15 European countries and Israel [47] showed that 19 of respondents over 18 years of age had suffered pain for more than 6 months, with pain intensity of 5 or more for the last episode, on a scale of 1 (no pain) to 10 (worst imaginable). Interviews of 4,839 of the respondents with chronic pain revealed that 66 scored their pain intensity to be of a moderate level (scores of 5–7), 34 at the more severe level (8–10 scores), 46 had constant pain, 56 had intermittent pain, and 49 had suffered pain for 2–15 years.

Pain, especially pathological pain, is often accompanied by a lowered tolerance for moderate painful stimulations and a prolonged sensation of pain after a brief pain stimulation (such as needle stick). This is known as hyperpathia. Another phenomenon that may occur together with pain is a sensation of pain from normally innocuous tactile stimulation such as touching of the skin. This is known as allodynia. These additional symptoms may contribute to the decrease in the quality of life from pain, but it is difficult to include such symptoms in epidemiological studies.

Table 2.2 shows the prevalence of pain as reported in a study of a general population in Canada, 1984. Table 2.3 shows how pain is related to the age of a person and Table 2.4 shows the prevalence of major pain disorders in Sweden.

## TABLE 2.2

## Age-Specific Pain Rates

| CHARACTERISTICS | NO PAIN N | % | PERSISTENT PAIN N | % | TEMPORARY PAIN N | % | TOTAL N | % |
|---|---|---|---|---|---|---|---|---|
| **Sex** | | | | | | | | |
| Males | 335 | 50.4 | 49 | 43 | 13 | 30.2 | 397 | 48.2 |
| Females | 331 | 49.6 | 66 | 57 | 28 | 65.1 | 425 | 51.7 |
| | | | | | | | 822 | |
| **Mean age by sex[a] (years)** | X | S.D. | X | S.D. | X | S.D. | X | S.D. |
| Males | 40.77 | 15.68 | 47.23 | 16.77 | 44.76 | 14.99 | 41.57 | 15.88 |
| Females | 39.77 | 15.75 | 49.95 | 17.26 | 39.78 | 16.56 | 41.06 | 16.34 |
| **Marital status** | | | | | | | | |
| Married / common-law | 471 | 70.4 | 85 | 73.6 | 32 | 74.4 | 588 | 71.6 |
| Single | 152 | 22.7 | 11 | 10.3 | 7 | 16.3 | 170 | 20.7 |
| Divorced / separated | 23 | 3.4 | 7 | 5.8 | 1 | 2.3 | 31 | 3.7 |
| Widowed | 20 | 3.0 | 11 | 10.3 | 1 | 2.3 | 32 | 3.8 |
| | | | | | | | 821 | |
| **Employment** | | | | | | | | |
| Full-time | 376 | 56.2 | 46 | 40.0 | 19 | 44.2 | 441 | 53.5 |
| Part-time | 53 | 7.9 | 10 | 8.0 | 5 | 11.6 | 68 | 8.2 |
| Housewife | 114 | 17.0 | 35 | 30.4 | 10 | 23.3 | 159 | 19.2 |
| Student | 63 | 9.4 | 1 | 0.01 | 3 | 7.0 | 67 | 8.1 |
| Retired | 46 | 6.9 | 21 | 18.0 | 2 | 4.7 | 69 | 8.3 |
| Unemployed / disabled | 16 | 2.3 | 2 | 2.0 | 2 | 4.7 | 20 | 2.4 |
| **Income[b] ($)** | | | | | | | | |
| Under 10,000 | | | 12 | 15.8 | 1 | 2.9 | | |
| 11,000-20,000 | | | 19 | 25.0 | 2 | 20.0 | | |
| 21,000-30,000 | | | 22 | 28.9 | 8 | 22.9 | | |
| 31,000-40,000 | | | 12 | 15.8 | 11 | 31.4 | | |
| 40,000 + | | | 11 | 14.5 | 8 | 22.9 | | |

[a] There are no significant differences on age by sex using ANOVA

Table 2.2. Selected Demographic Characteristics of General Practice Sample

Data from Crook, J., E. Rideout, and G. Browne, The prevalence of Pain Complaints in a General Population. Pain, 1984. 18: p. 299---314[90].

## TABLE 2.3

| Age (years) | Standard Population N | Persistent pain rate N | Per 1000 pop. |
|---|---|---|---|
| 18-30 [a] | 264 | 20 | 76 |
| 31-40 | 162 | 17 | 105 |
| 41-50 | 124 | 16 | 129 |
| 51-60 | 166 | 33 | 199 |
| 61-70 | 64 | 16 | 250 |
| 71-80 | 38 | 11 | 290 |
| 81+ | 5 | 2 | 400 |

[a] Twelve years

Table 2.3: How pain is related to age. Data from Cook, J., E. Rideout, and G. Browne, The Prevalence of Pain Complaints in a General Population. Pain, 1984. 18: p. 299-314[90].

## TABLE 2.4

| | > 6 months (%) | 1-6 months (%) | < 1 month (%) | Total prevalence ($) |
|---|---|---|---|---|
| Head, face, mouth | 8.9 | 1.0 | 4.7 | 14.6 |
| Neck | 19.3 | 2.3 | 4.6 | 26.2 |
| Shoulders, arms | 23.2 | 2.8 | 4.7 | 30.7 |
| Chest | 6.5 | 1.1 | 1.8 | 9.4 |
| Abdomen | 6.0 | 0.8 | 1.2 | 8.1 |
| Pelvis | 3.6 | 0.2 | 1.3 | 5.2 |
| Upper back | 10.2 | 1.3 | 1.9 | 13.4 |
| Lower back | 20.3 | 3.0 | 8.0 | 31.3 |
| Hips | 10.4 | 1.6 | 2.4 | 14.4 |
| Legs | 20.1 | 1.8 | 3.3 | 25.2 |
| Any pain or discomfort | | | | 65.90% |

Table 2.4: The prevalence of major disorders with central pain in Sweden, 1989. Data from Brattberg, G., M. Thorslund, and A. Wikman, The Prevalence of pain in a general population. The results of a postal survey in a county of Sweden. Pain, 1989. 37: p. 215-222.

Studies of the prevalence of different kinds of pain show considerable variations. The variation has different sources [242]. One is that diseases are not counted because people do no not seek medical assistance and even for those who do, the diseases may not be reported. The epidemiology is best known for diseases where there are legal obligations to report incidence, such as cancer in the USA. Data for many other diseases, such as low back pain, underestimate the real incidence and prevalence. Low back pain is a good example of several uncertainties. One source of uncertainty in the results of different epidemiologic studies of pain is shared with other voluntary studies, namely that not all persons selected for a study respond. Normally, epidemiologic studies will spend a considerable effort finding out if the people in the group of non-responders are different from those enrolled in the group that respond. This may not have occurred in all studies on the prevalence of pain.

The participants in some studies may have been selected in one way or another and the results may, therefore, not be representative of the general population. This also means that the epidemiology of self-reported pain, in fact, is not a valid measure of the epidemiology of pain, but it is rather the epidemiology of reported pain [242].

It was mentioned above that the effect of pain on a person's quality of life depends more on the distress or suffering (troubled pain) it causes and less on how strong a person perceives his or her pain. When discussing the prevalence of pain, it is the troubled pain that is of the greatest interest because that is the form of pain that affects the quality of life. Troubled pain may result in the inability to work and may have such a severe effect on a person that a person may commit suicide.

The incidence of only a few of the rare pain disorders is known with some accuracy. Examples are trigeminal neuralgia (TGN) which has an incidence of 5.9 per 100,000 women and 3.4 per 100,000 men (in a white population in the USA [202]). Glossopharyngeal neuralgia (GPN) has an incidence of 0.7/100,000/year.

The prevalence of distress from pain is poorly known and few epidemiological studies have taken quality of life as the object of study. (We will discuss the neurophysiologic basis for fear and distress in Chapter 3 in connection with physiological pain).

# Chronic widespread pain (CWP)

The prevalence of some specific disorders with pain is known in more detail than pain in general. One example is chronic widespread pain (CWP), which is an entity that includes fibromyalgia [77]. It is interesting that the prevalence of CWP is largest in the age interval of 60-69 years and that it is almost twice as frequent in females compared with males [77] (Figure 2.6).

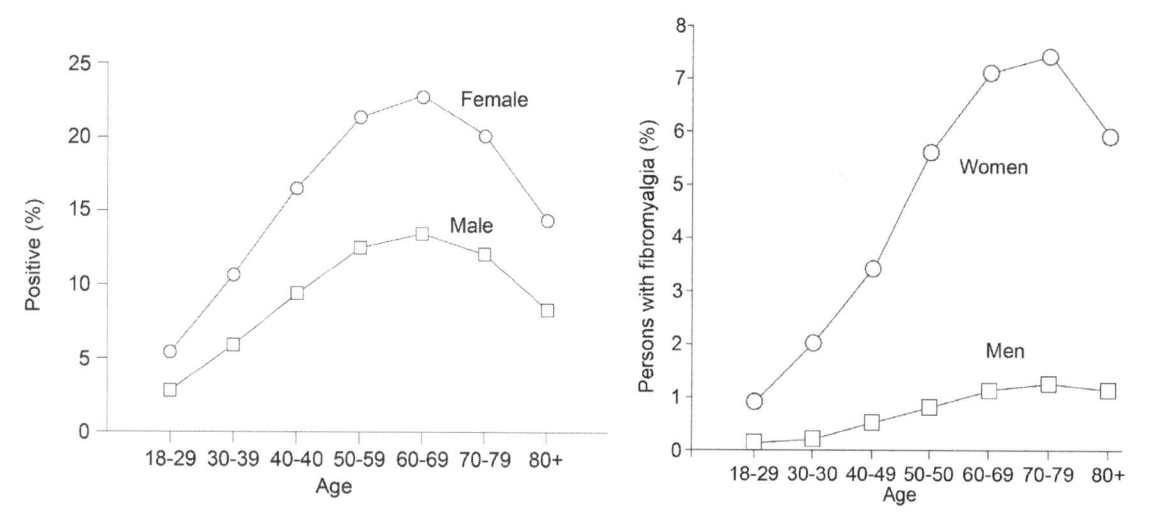

Figure 2.6 Prevalence of chronic widespread pain (CWP) by age and sex for the Wichita population ages 18 and above. (From Wolfe, F., K. Ross, J. Anderson, and et al, The prevalence and characteristics of fibromyalgia. Arthritis and Rheumatism, 1995. 38: p. 18-18. [484].) (Artwork by Monica Javidnia.)

Figure 2.7. Prevalence of fibromyalgia. Notice the difference between men and women. (Modified from Wolfe, F., K. Ross, J. Anderson, and et al, The prevalence and characteristics of fibromyalgia. Arthritis and Rheumatism, 1995. 38: p. 18-18. [484]. (Artwork by Monica Javidnia.)

It is seen from Figure 2.6 that the prevalence of CWP is approximately 12 of adult populations [242]. The pain in all of these studies was defined according to one standard, the one by the American College of Rheumatology, and that is one of the reasons for the lower variations in the results. The difference between the prevalence of fibromyalgia (alone) in women and men is even larger than it is for CWP (Figure 2.7).

Studies of the prevalence of these kinds of complex symptoms are complicated by the contribution from pain caused by neurobiological, psychological, and behavioral factors that all can cause chronic central pain

# How reliable are epidemiological data?

The prevalence of chronic pain has been reported for adult populations in the range from 2 to 40 [244]. As mentioned above, this wide variation in the reported prevalence has several causes.

Some of the most important factors that contribute to the variations are the way questions for studies of the prevalence of pain are formulated. This varies among studies. Some studies have used written questions distributed to groups of people more or less representative of the general population. The participants in some studies have been selected with regards to age, gender, ethnicity, and other criteria and, therefore, may not be representative of the general population.

Pain varies widely among individuals, not only in strength, but also in character and an individual's pain can vary widely from time to time. Many forms of chronic pain change from day to day and even change over the course of one day. Few epidemiologic studies have attempted to distinguish between the different origins of the pain.

The perceived severity of chronic pain depends on many different factors; one being a person's personality. The perception of pain is also influenced by external circumstances. These factors all make it difficult to obtain an accurate estimate of the prevalence of pain that affects a person's life, which is one of the reasons that the results reported by different epidemiologic studies differ considerably.

# Pain and affective disorders

Affective disorders, such as depression, are more common in individuals with chronic pain than in people who do not have extensive pain. Affective (mood) disorders occur more frequently in individuals who have pain over long periods of time [143, 320, 362].

Specifically, depressive symptoms occur frequently together with many chronic pain conditions such as rheumatoid arthritis (RA). Studies have found that depression occurs with at least mild severity in up to 42 of individuals with RA and depression contributes to mortality, decreased quality of life, increased health care costs, and disability [53].

A study by Breivik, 2006 [47] showed that 21 had been diagnosed with depression due to the pain and 61 were unable or less able to work outside the home, 19 had lost a job, and 13 had changed jobs due to their pain. Assessment of their treatment for the pain showed that 40 had inadequate pain management and less than 2 were seeing a pain management specialist.

A large study used random samples of 18,980 individuals aged between 15 and 100 years who were representative of the general population of 5 European countries (the United Kingdom, Germany, Italy, Portugal, and Spain). The results of the study showed that 4 (95 confidence interval of 3.7 to 4.3) of the sample had depression at the time of the interview.

Nearly half of the participants (43) in the study who had depression also reported having pain. The participants who had depression and chronic pain had a longer duration of their depressive symptoms than those who did not have pain (7 months longer) and were more likely to report severe fatigue, insomnia nearly every night, severe psychomotor retardation, weight gain, severe difficulty concentrating, and severe feelings of sadness or depressed mood [320]. The study was based on telephone interviews done between 1994 and 1999. The questions were designed to make it possible to make differential diagnosis according to the DSM-IV for mental disorders. The questionnaire also included questions about the individual's painful physical conditions, medical treatment, consultations, hospitalizations for medical conditions, and a list of diseases. Failure in the treatment of pain is known to promote depression.

# SECTION II
# PHYSIOLOGICAL PAIN

Physiological pain is pain caused by stimulation of pain receptors (nociceptors). This form of pain is, therefore, also known as receptor (or nociceptor) pain. Pain that is not caused by stimulation of receptors is referred to as pathological pain (see Section III). There are many different forms of physiological pain; therefore, there are many different causes (pathologies) of physiological pain. Pain is far more complex than normally assumed, involving many structures in the spinal cord and the brain.

There are two main forms of physiological pain, namely somatic pain and visceral pain. Somatic pain is caused by the stimulation of pain receptors and may be caused by trauma to the skin, ligaments, joints, and muscles, or by inflammatory processes (discussed in Chapter 10). Pain associated with peripheral nerves and cranial nerves is regarded to be physiological pain. There are no pain receptors in brain tissue, but the outer lining of the brain (dura mater) and its large arteries have pain receptors and thus, can elicit physiological pain. These pain receptors are innervated by the trigeminal nerve (CNV).

In this section, we will first discuss (in Chapter 3) the ascending and descending neural pathways that are activated in acute pain and that are elicited by the activation of pain receptors in the skin, joints, tendons, muscles, and in peripheral and cranial nerves. The various receptors involved will be described, together with the different kinds of nerve fibers that carry pain signals, and the neural circuits in the spinal cord, brainstem, and brain that process pain signals.

Itching has many similarities with pain and similar receptors and pathways mediate the sensation as pain. It is discussed at the end of Chapter 3. We will consider pain elicited from internal organs (visceral pain) in Chapter 4. Pain from peripheral and cranial nerves is discussed in Chapter 5. Modulation of pain will be discussed in Chapter 6 and Chapter 7 will discuss treatment of physiological pain.

# CHAPTER 3
# Somatic Pain

# Abstract

1. Somatic pain is caused by stimulation of specific receptors known as pain receptors (nociceptors).

2. Pain receptors (nociceptors) have many forms and are found in the skin, tendons, joints, ligaments, and muscles.

3. Pain receptors are innervated by C fibers and by Aδ fibers.

4. Trauma and inflammation can provide stimulation of pain receptors

5. Stinging (shooting) pain is mediated by small myelinated fibers (Aδ) and burning sensations are mediated by unmyelinated fibers (C-fibers).

6. Activation of pain receptors has a local effect on the skin leading to release of neuropeptides such as substance P, calcitonin gene-related peptides (CGRP), and neurokinase A (NKA).

7. Cells in the dorsal horn of the spinal cord and the trigeminal nucleus are the targets of pain fibers, and some processing of pain information occurs in these structures.

8. Aδ fibers project to cells in lamina I and C-fibers project to cells in lamina II of the dorsal horn of the spinal cord. Cells in lamina II send axons to terminate on cells in lamina I. Lamina I and II are known as substancia gelantinosa.

9. From the spinal cord, there are three ascending pathways for pain; the spinothalamic tract (STT) is the best known; it has two parts, a lateral and a ventral part. The two other tracts are the spinomesencephalic tract and the spinoreticular tract.

10. The spinotrigeminal tract carries pain information to the thalamus from the trigeminal nucleus.

11. The thalamus plays an important role in processing of pain signals. As is the case for sensory systems, the ventral and the dorsal-medial portions of the thalamus have different roles in processing pain signals from the dorsal horns of the spinal cord and from the trigeminal nucleus.

12. Axons of cells in lamina I cross the midline and form the lateral spinothalamic tract (STT) while the axons of cells in deeper lamina (lamina III-V) form the anterior STT.

13. The targets of the lateral STT axons are cells in the periaqueductal gray (PAG), the somatosensory cortex (3a), the intralaminar thalamus, cells in the anterior insula, the anterior cingulate cortex, the nucleus of the solitary tract (NST), and the lateral parabrachial area (LPb).

14. The axons of the anterior STT tract terminate on cells in the ventral posterior lateral (VPL) and ventral posterior inferior (VPI) thalamic nuclei. The axons from cells in the VPL and VPI project to the primary somatosensory cortex (SI) and secondary cortices (SII).

15. Both divisions of the STT give off branches that terminate in cells in the reticular formation.

16. The spinoreticular tract originates in the dorsal horn and ascends bilaterally. It has branches that terminate in cells in the reticular formation, and some of its fibers are interrupted in cells in the reticular formation. The thalamic target is the dorsal division; the cells of which project to secondary and association cortices and subcortical to many targets such as the lateral nucleus of the amygdala.

17. The main targets of the axons of the spinomesencephalic tract that originate in cells in the spinal cord are cells in the periaqueductal gray. The pathway crosses the midline.

18. There is extensive communication between the different segments of the spinal cord. For example, interneurons in lamina I send fibers to spinal segments above and below their own segment traveling in the tract of Lissauer.

19. Axons from cells in the caudal trigeminal nucleus that are targets of axons from pain receptors in the head form the trigeminothalamic tract (TTT).

20. The vagus nerve plays an important role in many forms of pain and it may be regarded to be a separate ascending pathway in addition to those in the spinal cord for pain.

21. The afferent fibers of the vagus nerve terminate in the nucleus of the solitary tract (nucleus tractus solitarious) (NST), the cells of which send axons to terminate on cells in many parts of the brain.

22. In addition to mediating pain from internal organs, the vagus nerve is also important in immune responses and it provides the feeling of illness.

23. As in sensory systems, pain pathways include abundant descending pathways.

24. Two major descending systems have been identified; one involving the periaqueductal gray (PAG) and the other is the noradrenalin-serotonin pathway. The PAG system again has two parts, the rostral ventromedial medulla (RVM) and the dorsolateral pontine tegmentum (DLPT).

25. The PAG receives input from many parts of the brain, such as the frontal lobe, the amygdala, the hypothalamus, the pontomedulary reticular formation, and the locus coeruleus.

26. The RVM has both inhibitory and facilitatory influence on cells in the dorsal horn of the spinal cord.

27. The raphe nucleus (nor-adrenalin-serotonin pathway) also influences excitability of cells in the dorsal horn of the spinal cord.

28. The ascending-descending pathways can be viewed as forming loops where information can circulate.

29. Itching (puritus) has many similarities with pain. The receptors for pain are sensitive to histamines and they are innervated by C-fibers.

30. Itching can be suppressed by painful stimuli.

31. Central representation of itching includes the ventro-medial posterior (VMpo) thalamus. A sensation of itching can be initiated by the central nervous system.

# Introduction

Somatic pain has an important protective role as a warning about trauma and diseases and it serves to discourage manipulation of injured tissue during healing. It is a normal sensation that alerts on injury or disease. Acute pain from an injury to an extremity elicits the withdrawal reflex that is aimed at moving the extremity away from danger. Somatic pain may be an indicator of illness and it may signal chronic injury. Pain can be caused by diseases, such as rheumatoid arthritis (RA), or other forms of inflammation. The different forms of cancer pain are yet another group of pain conditions caused by diseases. Trauma of various kinds can cause pain; ischemia is a common cause of pain. Almost all forms of surgical operations cause physiological pain that lasts for a short or long time. Some diagnostic tests are also common causes of pain.

While there are many similarities between sensory systems and pain systems, there are also many differences. One difference is that the sensation of pain from the stimulation of pain receptors is not as constant as the sensation of sensory stimuli, such as touch, sound, and light. The sensation of pain and the perceived strength of the stimulation of pain receptors by the same physical stimulation can change (be modulated) by internal and external factors (see Chapter 6). One cause of such variations is sensitization that may occur at the receptor level (peripheral sensitization) or in the central nervous system (central sensitization). Decreased pain sensitivity may also occur either because of peripheral or supraspinal influence on neurons in the dorsal horn of the spinal cord or in the trigeminal nucleus.

# Nature of somatic pain

Somatic pain elicited by the sudden stimulation of pain receptors typically has two components, a stringent pain sensation followed by a slower burning sensation. The first sensation of pain, such as that from stepping on one's toe, is a sharp, stingy pain followed by a burning pain (Figure 3.1). The initial and distinct sensation is precisely referred to the location on the body from where the pain stimulation occurs while the burning sensation that follows is poorly localized.

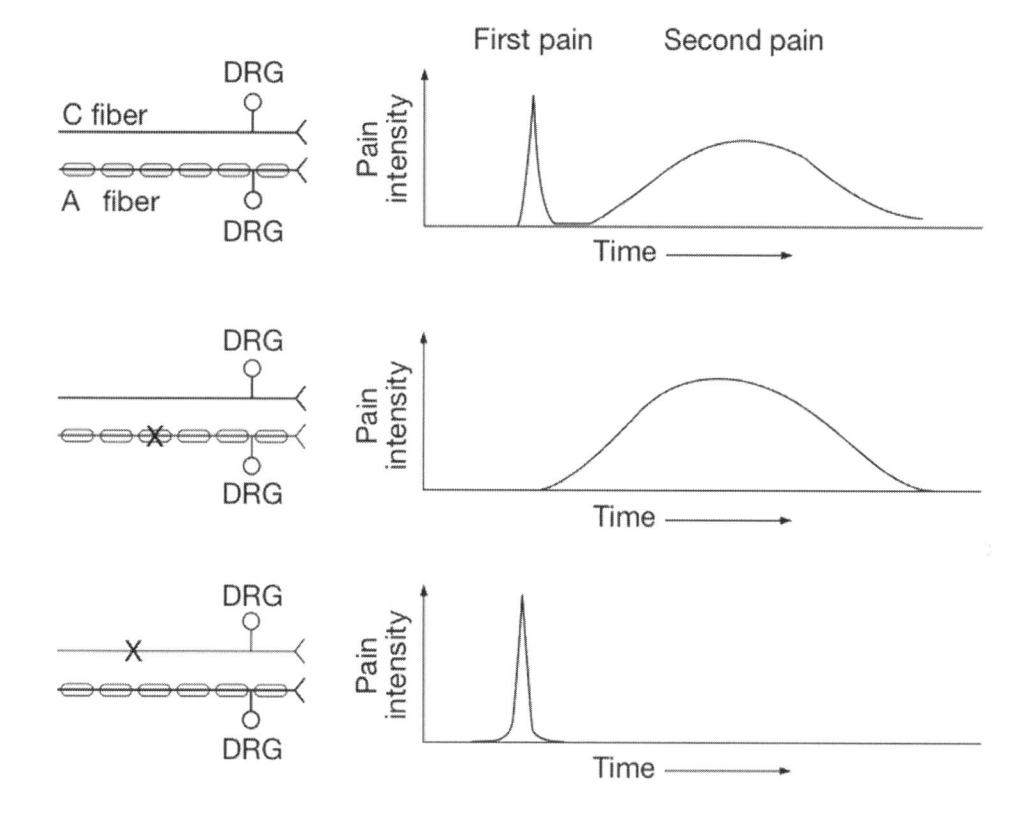

Figure 3.1 Stimulation of pain receptors causes an initial fast and a later slow component of pain sensation. The pain signals that cause these two different types of sensation are carried in two different types of nerve fibers (Aδ and C-fibers) (From Møller, A.R., Sensory Systems: Anatomy and Physiology. 2003, Amsterdam: Academic Press. Reprinted with permission by Elsevier [288].)

The stingy pain sensation is mediated by small diameter myelinated nerve fibers, type Aδ. The slow pain has an aching and burning character and it comes later than the initial pain's sensation. It is poorly localized anatomically and it is difficult to estimate its strength, which is poorly defined and subject to change by many factors. The slow aching pain sensation is mediated by C-type unmyelinated fibers.

Most anatomical regions on the surface of the body are supplied by both Aδ and C-fiber innervated pain receptors, so the anatomical location of pain is usually well defined. However, with one clear exception, namely the teeth, where the tooth pulp lacks Aδ innervated receptors and only C-fiber receptors are present. This explains why it is difficult to determine from which tooth the pain comes.

Compressing a peripheral nerve that contains Aδ and C-fibers affects the myelinated fibers more than the unmyelinated fibers; thus, impairing neural conduction in Aδ fibers more than in the C-fibers (Figure 3.1). Compressing a peripheral nerve may produce numbness with pain sensations preserved. Application of local anesthetics has the opposite effect by affecting C-fibers more than myelinated fibers, abolishing pain sensation while preserving the sharp phase of pain and sensation of touch that is mediated by larger myelinated fibers (Aβ).

# Painful stimuli have a local effect

Branching of nerve fibers that innervate pain receptors is abundant as it is of many other nerve fibers. Some of these branches innervate structures in the skin close to the pain receptors from where the fibers originate (Figure 3.2). These branches innervate structures, such as vascular structures, causing redness (giving it the name inflam-mation) by increasing blood flow. Action potentials propagate both centrally and peripherally in nociceptive fibers releasing substance P, calcitonin gene-related peptides (CGRP), and neurokinase A (NKA). These substances stimulate epidermal cells and immune cells causing vasodilatation, transport of plasma, and contraction of smooth muscles.

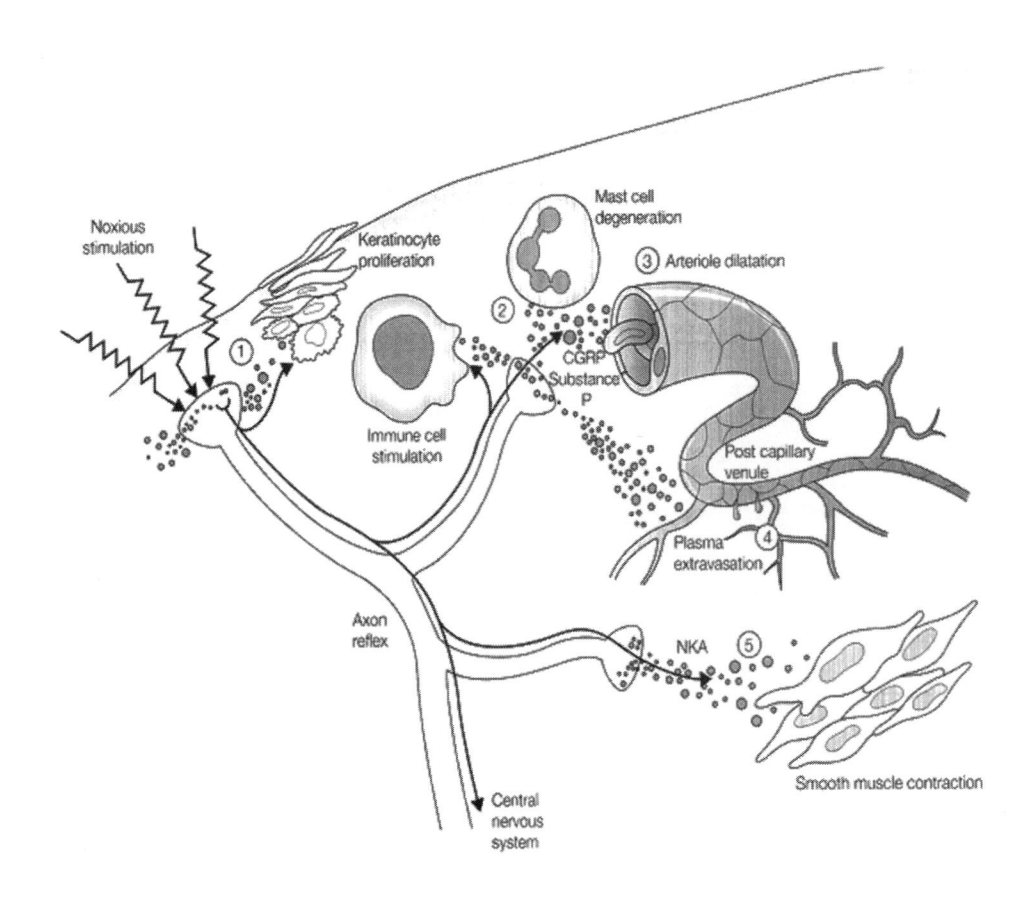

Figure 3.2 Local effects on the skin of stimulation of pain receptors. The antidromic activation of structures in the skin leads to the release of neuropeptides such as substance P, calcitonin gene-related peptides (CGRP), and neurokinase A (NKA). These substances can stimulate epidermal cells (1) and immune cells (2), or lead to vasodilatation (plasma extravasation) (4) and smooth muscle contraction (5). (From Meyer, R.A., et al., Peripheral mechanisms of cutaneous nociception, in Wall and Melzack's Textbook of Pain, S.B. McMahon and M. Koltzenburg, (Eds.), Editors. 2006, Elsevier: Amsterdam. p. 3-34, Artwork by Ian Suk, Johns Hopkins University. Reprinted with permission from Elsevier [274]).

# Tissue damage

An important and frequent cause of pain is tissue damage. The effect of tissue damage has been divided into three phases. The immediate, later, and long-term events that occur after traumatic injury involve distinctly different processes. In the immediate phase, there is a feeling of pressure, heat, or cold, and chemicals of various kinds are liberated.

Withdrawal reflexes may be activated immediately if the pain is transient and comes from the extremities. Depending on the strength of the pain, increased muscle tone may be initiated and the sympathetic nervous system may be activated causing increased blood pressure and heart rate, etc. Limbic structures of the brain may be activated creating emotional (fear) reactions. Plastic changes may begin to take effect in the spinal cord (trigeminal nucleus, if the pain comes from structures of the head) and/or the brain. Under certain circumstances, strong descending activity may act on pain circuits in the spinal cord to suppress transmission of pain signals; thus, abolishing pain sensation. This may be the result of the "fight and flight" reaction and it may abolish pain sensations for a short time, even from serious trauma.

In the second stage of tissue damage, events occur, such as the liberation of different peptides, causing dilation of blood vessels at the location of the trauma, which cause a feeling of heat from an increase in blood flow. Enzymes break down molecules of debris into smaller molecules and the created substances may stimulate pain fibers. Plastic changes in the spinal cord (or the trigeminal nucleus) and/or the brain may continue to develop. The effect of the descending activity that suppressed the pain sensation may begin to wear off and pain and awareness of the pain increases.

The last stage of changes that occur after trauma are long term changes that include plastic changes in the spinal cord and/or the brain, edema from leaking of fluid into tissue, further widening of blood vessels causing redness, feeling of heat from an increase in blood flow, invasion of white blood cells, and a feeling of tenderness from the sensitization of pain fibers (peripheral sensitization; primary hyperalgesia) and central sensitization (secondary hyperalgesia) also occurs. During that period, chemicals are transported in pain fibers to central structures causing central sensitization.

Severe pain reduces the quality of life and it may cause hypertension, resulting in an increased risk of stroke and myocardial infarction. Suffering from affective (psychiatric) disorders, such as depression, may develop with an increased risk of suicide.

# Receptors for pain, heat, and cold and their innervation

Pain receptors (nociceptors) are special receptors, so named because they respond to harmful stimulation such as certain chemicals, heat and cold, and to mechanical stimulation. Two kinds of temperature receptors, hot and cold receptors, belong to the pain receptor category of sensory receptors. Two other kinds of temperature receptors, sensing cool and warmth, are regarded to be sense organs for innocuous sensations.

Pain receptors are especially abundant in the skin and joints, but less so in muscles. Joints, tendons, and visceral organs also have pain receptors. Coverings of peripheral nerves, the dura mater, and certain cerebral vessels have pain receptors (not the brain itself, nor the spinal cord) that mediate harmful stimulations. Trauma of various kinds may cause mechanical stimulation of pain receptors, but most important, are chemicals that are released in connection with tissue damage.

The sensitivity of most pain receptors may be increased by the secretion of norepinephrine from sympathetic nerve endings; thus, providing control of pain sensitivity from the sympathetic nervous system (known as peripheral sensitization). Sympathetic activation has many other effects on pain, as discussed later in this chapter.

Under pathological circumstances, not only can pain receptors mediate the sensation of pain, but also receptors that normally mediate the sensation of touch can cause pain sensation when overstimulated.

# Innervation of pain receptors

Pain information is mediated by nerve fibers of two types according to the classical classification, Aδ fibers and C-fibers. Aδ fibers are myelinated and have axon diameters in the range of 1-5 μm and a conduction velocity from 5 to 30 m/sec. C-fibers are unmyelinated and the axons have diameters between 0.2 and 2 μm and a conduction velocity of between 0.5 and 1 m/sec.

These are classified as polymodal fibers because they respond to several different modalities of stimulation. Both Aδ and C-fibers respond to mechanical stimulation and to temperature (hot and cold) (3.3).

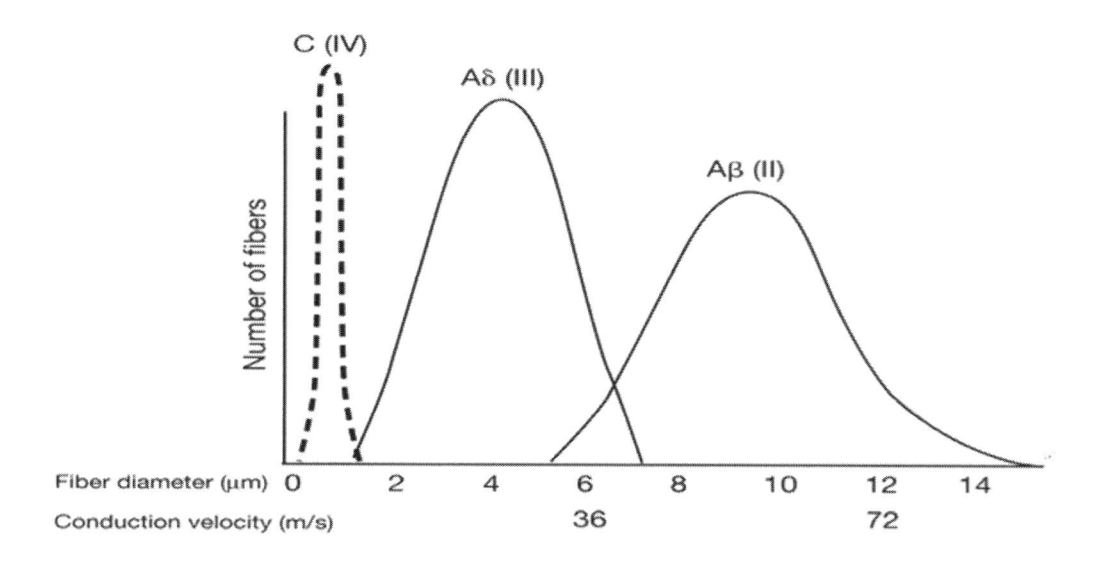

Figure 3.3 Axon diameters and conduction velocity of different classes of nerve fibers. (Modified from Møller, A. R. (2006) Neuroplasticity and disorders of the nervous system. Cambridge University Press Cambridge. Reprinted with permission from Cambridge University Press [288].)

The conduction velocity of nerve fibers within the same group (such as Aδ or C-fibers) varies (Figure 3.3). In particular, the conduction velocity decreases along a nerve fiber being fastest (largest axon diameter) near the axon's cell body. Decreasing conduction velocity with the distance away from the cell body is caused by decreasing axon diameters. Also, the part of Aδ nerve fibers that is far away from the cell body is more susceptible to nerve diseases (peripheral nerve neuropathy) and to age related changes than the parts that are close to the cell body.

The cold and heat receptors are innervated by unmyelinated C-fibers. The threshold for heat sensation (pain) is approximately 45 degrees centigrade and the threshold for cold sensation is around 14 degrees centigrade for hairy skin.

Thus, cold pain is caused by temperatures that are further away from normal skin temperature than heat. There is evidence that heat receptors are located close to the surface while cold receptors are located deep in the skin. The sensation of heat pain rises much faster than the sensation of cold pain when the temperature is changed away from the threshold. Most pain receptors respond when the skin temperature drops below 0 degrees centigrade.

Not all C-fibers mediate pain. Some low threshold mechano-receptors that are innervated by C-fibers respond to innocuous stimulation (pleasant touch).

# Aδ and C-fibers carry different kinds of pain sensations

The pain signals carried by Aδ fibers cause a pricking pain and provide accurate information about the anatomical location of the pain. This sensation is more robust than that carried by C-fibers, which is burning in nature and poorly localized. There are two kinds of Aδ fibers [274], type I and II. Type I Aδ fibers carry the response to heat, mechanical, and chemical stimuli and their mean conduction velocity is 25 m/sec. Type II Aδ fibers have a mean conduction velocity of 15 m/sec. These fibers have a high threshold and are rare.

Neural activity in C-fibers causes burning pain sensations. The slow conduction of C-fibers delays the burning sensation relative to the sensation medicated by Aδ fibers. The longer duration of the burning sensation (see Figure 3.3) is partly due to the variation in the conduction velocity of different C-fibers. This causes a spread in time of the activity that arrives at the target cells in the spinal cord or the trigeminal nucleus.

# Bottom-up and top-down communication of pain signals

Descartes assumed that there were only bottom-up connections to the brain from pain receptors, but we now know that there are also top-down connections; thus, a feedback from the brain to the periphery of the nervous system. Descartes also regarded the brain to have two different kinds of functions: one that was automatic and one that was complex. The automatic function he illustrated by the withdrawal reflex and the complex part was, in his words, the "soul".

Although the Cartesian view of dualism is still regarded as valid to some extent, we now regard what he called the "soul" or "matters of the mind" to also be a product of physical matter such as structures of the nervous systems.

# Neuroanatomy of somatic pain

Considerable processing of pain signals occurs in the spinal cord and the caudal trigeminal nucleus. From there, pain signals reach many parts of the brain through several ascending tracts, of which the anterior and lateral spinothalamic tracts (STT) are the most important. Pain signals can reach the "emotional brain," mainly the amygdala and the anterior cingulated cortex, through two routes.

One route is via the ventral thalamus and a chain of cortical structures and the other is via the dorsal and medial thalamus and directly to the lateral nucleus of the amygdala (high route and low route, respectively, Le Doux, 1992, [227]). There are several descending tracts that target cells in the dorsal horn of the spinal cord and through which modulation of pain signals occur (described in Chapter 6).

# The dorsal horn

Pain signals are extensively processed in the dorsal horn of the spinal cord and pain from the head is processed in the trigeminal nucleus before entering the brain. Pain signals reach the dorsal horn through dorsal roots of spinal sensory nerves and pain signals from the head reach the trigeminal nucleus through the trigeminal nerve (CNV), the glossopharyngeal nerve (CNIX), and the vagus nerve (CNX) [497]. These are bipolar axons that have their cell bodies in the dorsal root ganglia (DRG).

The axons that are of two types, Aδ and C, terminate on cells in the dorsal horn of the spinal cord (Figure 3.4).

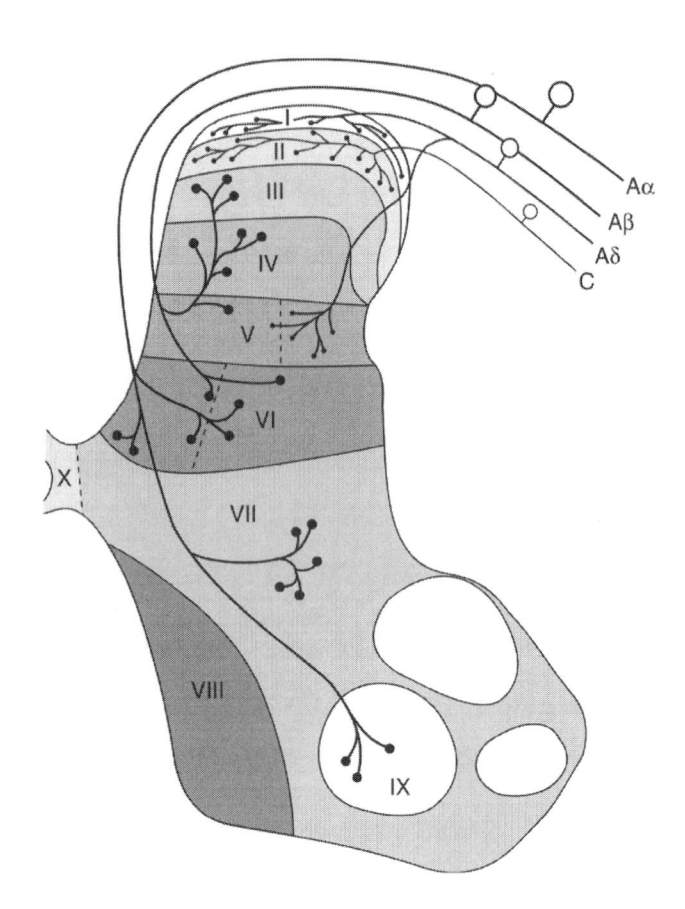

Figure 3.4 Different types of sensory nerve fibers terminating on cells in the horn of the spinal cord. (Modified from Brodal, 1998.)

The gray matter (horn) of the spinal cord is divided into lamina, each of which is usually labeled with a Roman numeral (Rexed's classification [356]).

The Aδ fibers that mediate sharp pain terminate on cells in lamina I of the dorsal horn and the C-fibers that mediate slow burning pain terminate on cells in lamina II. The short axons of these cells make synaptic contact with cells in lamina I (Figure 3.5). Lamina I and II are also known as substantia gelantinosa after its galantine-like appearance when observed in a microscope. Aδ fibers branch and make contact with other cells in lamina I. Other collateral fibers of the Aδ fibers terminate in lamina IV and V (Figure 3.4).

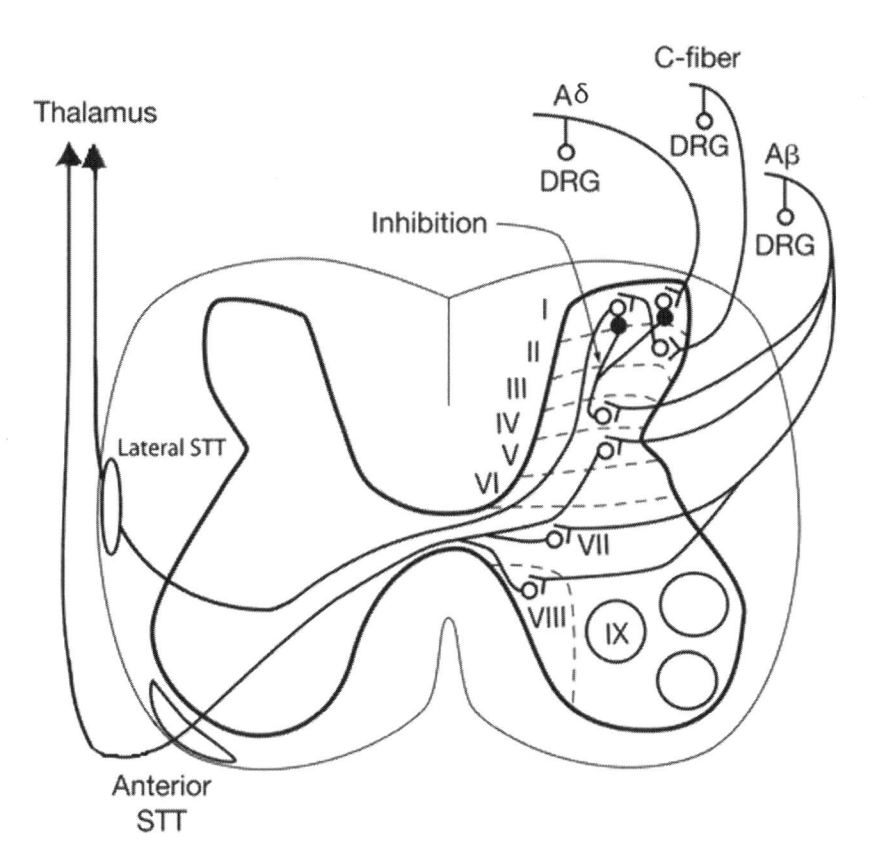

II PHYSIOLOGICAL PAIN  Chapter 3 Somatic Pain  77

Figure 3.5 Schematic illustration of the connections through which innocuous sensory input mediated by large myelinated (Aβ) fibers can inhibit pain cells in lamina I that receive harmful input from Aδ fibers and C-fibers via interneurons and which give rise to axons of the STT. (Modified from Møller, A. R. (2006) Neuroplasticity and disorders of the nervous system. Cambridge University Press Cambridge. Reprinted with permission from Cambridge University Press [288].)

The cells in the dorsal horn provide the first stage of processing of pain information from the body and the trigeminal nucleus in a similar way and provide the earliest processing of pain signals from the head.

The cells of the DRG were earlier believed to (only) serve the purpose of providing nutrients for the axons, but the DRG is now known to be involved in the function of the axon. Thus, the DRG cells play a far more important role than earlier believed [241].

Some of the interneurons in lamina I send fibers to spinal segments above and below their own segment traveling in the tract of Lissauer [108]. Similar circuits exit in the caudal trigeminal nucleus. Most of the axons of the cells in lamina I of the spinal horns cross the midline at the segmental level and ascend in the lateral tract of the spinothalamic tract (STT).

There are also connections from the sympathetic nervous system to some cells in the dorsal horn. Descending fibers from the brainstem terminate on cells in the dorsal horn whereby extensive control of pain signals occur (see Chapter 6).

# The trigeminal nucleus

Pain fibers from the head travel in the fifth, ninth, and tenth cranial nerves to terminate in the caudal (spinal) part of the trigeminal nucleus. These pain fibers innervate pain receptors in the head, including the mouth, the dura mater, and large vessels in the brain. The fibers that carry pain information in these cranial nerves terminate in the caudal (or spinal) portion of the trigeminal nucleus.

The trigeminal nucleus has similarities with the dorsal horn of the spinal cord. It is an elongated structure in the brainstem that reaches from the midbrain into the upper part of the spinal cord (Figure 3.6). Its rostral parts are concerned with innocuous stimulation of the skin in the face and mucosa in the nose, mouth, and the throat. The caudal part is mostly involved with harmful stimulation of the skin on the face, the mucosa of the mouth, pharynx, and throat, the dura mater, and some large vessels of the brain.

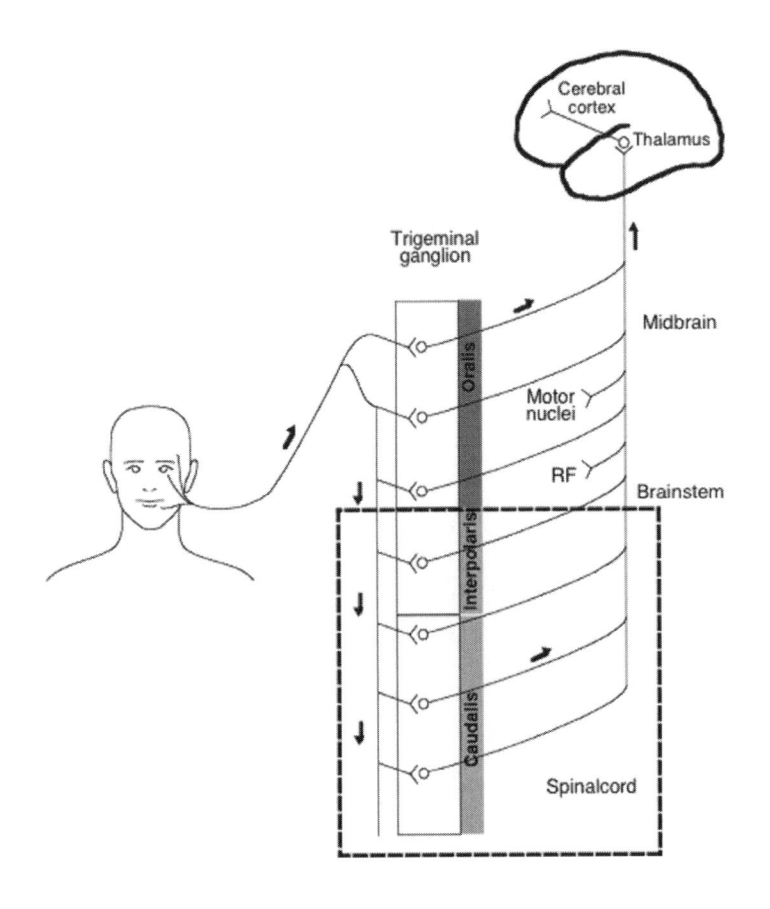

Figure 3.6. Pain pathways from the head of the trigeminal nucleus (indicated by dashed rectangle). RF: Reticular formation. (Adapted from Sessle, 1986 [387].) (From Møller, A. R. (2006) neuroplasticity and disorders of the nervous system. Cambridge University Press Cambridge. Reprinted with permission from Cambridge University Press [288].)

The axons from cells in the caudal trigeminal nucleus terminate on similar cells in the thalamus as those that the axons of the STT terminate on. The cells in the trigeminal nucleus also have connections to the dorsal cochlear nucleus [235, 497, 503], making this a structure of importance for tinnitus [301] (see Chapter 7).

The trigeminal nucleus is the site of pathologies that cause a particular kind of pain, trigeminal neuralgia, that consists of attacks of excruciating pain in one of the three radiations of the trigeminal nerve [426].

# Pain pathways

Like sensory pathways, pain pathways have both ascending (bottom-up) and descending (top-down) paths. The ascending pathways from the spinal cord and from the trigeminal nucleus reach many parts of the brain.

The ascending pathways for acute pain share some of the structures that are involved in somatosensory perception. The descending pathways originate in many structures in the brain, mainly the periaqueductal gray (PAG), and these pathways reach cells in the dorsal horn of the spinal cord and cells in the trigeminal nucleus.

Pain engages many parts of the brain. For example, the central pathways for pain reach structures that belong to the reward network. Ascending pain pathways are often regarded as part of the somatosensory system, known as the anterior lateral system.

# Ascending pain pathways

The ascending pathways for pain, heat and cold, and itching are known as the anterior lateral system. The anterior lateral system consists of three independent tracts: the spinothalamic tract (STT), spinoreticular and the spinomesencephalic tracts, and for the trigeminal system, the trigeminothalamic tract (TTT) [108, 480, 481] . The STT is the best known and probably the most important of these tracts. It has two parts, an anterior and a lateral tract.

There are two reasons for showing neural pathways. One reason is to describe which structures are involved and how the structures are interconnected. The other reason is to show the anatomical location of the structures that are involved. The anatomical location is important for the neurosurgeon who wants to operate upon the structures or for implanting electrodes to stimulate specific structures electrically (deep brain stimulation, DBS). However, the exact anatomical location of different structures is irrelevant for the neuroscientist and the physician or surgeon who wants to understand how different structures interact in the processing of pain signals or in the generation of phantom sensations such as pain.

While it is common in textbooks to combine these two ways of describing pathways, we will, in this book, focus on functional relationships that are illustrated without describing their anatomical location in the brain and spinal cord.

# Spinothalamic tract

The spinothalamic tract (STT) is the best known of the three ascending fiber tracts that communicate pain information to the brain. This tract consists of axons of cells in the dorsal horn that receives harmful input through Aδ and C-fibers.

The fibers cross the midline at the segmental level of the spinal cord and ascend in two separate tracts, the anterior (ventral) STT and the lateral STT.

One of the two parts of the spinothalamic tracts (STT), the lateral tract, originates in cells in lamina I, while the other part, the anterior STT tract, originates in cells in lamina IV and V (Figure 3.5). The cells in lamina I that contribute to the STT receive monosynaptic input from Aδ fibers and poly (di) synaptic input from C-fibers.

Both parts of the STT cross the midline at each segment of the spinal cord and ascend on the contralateral side of the spinal cord. This is different from sensory signals from innocuous stimulation that ascend on the same side of the spinal cord to reach the dorsal column nuclei from where axons cross the midline.

A simplified diagram, of the STT and its main projections, is shown in Figure 3.7. Central pain pathways project to primary cortices conveying spatial ("where") information. The dorsal/medial thalamus provides "what" information. Information that travels in the two tracts of the STT can also reach the reticular formation and thereby, contribute to arousal [287].

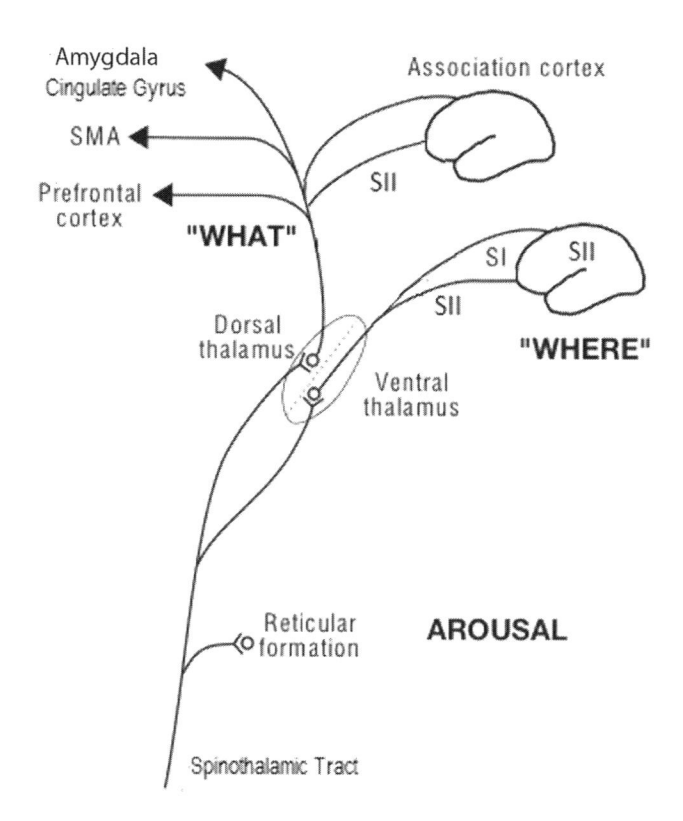

Figure 3.7. Simplified diagram of pathways involved in mediating the sensation of receptor pain. (Modified from Møller, Møller, A.R., Sensory Systems: Anatomy and Physiology. 2003, Amsterdam: Academic Press. Reprinted with permission from Elsevier [287].)

Most STT fibers (85-90 percent) originate in the contralateral spinal horn and 10-15 percent come from the ipsilateral side. Cells in the upper cervical ($C_1$-$C_2$) segments of the spinal cord contribute bilaterally to the STT [108]. In the brainstem, the STT is joined by axons from the caudal trigeminal nucleus (the trigeminothalamic tract, TTT).

# Lateral spinothalamic tract

The lateral tract of the STT (Figure 3.8) is responsible for communicating affective and emotional qualities of painful stimulation; thus, similar to the non-classical pathways of the auditory system that may evoke fear and other emotional reactions to sound in individuals with tinnitus (phonophobia) [295]. Its axons originate in cells in lamina I of the dorsal horn.

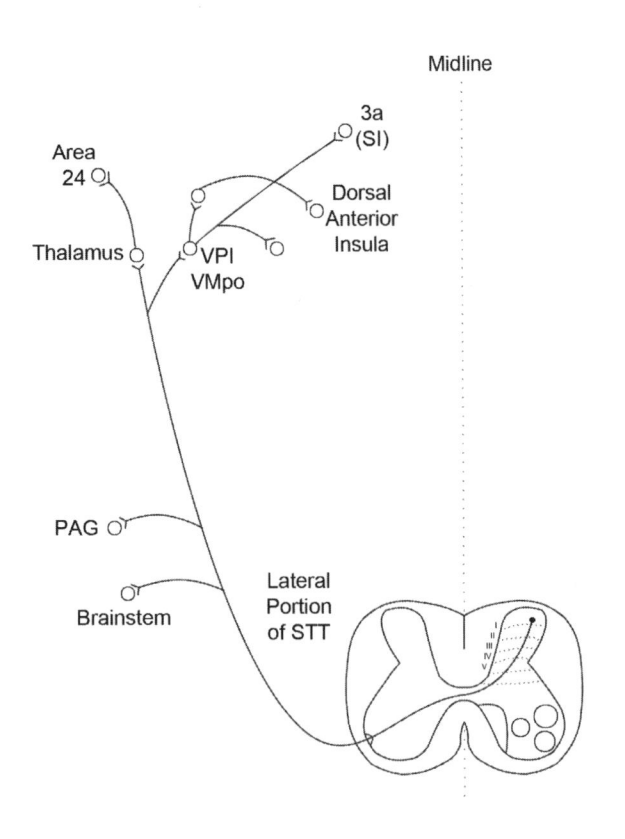

Figure 3.8 Connections from the lateral portion of the STT from cells in lamina I of the dorsal horn. VPI: Ventral posterior inferior (nuclei of the thalamus); VMpo: Ventromedial posterior oralis (nuclei of the thalamus); SI: Primary somatosensory cortex. (Modified from Møller, A. R. (2006) Neuroplasticity and disorders of the nervous system. Cambridge University Press Cambridge. Reprinted with permission from Cambridge University Press [288].) (Artwork by Monica Javidnia.)

Axons from cells that travel in the lateral tract of the STT, mainly originating in lamina I of the dorsal horn, project to the caudal ventrolateral medulla (CVLM), the nucleus of the solitary tract (NST), and the lateral parabrachial area (LPb). These tracts terminate in several nuclei of the somatosensory and intralaminar thalamus. The fibers of the STT terminate in several parts of the thalamus, as many as six areas have been identified [108].

Neurons in the CVLM give rise to a descending projection to the dorsal horn and may integrate nociceptive and cardiovascular responses.

The lateral tract of the STT also projects to many other parts of the brain, such as the anterior cingulate gyrus, Brodman area (BA) 24c, the BA 3a of the somatosensory cortex, and the dorsal anterior insula via the ventral posterior inferior (VPI) nucleus of the thalamus. The axons of the lateral tract terminate on cells in the ventral posterior lateral (VPL) and ventral posterior inferior (VPI) thalamic nuclei. The axons from cells in the VPL and VPI project to the primary somatosensory cortex (SI) and secondary cortices (SII). It has, however, been confirmed in studies in monkeys that activity in STT can reach multiple cortical areas located in the contralateral hemisphere [111]

Thus, this tract provides subcortical connections to many structures, but has minimal cortical projections. This part of the STT resembles the non-classical somatosensory pathways targeting the medial part of the thalamus, the cells of which send their axons to the secondary somatosensory cortex, bypassing the primary cortex, and instead, targeting SII.

The neurons in the superficial dorsal horn (lamina I) also project to forebrain areas such as the amygdala and hypothalamus [136]. These connections, the spinoparabrachial (SPb) pathway, are believed to be the basis for emotional (and aversive) and autonomic reactions to pain.

The lateral portion of the STT, originating in lamina I cells, provides information about the properties of the pain (object information, "what"). The spinoreticular tract is mainly bilateral and its main target is the reticular formation of the brainstem.

# Anterior spinothalamic tract

The fibers of the anterior STT tract originate in cells in deeper layers of the dorsal horn, mostly layers V and VII and also from layers VI and VIII. Cells in the intermediate zone of the dorsal horn also contribute to the anterior tract of the STT.

The cells in lamina IV-V that give rise to fibers of the anterior tract of the STT include cells that received A$\delta$ and C-fibers. Cells that receive signals from A$\beta$ fibers also contribute to STT axons (Figure 3.9). The cells in lamina VII-VIII (the intermediate zone) that contribute axons to the STT receive their input from large diameter fibers that innervate receptors in the skin, muscles, and joints. The receptors of these fibers respond to both innocuous and harmful stimuli, including proprioceptive and visceral input, and they are both inhibitory and excitatory [139].

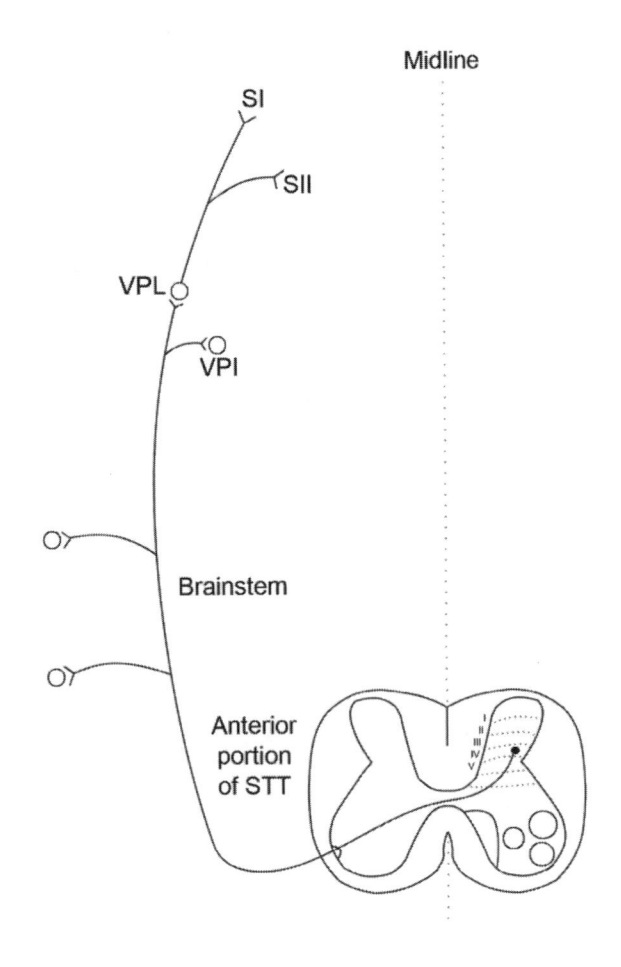

Figure 3.9 Connections from the anterior STT from neurons in lamina IV-V. VPI: Ventral posterior inferior (nuclei of the thalamus); VPL: Ventral posterior lateral (nuclei of the thalamus). (Modified from Møller, A. R. (2006) Neuroplasticity and disorders of the nervous system. Cambridge University Press Cambridge. Reprinted with permission from Cambridge University Press [288].) (Artwork by Monica Javidnia.)

The anterior portion of the STT projects to both primary and secondary somatosensory cortices via the ventral posterior lateral (VPL) thalamic nuclei. The anterior part has collateral fibers going to various parts of the brainstem, such as the reticular formation and some fibers, targeting cells in the VPL and the ventral posterior inferior (VPI).

The targets of axons of the cells of the anterior tract are the nuclei of the VPL and VPI of the thalamus, the neurons of which project to primary somatosensory cortices (Figure 3.9). The anterior part of the STT tract provides information about the anatomical location to which pain is referred (spatial information "where") and thus, resembles the somatosensory pathways that mediate innocuous receptor stimulation.

# Projections of C-fibers

Most of our understanding of the physiology of pain comes from studies in animals, and mostly subprimates. In a unique study, Kakigi and co-workers stimulated C-fibers selectively in human volunteers using a low intensity $CO_2$ laser beam to a tiny area of skin using a thin aluminum plate with holes as a spatial filter [197].

The response from the cerebral cortex was recorded from electrodes placed on the scalp (electroencephalography, EEG) and the magnetic response was recorded (magnetoencephalography, MEG). The results were interpreted to show that C-fiber stimulation performed in this way elicited responses from both primary and secondary somatosensory cortices (SI and SII) contralateral to the stimulation, and activation of SII on the side ipsilateral to the stimulation.

The pathways were assumed to be the lateral tract of the STT that project to the dorsal and medial portion of the thalamus from where axons project to secondary somatosensory cortices on both sides (Figure 3.10). The C-fibers of the lateral tract also project to the secondary somatosensory cortex (SII) on both sides and, to some extent, to area 3a (SI) [108] (Figure 3.10) [197]. The neurons in the dorsal and medial thalamic nuclei also send axons directly (subcortical) to many different structures.

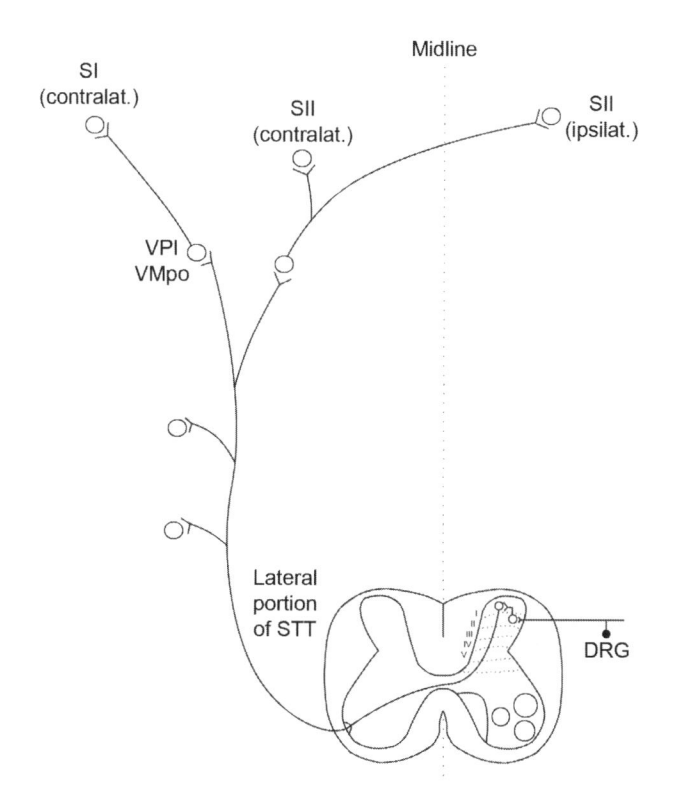

Figure 3.10 Schematic illustration of the projection of unmyelinated C-fibers through the lateral portion of the STT. Notice that the projections to SII are bilateral, but SI only receives input from contralateral receptors. Data from [197]. (Modified from Møller, A. R. (2006) Neuroplasticity and disorders of the nervous system. Cambridge University Press Cambridge. Reprinted with permission from Cambridge University Press [288].) (Artwork by Monica Javidnia.)

The same kinds of recordings also showed indications of activation of other structures including components of the limbic system such as the insular cortex and the cingulate cortex. It is interesting that the SII on both sides receives projections from the cells in the dorsal horn that receive C-fibers; thus, the lateral tract of the STT projects bilaterally to the SII, but only the contralateral SI receives input from C-fibers. (Data from Kagiki et al 2003, [197])

The fibers of many parts of the STT and the TTT send collateral fibers to many locations along their ascending paths. Many of these collaterals terminate in the reticular formation of the brainstem, thus affecting wakefulness.

# The spinomesencephalic and spinoreticular tracts

The spinoreticular tract is specifically important for the ability of pain stimulations to increase arousal. The spinomesencephalic pathway seems to only project to the PAG. The spinoreticular pathway (Figure 3.11) is mostly bilateral, targeting mainly the reticular formation where its fibers make synaptic contact with neurons.

The spinoreticular tract uses the dorsal thalamus as its target, but may also project to the primary somatosensory cortex (SI). Only the STT has connections to the ventral thalamus, the cells of which provide the main projection to the primary somatosensory cortex (SI).

The fact that pure C-fiber activation reaches the SI cortex through the spinothalamic tracts may explain why stimulation of C-fibers may produce a sensation of pressure or touch, in addition to a sensation of burning pain.

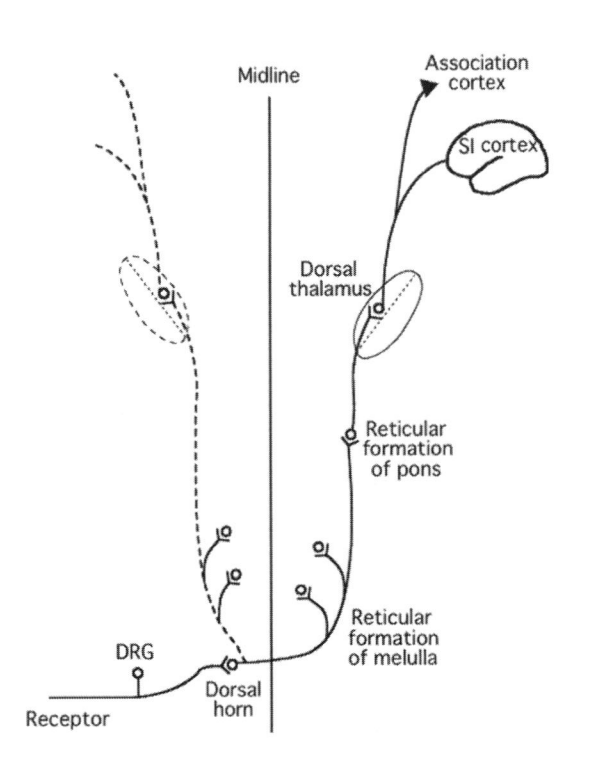

Figure 3.11 Spinoreticular pathways. VPI: Ventral posterior inferior (nuclei of thalamus); VPL: Ventral posterior lateral (nuclei of thalamus); SI: Primary somatosensory cortex; SII: Secondary somatosensory cortex. (Modified from Møller, Møller, A.R., Sensory Systems: Anatomy and Physiology. 2003, Amsterdam: Academic Press. Reprinted with permission from Elsevier [287].)

The spinomesencephalic tract (3.12) has as its main target the periaqueductal gray (PAG). The spinoreticular and spinomesencephalic tracts are important for the control of pain processing.

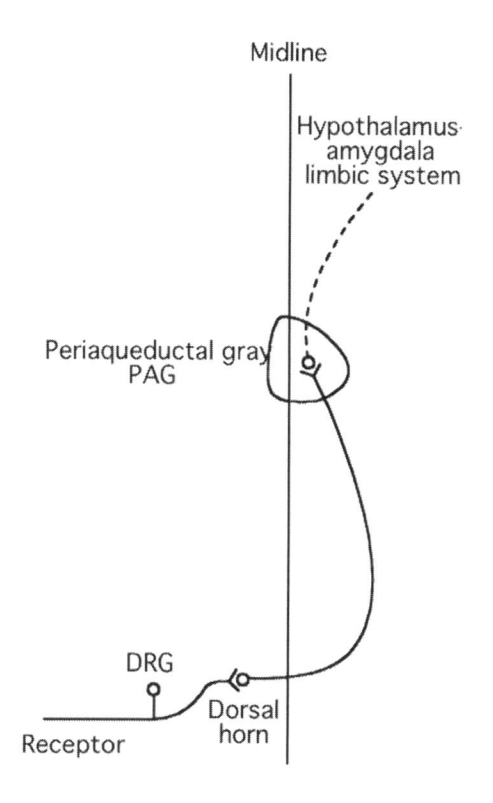

Figure 3.12 The mesencephalic tract. (Modified from Møller, Møller, A.R., Sensory Systems: Anatomy and Physiology. 2003, Amsterdam: Academic Press. Reprinted with permission from Elsevier [287].)

There is considerable individual variation in the pain pathways [177]; however, many of the studies of the neuroanatomy of pain have been done in animals and the results may not be directly applicable to humans. This is especially the case for the two tracts, the spinomesencephalic and the spinoreticular tracts. Some of the published results of anatomical studies seem contradictory.

# The role of the vagus nerve

The vagus nerve and its targets are not normally regarded as parts of pain circuits, but more recently, it has become evident that the vagus nerve provides a different route of sensory and pain information to the brain especially from viscera and also, to some extent, from the head.

The cells in the nucleus of the solitary tract, NST (nucleus tractus solitarii) are the main targets from the afferent fibers in the vagus nerve and they receive cardio-respiratory inputs through the vagus nerve. The NTS is believed to be involved in the reflex tachycardia that may result from harmful stimulation [43]. The axons from the NTS can reach many parts of the brain (Figure 3.13).

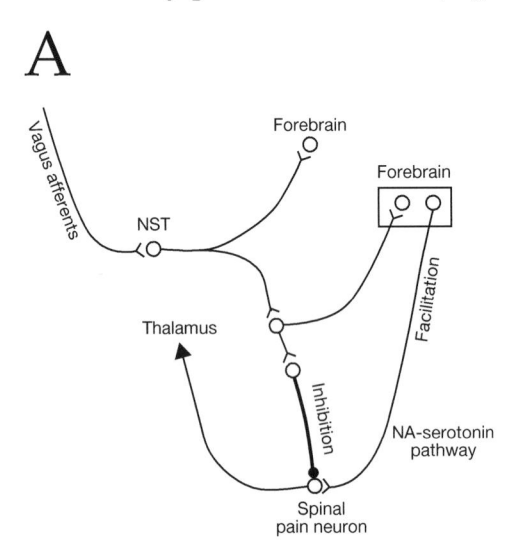

Figure 3.13 Central connections of vagus ascending fibers.

A. Simplified diagram of the central connections of the vagus nerve.

(Modified from Møller, A. R. (2006) Neuroplasticity and disorders of the nervous system. Cambridge University Press Cambridge. Reprinted with permission from Cambridge University Press [288], after [37].)

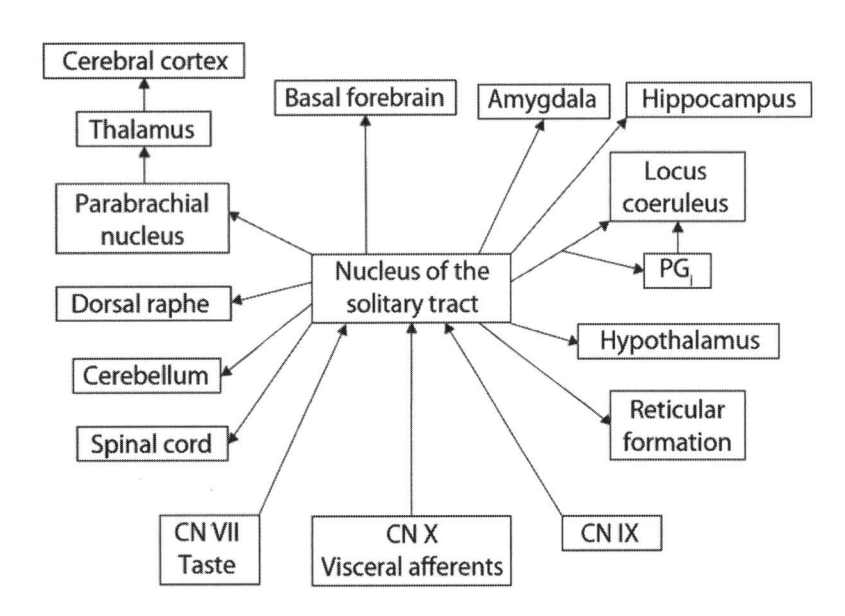

Figure 3.13 B. Projections from cells in the nucleus of the solitary tract, NST, to cells in structures in the brain. Modified from Ansari, S., K. Chaudhri, and K. Al Moutaery, *Vagus nerve stimulation: Indications and limitations.* Acta Neuroschir. Suppl, 2007. **97**(2): p. 281-286. (Artwork by Monica Javidnia.)

Cells of the NTS project to several central nervous system structures including the hypothalamus, the hippocampus, locus coeruleus, amygdala nuclei, the dorsal raphe nucleus, the mesencephalic reticular formation, the paraventricular hypothalamus nucleus [367], and possibly the nucleus basalis (or nucleus of Meynert). It provides adrenergic as well as cholinergic activation of the brain. Stimulation of the vagus nerve provides similar arousal of cerebral cortices and facilitation of plastic changes as stimulation of the nucleus of Meynert. The vagus nerve may be regarded as a separate ascending pathway for pain. The vagus nerve also has a very important function in controlling a cholinergic system of the brain, through the basal nucleus. This nucleus controls the excitability of neurons in the wide areas of the cerebral cortex and it promotes plastic changes [16, 206].

The territory of innervation of the afferent fibers of the vagus nerve is almost entirely from internal organs. There is evidence that vagal-solitary-parabrachial afferents are involved in visceral sensations. The role of the vagus nerve will, therefore, be discussed in more detail in Chapter 4 that concerns visceral pain.

The mouth and the esophagus, however, are also innervated by the vagus nerve, but the role of the vagus nerve in pain in the mouth is not known. It is well established that pain from these regions are mainly mediated through the trigeminal and glossopharyngeal nerves that project to the caudal trigeminal nucleus.

# Central projections of pain

Activation of pain receptors sends signals to many parts of the brain, including different parts of the thalamus, different regions of the somatosensory cortex, and the lateral nucleus of the amygdala.

Acute pain, elicited by the stimulation of pain receptors (physiological pain) may elicit activity in many structures in the brain (Figure 3.14).

The implications of that are incompletely known. Probably, the most important of these structures are the SII [368], the various nuclei of the amygdala, the anterior and posterior cingulate cortex, and the prefrontal cortex. Little is known about the role of the insula cortex [417] in general, but it may be a very important structure regarding neuropathic pain.

The insula lobe may be regarded as the fifth lobe of the brain, hidden under the temporal, frontal, and parietal opercula. It is the least known and functional data on this region in humans is scarce. New techniques used for the localization of the foci of severe epileptic seizures for surgical treatment have brought a wealth of information about the functional and somatotopic organization of the insula [417].

Some authors have stated that there are no specific somatosensory cortical representations of pain [345]. This means that in contrast to sensory modalities such as hearing, vision, somesthetics, and taste, the modality of pain does not have a specific cortical center. Other investigators find that cortical areas are activated by painful stimuli and that pain in these areas is distributed over large parts of the cortex surface [269].

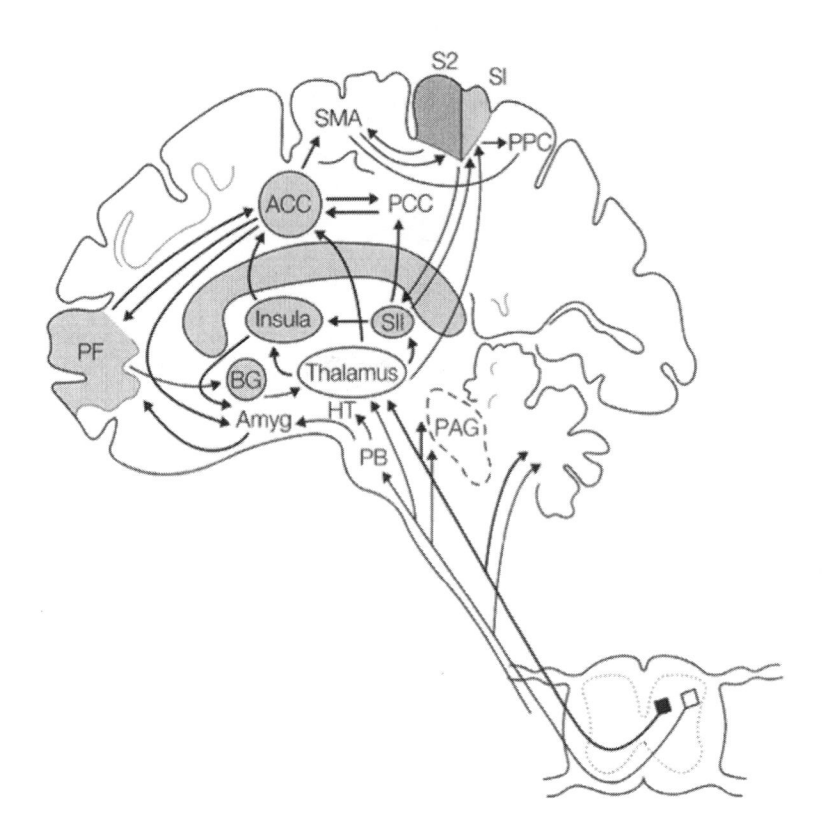

Figure 3.14 Central projections of the anterior lateral and ventral pain pathways indicating how activation of pain receptors may send signals to many parts of the brain. ACC: Anterior cingulate cortex; BG: Basal ganglia; HT: Hypothalamus; PB: Parabrachial nucleus of dorsolateral pons; PCC: Posterior cingulate cortex; PPC: Posterior parietal complex; SMA: Supplementary motor area. (From Price, D.D., Psychological and neural mechanisms of the affective dimension of pain. Science, 2000. 288: p. 1769-1772. Reprinted with permission from AAAS) [334]

The cerebral cortex is, however, known to be of importance in some forms of pain such as pain associated with amputations, where some of the symptoms are caused by faults in the mapping of the body on the cerebral cortex (discussed in Chapter 8). This is because the perception of pain and the generation of the sensation of pain make use of the somatosensory maps of the body surface that are created on the somatosensory cortex and on other structures of the brain.

These maps are normally updated regularly by somatosensory input and the perception of "self" is closely related to these maps (discussed in Chapter 12). Methods have been devised to correct such erroneous mapping of the body.

Stimulation of pain receptors also activates regions of the brain that are not normally associated with the somatosensory system as illustrated in Figure 3.14. These regions include the anterior cingulate cortex (ACC), the basal ganglia (BG), the parabrachial nucleus (PBN) of the dorsolateral pons, the hypothalamus (HT), the posterior cingulate cortex (PCC), the posterior parietal complex (PPC), and the supplementary motor area (SMA).

The major targets of pain information are parts of the insular cortex, secondary somatosensory cortex, and several cortical areas in the cingulate sulcus. Anatomical (tracer) studies in monkeys showed that neurons in the ventral premotor area project to the cingulate motor areas and each of the cingulate motor areas receives STT input [111]. The cingulate motor areas in the monkey project directly to the primary motor cortex. Thus, the substrate exists for the STT system to influence the cortical movement system. Imaging studies indicates that the human equivalents of the three cingulate motor areas also correspond to sites that are activated by painful stimulations.

The thalamic projections to somatosensory area 3a, which is anatomically close to the areas, may also explain why electrical stimulation of the premotor areas can suppress pain [275, 446]. There are, however, also other explanations. Other authors hypothesize that MI stimulation acts on pain circuits through superficial (layer I) axons in the primary motor cortex that connect to somatosensory cortices [12]. Many of these structures may also be activated in pathological pain such as central neuropathic pain (see Chapter 8), but little is known about the extension of involvement of the brain in these kinds of pain.

# The role of the thalamus

The thalamus plays key roles in both sensory systems [287] and motor systems and also in various forms of pain. All sensory information, except olfaction, is processed in the thalamus. The nuclei of the ventral and the dorso-medial parts of the thalamus have distinctly different functions in sensory systems [287] and in pain.

The ventral parts process sensory information with great accuracy and send the information to the primary sensory cortices and from there, information goes to other parts of the sensory cortices (secondary and association cortices). These parts of sensory systems provide accurate and detailed analysis of sensory information and are known as the classical systems, or the "slow and accurate" systems. The cells of the other system, the dorso-medial thalamus, send their axons to secondary and association cortices bypassing the primary cortices. These cells also send axons directly to many parts of the brain, most notably, nuclei of the limbic system such as the lateral nucleus of the amygdala, the anterior cingulate, and the hippocampus.

This part of sensory systems, known as the non-classical or extralemniscal system, provides less accurate and less detailed analysis of sensory signals than classical or lemniscal system ("slow and accurate"). Its analysis is, therefore, also called the "fast and dirty". With its subcortical connection to limbic structures, it activates parts of the brain that evoke emotional responses, as do the connections from the secondary sensory cortices [368]. Another important feature of the thalamus is the reticular thalamic nucleus that acts as a gatekeeper regarding neural traffic to and from the thalamus. Little is known about the exact involvement of this structure in neural processing of pain signals. (For more information about non-classical and classical sensory systems, see Møller 2003, [287].)

# The role of the dorsomedial thalamus

Many studies agree that the dorso-medial thalamus plays an important role in pain and that it provides objective information about many forms of pain. Its connections to the secondary somatosensory cortex (SII) and, in particular, its subcortical connections to many structures that are involved in the emotional reactions to pain, have recently directed attention to this part of the thalamus for treatment of pain.

Studies in the monkey show that the posterior portion of the ventral medial nucleus (VMpo) is a dedicated lamina I spino-thalamo-cortical relay for pain and temperature sensation [37]. There is evidence that the ventromedial posterior, (VMpo) region of the thalamus in primates relays information from lamina I in the dorsal horn that is important for pain, temperature, itching, muscle ache, sensual touch, and other feelings from internal structures of the body [85].

These studies have also provided strong evidence for the general hypothesis that the STT consists of several functionally and anatomically different components [87].

Studies in humans show that the dorsal-medial thalamic nuclei are the thalamic areas from which pain, temperature, and visceral sensations can be evoked by microstimulation, and from which nociceptive and thermoreceptive neurons have been recorded in humans [197]. The recent proliferation of surgical procedures for implantation of electrodes for deep brain stimulation (DBS) has provided opportunities for studies that previously could only be done in animals. Such studies have produced a wealth of new information, but these techniques also have disadvantages, for example, lack of histological verification of electrode positions. There are also ethical aspects that limit the time for such studies.

Infarcts in parts of the thalamus may cause analgesia and absence of sensation to heat and cold (thermoanaesthesia). Damage to these areas can also lead to the paradoxical development of central pain [37]. (Anesthesia dolorosa is another example of absence of sensation (numbness) and severe pain.)

The cells in the VMpo also have extensive subcortical connections to many parts of the brain (Figure 3.15). The medial dorsal (MDvc) part of the thalamus projects to area 24c (the anterior cingulate cortex) [86]. The VMpo nucleus, in addition to projecting to the secondary somatosensory cortex, also projects to the dorsal portion of the insula cortex and area 3a of the somatosensory cortex.

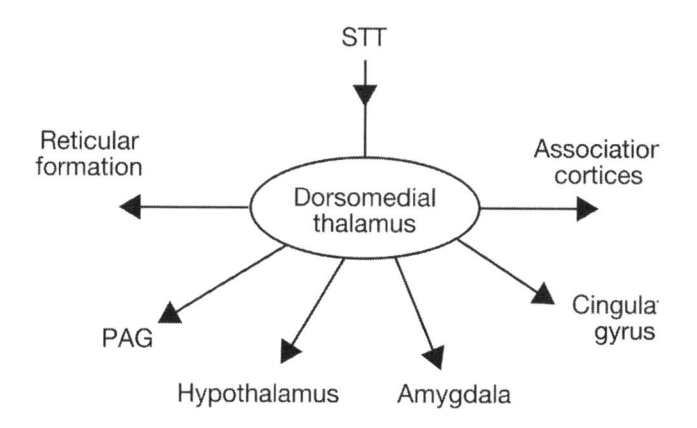

Figure 3.15 Connections from neurons in the dorsomedial thalamus that are activated by the lateral tract of the STT and originate in lamina I of the dorsal horn. (Modified from Møller, A. R. (2006) Neuroplasticity and disorders of the nervous system. Cambridge University Press Cambridge. [288].)

Ventral sensory nuclei of the thalamus have extensive projections to primary cortices and lack subcortical connections. The pain pathways that use the ventral thalamus provide information about the location of the pain on the body; thus, providing spatial ("where") information whereas the anterior pathway for the STT provides information about the character of the pain ("what") [108].

The ventral nuclei of the thalamus used by the classical sensory pathways are phylogenetically younger than the dorsal-medial thalamic pathways. The VPL of the thalamus that projects to the primary somatosensory cortex (SI) probably contributes to both sensory-discriminative and affective-motivational aspects of pain (through the somatosensory and insular cortex, respectively) [136].

# The amygdala

The amygdala is of particular interest in connection with pain because of its role in affective (mood related) symptoms.

The amygdala consists of three main nuclei. The lateral nucleus (AL) is the target for sensory and pain information, except olfaction. The lateral nucleus projects to the basolateral nucleus, which sends its output to the central nucleus which is the main output nucleus that connects to endocrine (hypothalamus), behavioral, and autonomic structures.

Axons from cells in the lateral nucleus of the amygdala project to the anterior cingulate, the insula cortex, the basal ganglia, the hypothalamus, the parabrachial nucleus (PBN) of the dorsolateral pons, the posterior parietal complex, the PAG, and the supplementary cerebral cortical motor area (Figure 3.16).

These structures also receive information from the ventral thalamus, but only through a long chain of neurons, including the primary cortex and association cortices.

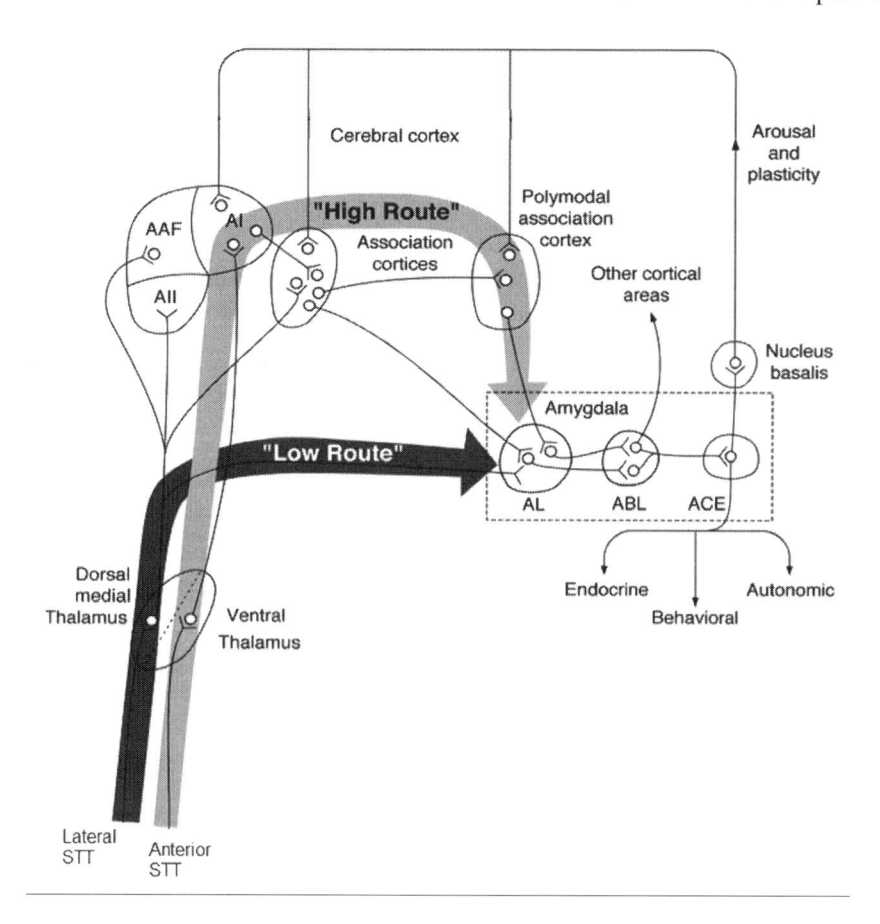

Figure 3.16 Two different routes to the amygdala (lateral nucleus) from the auditory system. Schematic drawing illustrating the "high route" and the "low route" from sensory systems to the lateral nucleus of the amygdala. The drawing shows connections from the auditory system to the lateral nucleus of the amygdala. ABL: Basolateral nucleus of the amygdala; ACE: Central nucleus of the amygdala; AL: Lateral nucleus of the amygdala. Connections between the different nuclei of the amygdala and connections from these nuclei to different parts of the central nervous system are also shown. (Modified from Møller 2003 [287], based on LeDoux [227].)

The basolateral nucleus (ABL) also receives input from many parts of the cerebral cortex and the central nucleus is the main target of olfactory information. The ABL sends information to the central nucleus (ACE), which is the main output nucleus of the amygdala that connects to endocrine, behavioral, and autonomic regions of the brain. The output of this nucleus serves as the input to the nucleus basalis (nucleus of Meynert) that has two main functions, namely arousal of the cerebral cortex and facilitation of neuroplasticity.

The amygdala nuclei receive input from many parts of the brain and send information to many parts. There are, therefore, many possibilities for many parts of the brain to receive information about pain in addition to direct information from the STT and TTT that also can reach different parts of the brain. This could explain the affective reactions to pain including depression [312, 362], increased fear, etc. (see discussion about depression and chronic pain in Chapter 8).

In general, sensory information, including pain, can reach the lateral nucleus (AL) of the amygdala through two different sensory routes, namely through primary, secondary, and association cortices to the lateral nucleus of the amygdala and through a short subcortical route from the dorsal and medial nuclei of the thalamus. These two routes are known as the "high route" and the "low route", respectively [227] (Figure 3.16).

Information that travels through the "low route" is not highly processed and is primarily projected directly to the lateral nucleus of the amygdala from the medial/dorsal thalamus. This projection is fast and it is often very difficult, if not impossible, to block information traveling in this route.

# Anatomical basis for central modulation of physiological pain

Sherrington showed in 1906 that nociceptive (pain elicited) reflexes were enhanced after transection of the spinal cord; thus, evidence that spinal cord transmissions of pain can be modulated via descending influences from the brain and that this influence was (mainly) inhibitory [391].

The discovery of the descending pathways that could modulate pain was an important contribution to our understanding of the neurophysiologic basis for pain. Descending control of transmission and processing of pain signals in the spinal cord originates from many regions in the brain and it plays important roles regarding the experience of both acute and chronic pain.

Shifts in the balance between inhibiting and facilitating outflows from the brainstem play a role in setting the gain of pain signal processing in the spinal cord. These relationships between inhibition and facilitation are controlled by different regions of the brain and related behavioral priorities and they are strongly affected by neuroplasticity.

In general, the processing that occurs normally in the spinal cord and the trigeminal nucleus is not constant and can change as a result of activation of neuroplasticity (discussed in Chapters 8 and 12, see also Appendix A).

# Descending systems

Similar to sensory systems, pain systems have massive descending pathways and are generally parallel to ascending pathways [287]. It is, therefore, more appropriate to regard the descending pathways to be reciprocal pathways to the ascending pathways. Also, regarding pain pathways, the ascending-descending pathways form loops where information may circulate.

Three or four separate descending systems, which can modulate the transmission of pain signals in the spinal cord, have been identified [120, 163]. In addition, the vagus nerve may also be regarded as a part of the descending pathways that can modulate pain [137, 209].

It was mentioned earlier that the cells in the dorsal horn that receive pain signals have synaptic contact with larger myelinated sensory fibers (A$\beta$ fibers) that innervate sensory receptors of innocuous stimuli (Figure 3.5). This input from the periphery is inhibitory and it can modulate the transmission of pain signals. It is a part of the gating of pain signals described by Melzack and Wall (1965). The so-called "intermediate zone", consisting of cells in lamina VI, VII, and VIII, has cells that receive input from large diameter fibers (mainly A$\beta$ fibers) that innervate receptors that respond to innocuous and nocuous (painful) stimulations from large areas of skin.

In the dorsal horn, pain signals can not only be affected by signals from such innocuous stimulation (Figure 3.5), but pain signals can also be modulated by descending activity from the brain that affects neural processing in pain circuits in the dorsal horn of the spinal cord. Input from the periaqueductal gray (PAG) is prominent in modulation transmission of pain signals in the dorsal horn. Also, influence from the raphe nucleus (NA-serotonin pathway) can exert inhibition on some of the cells in lamina I of the dorsal horn through interneurons that connect the axons of the descending pathways to cells in lamina I of the dorsal horn.

Descending systems can modulate traffic in ascending pain pathways and thereby, cause suppression and enhancement of pain sensations. The main targets of the descending pathways are cells in the dorsal horn and the caudal part of the trigeminal nucleus.

98  PAIN Its Anatomy, Physiology and Treatment

Figure 3.17 shows a simplified schematic of the organization of the descending pathways. The drawings are superimposed on their respective anatomical structures. In the subsequent illustrations, the individual parts of the descending system are shown as diagrams of the most important connections without showing their anatomical locations.

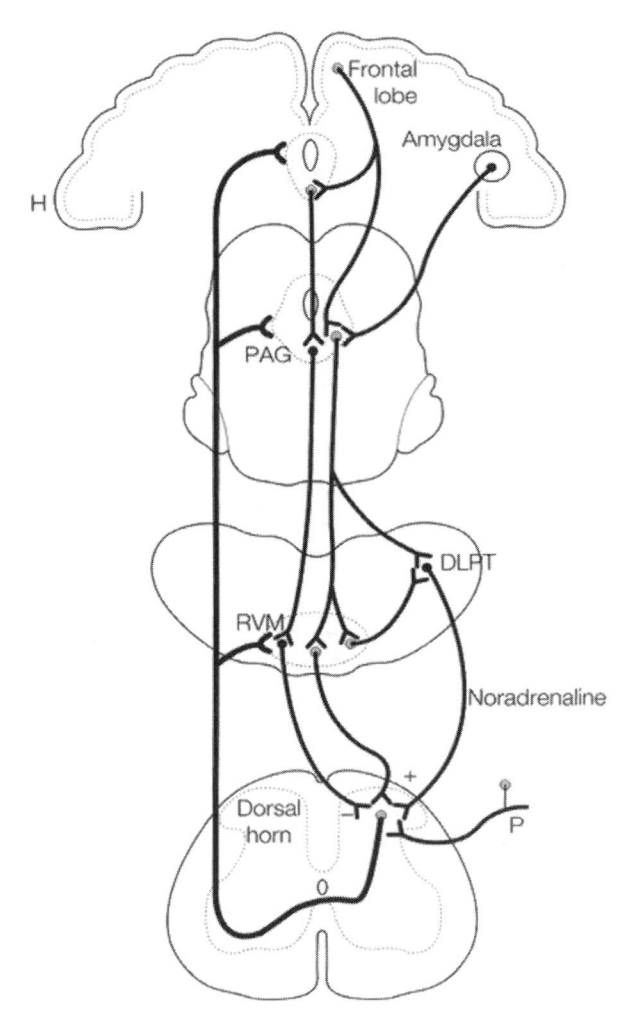

Figure 3.17 Summary of the major pain modulating pathways, involving the periaqueductal gray (PAG), rostral ventromedial medulla (RVM), and the dorsolateral pontine tegmentum (DLPT). (Reproduced from Fields, H. L., Basbaum, A. I., & Heinricher, M. M. (2006). Central nervous system mechanisms of pain modulation. In S. B. McMahon & M. Koltzenburg (Eds.), Wall and Melzack's Textbook of Pain (pp. 125-142). Amsterdam: Elsevier [120].) Reprinted with the permission of Elsevier.

There are three main descending systems that project to the dorsal horn of the spinal cord. Two of these, the rostral ventromedial medulla (RVM) and the dorsolateral pontine tegmentum (DLPT), originate in the PAG and the third (not shown in Figure 3.17) is the noradrenalin (NA) serotonin pathway. The PAG together with the nucleus cuneiforms (not shown in Figure 3.17), located adjacent to the PAG, control spinal nociceptive neurons via RVM and DLPT neurons.

The major pain modulating pathways involve the periaqueductal gray (PAG), the rostral ventromedial medulla (RVM), and the dorsolateral pontine tegmentum (DLPT). In principle, the PAG controls spinal nociceptive neurons via the RVM and the DLPT. The RVM provides both serotonergic and non-serotonergic innervations to the dorsal horn and the DLPT provides noradrenergic innervations to the dorsal horn.

# Periaqueductal grey (PAG)

The involvement of the periaqueductal gray (PAG) in pain is extensive. It is located in the midbrain and it was shown early in animal experiments that electrical stimulation of the PAG could reduce pain; that was one of the first signs of influence on pain from the brain. The role of the PAG in pain, especially in the modulation of pain, is now confirmed in many studies.

The periaqueductal gray matter (PAG) [203, 240, 436] is an important structure for processing pain signals. In particular, it is an important source of descending activity that can modulate transmission of pain signals in the dorsal horn of the spinal cord and in the trigeminal nucleus.

The PAG controls spinal nociceptive neurons in the dorsal horn via the RVM and DLPT networks. Descending signals that can modulate pain transmission in the dorsal horn of the spinal cord come from the PAG. The PAG provides important input to the RVM circuit where serotonergic and non-serotonergic innervations exert bidirectional control of neural traffic that is related to pain. The PAG also plays a role for another important network, the DLPT, which provides noradrenergic innervations of the dorsal horn. Thereby, the RVM and DLTP are important descending circuits that modulate pain signals in the dorsal horn (see Chapter 6).

The PAG receives information from the frontal lobe, hypothalamus, amygdala, locus coeruleus, nucleus cuneiforms, and pontomedullary reticular formation and relays it to the RVM and the DLPT (Figure 3.18). There is a direct connection from the medial prefrontal and insular cortex to the PAG.

The amygdala also provides input to the PAG as well as receives signals from the PAG. As in so many other systems, these connections are mostly reciprocal, forming loops. The connections from different brain regions to the PAG are described in Figure 3.18.

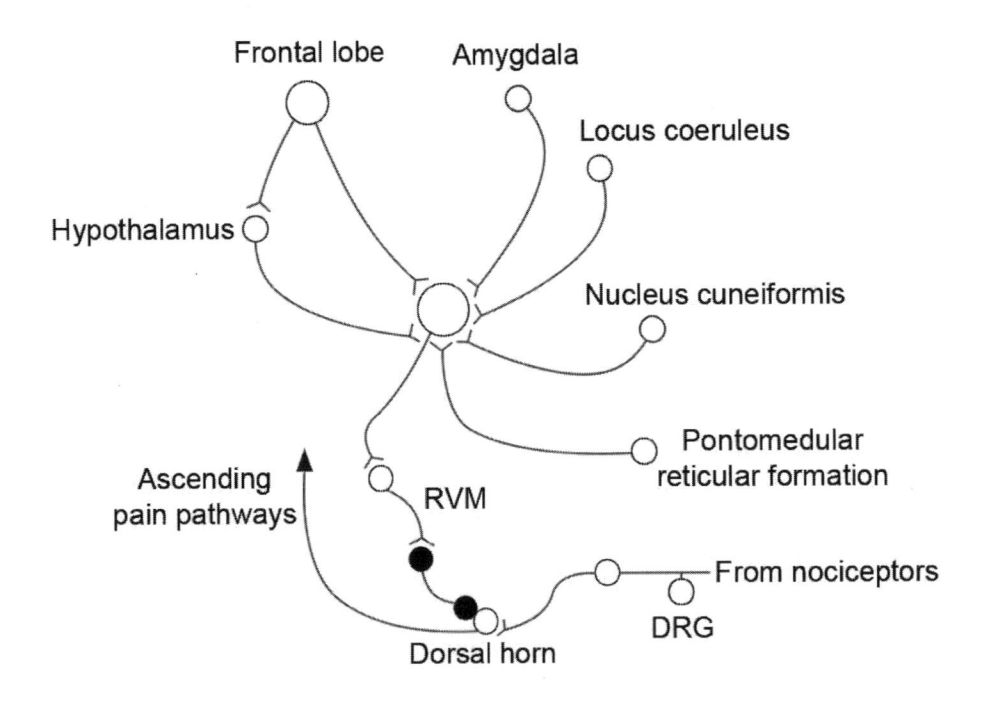

Figure 3.18 Input to the PAG and pathways through which modulation of transmission of pain signals by the PAG occur through the RVM pathway. (Modified from Møller, A. R. (2006) Neuroplasticity and disorders of the nervous system. Cambridge University Press Cambridge. Reprinted with permission from Cambridge University Press [288].) (Artwork by Monica Javidnia.)

# The rostral ventromedial medulla (RVM)

The RVM may be regarded to be the final common output for descending influences from rostral brain sites [118, 280] (Figure 3.7, 3.18). There are three types of RVM neurons: on-cells, off-cells, and neutral cells. There are dual inputs to dorsal horn cells from the RVM that provide the effect of on and off neurons on the transmission of pain signals in the dorsal horn. The RVM has two kinds of cells.

One type of cell, "on-cell", excites dorsal horn cells and the other type, "off-cell", inhibits dorsal horn cells (Figure 3.19).

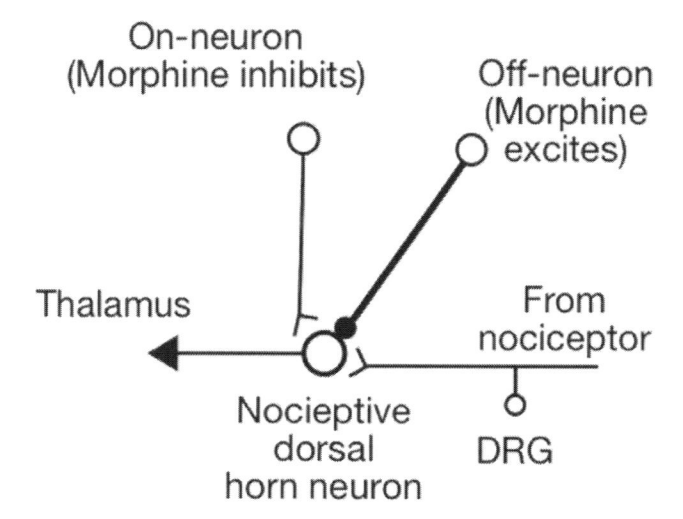

Figure 3.19 Illustration of the dual inputs to dorsal horn cells from the RVM that provide the effect of "on" and "off" neurons in the transmission of pain signals in the dorsal horn. (Modified from Møller, A. R. (2006) Neuroplasticity and disorders of the nervous system. Cambridge University Press Cambridge. Reprinted with permission from Cambridge University Press [288]).

It is worth noting that the RVM descending systems have two parts, an inhibitory and an excitatory part. This means there are parallel inhibitory and excitatory descending pathways and at least the RVM and DLTP can both enhance and suppress impulse traffic in pain circuits in the dorsal horn and the trigeminal nucleus. It was shown many years ago that electrical stimulation of the PAG can cause a decrease in pain sensation (analgesia), but more recently, it has become evident that activation of these same circuits can have the opposite effect [354]. If the PAG-RVM-DLPT malfunctions, an increase in pain sensation may occur. Such lack of inhibition can lead to more severe states of chronic pain such as complex regional pain syndrome (CRPS) type I and II and it can exaggerate the "wind-up" phenomenon. The net effect of the activation of these descending systems depends on the balance between the activity in the inhibitory and in the excitatory paths.

Inhibitory control from the PAG-RVM system preferentially suppresses nociceptive inputs mediated by C-fibers, preserving sensory-discriminative information conveyed by more rapidly conducting A-fibers. The on-cells that excite dorsal horn pain cells are inhibited by opioids and the off-cells that are excited by opioids inhibit pain cells in the dorsal horn.

The neutral cells are producers of serotonin; in fact, the RVM is the main source of serotonin in the brain. The descending system can modulate the functions of neurons in lamina I and II of the dorsal horn as shown in Figure 3.19. Many electrophysiological and pharmacological studies have later contributed to the understanding of how the descending influences on spinal nociceptive processing involve the PAG. As seen in Figure 3.19, the RVM is closely related to the function of opioids as pain relievers (see Chapter 7).

The on-cells and off-cells are differentially activated from higher regions of the brain that are involved in fear reactions, illness, and psychological stress reactions to enhance or inhibit pain.

The way the RVM modulates the excitability of nociceptive cells in the dorsal horn is illustrated in Figure 3.19. Neural activity in the RVM circuit can both inhibit (via an interneuron) and enhance excitability of the nociceptive neurons. This is important for understanding the action of opioids as pain suppressors (see Chapter 6).

# The dorsolateral pontomesencephalic tegmentum pathway (DLPT)

The PAG connects to the dorsolateral pontomesencephalic tegmentum pathway (DLPT) through which it can modulate impulse traffic in the neurons that receive input from pain receptors, in a similar way as the RVM circuits do.

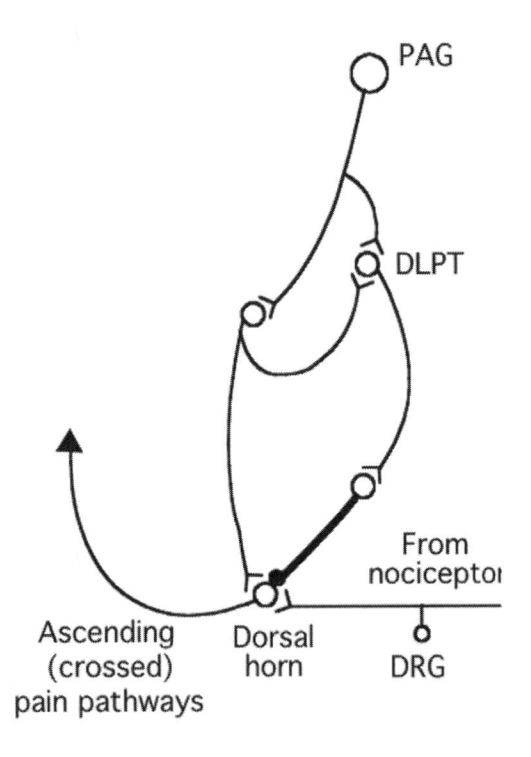

Figure 3.20 Schematic diagram showing the dorsolateral pontomesencephalic tegmentum pathway (DLTP). (Modified from Møller, A. R. (2006) Neuroplasticity and disorders of the nervous system. Cambridge University Press Cambridge. Reprinted with permission from Cambridge University Press [288].)

The loop-like appearance of the ascending-descending pathways is illustrated in Figure 3.21 and Figure 3.22, which serve as a summary of the pathways between the PAG and the dorsal horn.

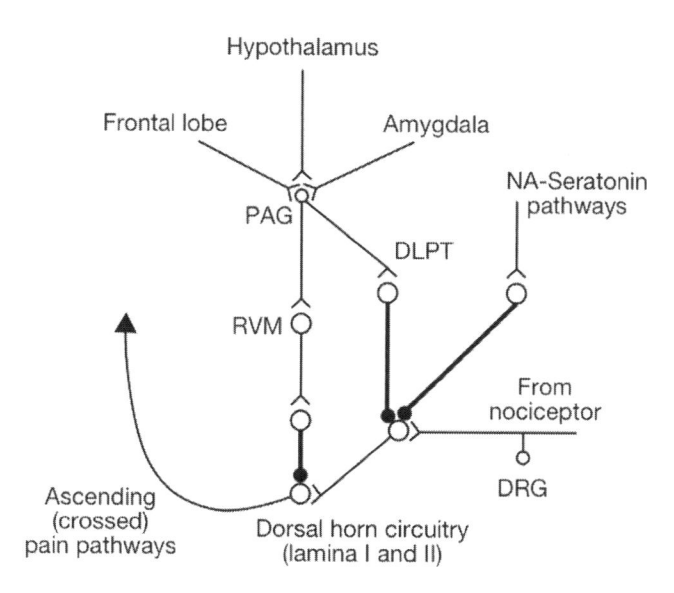

Figure 3.21 The three different descending spinal tracts to cells in lamina I and II of the dorsal horn (RVM, DLPT, and NA-Serotonin pathways), showing the sources of input to the PAG. (Modified from Møller, A. R. (2006) Neuroplasticity and disorders of the nervous system. Cambridge University Press Cambridge. Reprinted with permission from Cambridge University Press [288].)

The RVM and the DLTP pathways originate in the brainstem and the modulation occurs mainly by influencing neurons in lamina I and II of the dorsal horn [29, 119] . The DLPT also targets neurons in the dorsal horn, but it is mainly excitatory (facilitating). These are some of the anatomical substrates for the complex modulation of pain sensations. (For a review, see [35].)

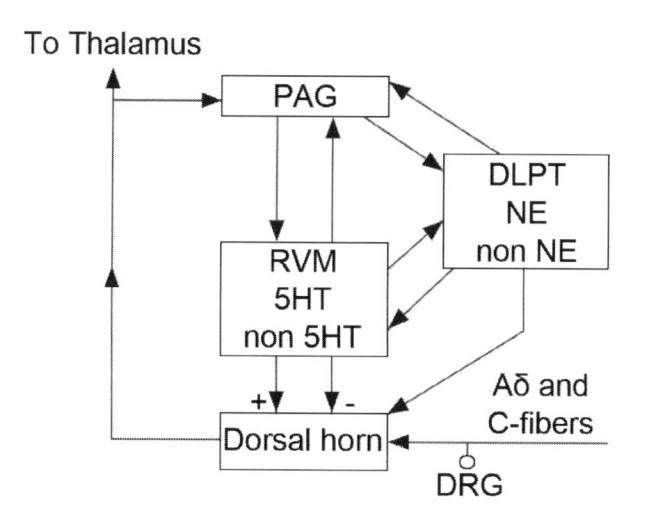

Figure 3.22 Summary illustration of the two-way connections between PAG, DLPT, and RVM and their connections to the dorsal horn (Adapted from Fields and Basbaum, 1999 [119]. (Artwork by Monica Javidnia.)

# Other descending pathways

In addition to the specific brainstem circuits, RVM and DLPT, the norepinephrine (NA) - serotonin pathway originating in the brainstem reticular formation can influence the transmission of pain signals in the dorsal horn of the spinal cord (Figure 3.23).

The axons in this pathway have cells in lamina II of the spinal horn as their target. Neural activity in this pathway can, therefore, modulate transmission of pain signals in the dorsal horn of the spinal cord (and the caudal nucleus of the trigeminal nucleus). Several higher-level areas of the brain, such as the cingulo-frontal regions, the amygdala, and the hypothalamus [152], also provide control over the processing of pain signals from the interaction with nociceptive processing from cognitive and emotional variables, thereby influencing the experienced pain.

Descending monoaminergic connections from the reticular formation to the dorsal horn may also suppress pain impulses in the dorsal horn, preventing pain from reaching higher brain structures.

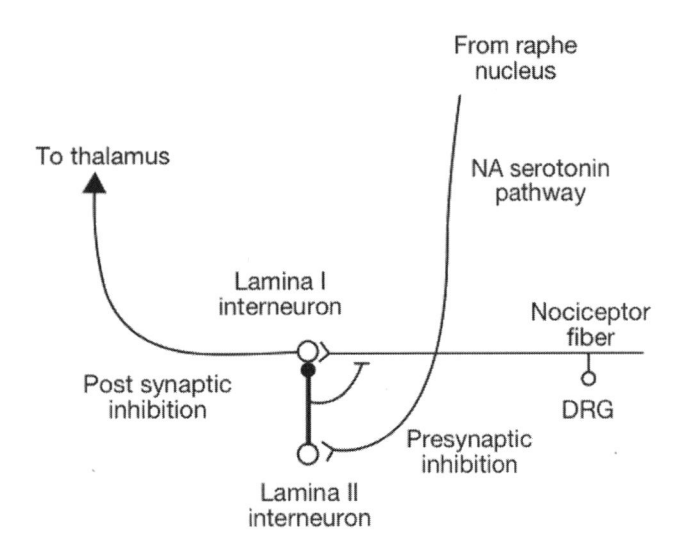

Figure 3.23 Schematic diagram showing the descending pathways from the raphe nucleus (NA-serotonin pathway) that terminates on pain neurons in the dorsal horn. (Modified from Møller, A. R. (2006) Neuroplasticity and disorders of the nervous system. Cambridge University Press Cambridge).

# Itch

Itching (puritus) has many similarities with pain. Like pain, itching is an unpleasant sensation that can have many causes. Like pain, itching is many different things. There are many forms and causes of itching. Itching can be caused by peripheral stimulation [194] and from central disturbances [110, 439, 463].

It can be caused by something irritating the skin locally, it can be chemical applied locally to the skin, and it can be caused by disorders of the skin, such as eczema (atopic dermatitis, a systemic disease that causes uremia, etc.).

There are other differences between pain and itching. While painful stimuli applied to the extremities elicit a withdrawal reflex, substances that cause itching elicit a scratching reflex, and scratching is often associated with pleasure. Insect bites are perhaps the one that affects most people. The common forms of itching, such as from mosquito bites, are associated with the release of histamine in the skin. Similar releases of histamine can occur as an allergic reaction causing redness of the skin. Allergic reactions can cause itching by similar mechanisms. Disorders of the skin are probably the most common disorders that cause itching, and that is, perhaps, the reason that itching is mainly treated by dermatologists.

Dry skin is perhaps not regarded as a disease, but it is a common cause of itching, often caused by dry air and frequent showering. These are benign forms of itching, but pathologies that cause constant itching severely affect the quality of life. Allergies of various kinds (hives) and various forms of dermatitis are common causes of persistent itching. Wound healing is a common cause of itching and scratching can prolong healing.

There is some clinical evidence that itching can occur together with peripheral nerve disorders [78, 253, 499]. For example, itching may occur as a side effect to the administration of opioids [210]. This form of itching is not caused by the release of histamine. It cannot be reduced by antihistamines, but antagonists to opioids (naloxone and Naltrexone that inhibit μ and κ receptors) [222, 437] can reduce this form of itching, thus indicating that opioid receptors are involved in itching.

Itching can be caused by disorders of the nervous system (neuropathic itch). It can, in rare incidents, be psychogenic; it can be a neurotic scratching. Several medical disorders are associated with itching. Uremia, jaundice, and thyroid illness are common causes of general itching [372]. It has recently been found that the two modalities of the stimulation of pain receptors, itching and pain, use two different neural pathways [94].

# Itch receptors

The receptors in the skin that mediate itching are specialized chemoreceptors innervated by unmyelinated nerve fibers and specialized circuitry in the spinal cord processes the information from these receptors [156, 381, 496].

Histamine and serotonin can activate neurons in lamina I and II of the dorsal horn [66] and these neurons may mediate the scratching behavior in response to itching [194].

The receptors that are sensitive to histamine are innervated by C-fibers, they are not mechanosensitive, and they have very large receptive fields. These receptors are specialized chemoreceptors and specialized circuitry in the spinal cord processes the information from these receptors [156, 381, 496].

# Neural pathways

Neural activity that is elicited by the stimulation of "itch" receptors travels in similar ascending pathways as pain impulses [194, 381]. A specific class of cells of STT neurons in lamina I of the spinal horn have been found to respond selectively to histamine applied iontophoretically, simulating the cause of (peripheral) itching [5].

Prostaglandins enhance the sensitivity of pain receptors to histamine. They can become sensitized to mechanical stimulation by the presence of inflammation. When inflammatory processes cause itching, they seem to do that by activating histamine-positive mechanosensitive pain receptors that are innervated by C-fibers [383].

Specific pathways of "pure" histaminergic itching have been identified and traced from the mechano-insensitive nerve fibers in the skin to their central cortical projections [463]. Histamine and serotonin can activate superficial neurons in the dorsal horn [66]. These neurons may mediate the scratching behavior in response to itching [194]. There is evidence that peripheral and central sensitization occurs in chronic itch conditions that are similar to that in chronic pain [382]. It will be of major interest to reveal whether the underlying mechanism for sensitization in the itch and pain pathways are also similar, as this might have major implications for therapy.

Activating pain receptors can decrease itching, which means that itching depends on the absence of activation of mechanosensitive pain receptors.

# Central representation of itching

There is considerable evidence of the existence of specific itch neurons in the spinal cord and these cells have been shown to project to the thalamus [463]. Studies have shown that these neurons that are located in lamina I of the dorsal horn were excited by iontophoretic histamine and the physiological response paralleled the pure itching sensation this stimulus elicits in humans.

The response also matched that of the responses of peripheral C-fibers that have similar selectivity; there were indications that these cells represent a unique subset of lateral STT neurons [5]. Other studies have found that a lesion of the lateral STT disrupts itching along with pain and temperature sensations.

The axons of itch sensitive cells in lamina I project to the ventromedial thalamus that, in turn, project to the insular cortex [85]. There is evidence that VMpo in primates relays information from lamina I in the dorsal horn that is important for itching, in addition to pain, hot, and cold, and is mediated by the lateral spinothalamic tract [85]. These studies have also provided strong evidence for the general hypothesis that the STT consists of several functionally and anatomically differentiable components [87].

Thus, there is evidence that itching activates specific neural elements, both peripherally and centrally [5]. It has been shown that itching employs specific pathways [94, 382]. Other studies have found that the induction of itching using the application of histamine also activates motor areas, which may explain the scratch reflex.

There is considerable overlap between regions of the brain that are activated by itching and those that are activated by pain. Some classical pain structures, such as the PAG, seem to inhibit itch responses. The involvement of the insular cortex is interesting. Little is known about the function of the insular cortex regarding itching, but recent studies in humans that were done in connection with diagnostic work-up for epilepsy surgery have lent some important information about the function of the insular cortex.

The development of these methods gives hope for better understanding of the function of the insular lobe [417].

Itching can be elicited from the central nervous system as indicated by the fact that itching of the face often occurs when sleepy or just before sleep. Itching is also associated with depression and other affective disorders.

Itching induces scratching; therefore, the central projection of nerve fibers that mediate itching must be different from that of fibers that mediate the sensation of pain. The motor commands that are elicited in connection with itching (scratching) may be initiated at subcortical levels as indicated by the fact that people scratch in their sleep. Motor activity can be highly coordinated indicating that it involves cerebral activity.

There is a certain pleasure associated with scratching which indicates association with the old part of the brain such as limbic structures and the cingulate gyrus. It is known that pain under certain circumstances can suppress itching. Itching, like pain, is subject to both peripheral and central sensitization. The neural circuits that generate the activity that cause the sensation of itching are complex and the anatomical and physiological bases of itching are poorly understood.

# Discrimination between pain and itching

It is evident from many studies that there are great similarities between itching and pain. The question is, therefore, how do people so distinctly differentiate between these two harmful stimulations that engage many similar receptors and share neural structures from the periphery to the central portions of the brain?

Itching uses similar pathways as used by harmful (physiological pain) stimulation, but different receptors. Itching rarely occurs together with pain and pain can inhibit itching [194]. The receptors for itching have similarities with those that are activated by capsaicin, but the targets for the nerve fibers from the itch receptors are different from that of the capsaicin receptors. Capsaicin, like other pain stimulants, causes a burning sensation, but itching creates a desire to scratch.

In a fMRI study of the neural substrates of perceptual differences between itching and pain, Mochizuki et al (2007) [282] showed that the anterior cingulate cortex, the anterior insula, the basal ganglia, and the pre-supplementary motor area were commonly activated by itching and pain. The neural activity, however, in the posterior cingulate cortex (PCC) and the posterior insula associated with itching was significantly higher than that associated with pain and significantly proportional to the itching sensation. This means that the difference in the sensitivity of PCC, the posterior insular cortex, and the thalamus between itching and pain would be responsible for the perceptual difference between these sensations.

Earlier, other investigators had shown that the secondary somatosensory cortex (SII) was not activated by itching, but Mochizuki and co-workers showed activation of SII by pain that was not significantly different from that by itching [282]. Secondary sensory cerebral cortices have recently been shown to be involved in the memory of an emotional event and fear [368]. This may explain some of the features of itching.

The generation of the neural activity that causes the sensation of itching is complex and the anatomical and physiological bases of itching are poorly understood. People can scratch in their sleep. Therefore, it may be assumed that the motor commands elicited by itching for scratching are initiated at subcortical levels. Scratching can also be a highly coordinated motor activity indicating it requires involvement of cerebral activity. There is a certain pleasure associated with scratching which indicates association with the old part of the brain such as limbic structures and the cingulate gyrus.

# Itching as a side effects of administration of opioid

Administration of opioids can have beneficial effect on itch but itch can also be a side effect of opioids. Whichever one of these opposite effects is greatest will dominate, and there is no doubt that the analgesic and anti pruritic effect of opioids normally is the dominating effect. However, this balance between beneficial and non-beneficial effects may be shifted for unknown reasons and individual variations so that the paradoxical effects may become noticeable in some individuals under certain circumstances. If that occurs, effect of treatment of pain or itch may appear confusing both to the patient and the physician.

# CHAPTER 4
# Visceral Pain

## Abstract

1. Pain from viscera (internal organs) is caused by stimulation of receptors, but is different from somatic pain in many ways.

2. Visceral pain is less distinct than somatic pain and it is felt as coming from the surface of the body (referred pain).

3. Visceral pain is less precisely localized and it varies between individuals; it has strong emotional components.

4. Innervation of pain receptors in viscera is sparse compared with that of receptors in the skin.

5. Nerve fibers that innervate abdominal organs project to cells in the dorsal horn of the spinal cord.

6. Visceral receptors respond to distension of hollow organs and stretching of structures.

7. Pain receptors in internal organs are mostly chemoreceptors.

8. Visceral receptors respond to ischemia, but are generally insensitive to cutting and burning of tissue.

9. Ischemia, such as that of the heart, gives diffuse symptoms and there are great individual variations.

10. The vagus nerve plays an important, but poorly understood role in visceral pain.

11. Afferent fibers of the vagus nerve that project to the nucleus of the solitary tract (nucleus tractus solitarius) mediate at least partly the illness response that is typical for disorders of visceral organs.

12. Referred pain may be a result of shared targets of innervation of visceral and somatic (skin) receptors in the dorsal horn of the spinal cord. Other theories ascribe the phenomenon to overlapping innervation in the brain.

13. The insula plays an important role in mediating sensations from internal organs.

# Introduction

Pain from internal organs (visceral pain) is different from pain from peripheral structures (somatic pain). (Viscera means internal organs of the body, but the common usage of the word refers to organs of the chest and abdomen.) Pain from internal organs is less distinct than somatic pain. Visceral pain is felt as coming from the surface of the body (referred pain); localization varies from individual to individual.

All forms of pain can have emotional components, but pain from viscera and other deep structures differs from pain evoked by stimulation of pain receptors in superficial structures in that deep pain evokes passive emotional coping to a greater extent than somatic pain.

Clinically, visceral pain is usually regarded as a sign of disease processes that must be remedied. Therefore, treatment of visceral pain is focused on treatment of the underlying cause of the pain to a greater extent than somatic pain. Visceral pain, where the cause cannot be found (idiopathic pain) or where treatment of the underlying cause is not effective in relieving the pain, is more difficult to treat than somatic pain. These unique features of visceral pain are often overlooked and the management of visceral pain is typically poor. Drugs that are used with some efficacy to treat somatic pain often present unwanted effects on the viscera.

Pain from different internal organs has its own specific character, but that varies from individual to individual [81]. The emotional components of visceral pain tend to be greater than for pain caused by activation of nociceptors in the skin and muscles. Pain from internal organs may be perceived as inescapable to a greater extent than other forms of pain [36]. Pain from deep structures typically evoke passive emotional coping while pain from superficial structures normally evokes active emotional coping reactions such as the "fight and flight" response [203, 240].

Painful stimulation of the viscera is likely to produce referred pain and other sensations, such as nausea and a generally feeling of being unwell [336, 338]. The autonomic nervous system is often activated causing a change in the heart rate, paleness, etc.

For example, it is not generally recognized that ischemia of the heart can occur without pain in many individuals [198], but with symptoms such as nausea and vomiting or just feeling ill [336, 337]. Often, people are recommended to watch for pain in the left side of the body as an indication of a heart attack while only about half of heart attacks have these signs. The other half of heart attacks, often known as silent heart attacks, have symptoms that are general symptoms of an illness similar to what commonly occurs in connection with influenza, for example, instead of pain.

In fact, much regarding pain from the heart and viscera is unknown; in particular, it is unknown why there is such a great individual variation in the symptoms of insults to internal organs [198]. Some investigators have ascribed the variation to individual differences in anatomy and to biochemical differences [311], especially in the heart. The differences in the symptoms and signs of ischemia may also be explained by the fact that two different afferent systems mediate responses from visceral receptors, namely spinal nerves and the vagus nerve.

Variations in central processing of pain signals may also contribute to the differences in the expression of visceral pain [336]. These matters are naturally of great importance for diagnostics, but they are also of importance for individuals who need to know which signals should be interpreted as being indications of a serious condition that need prompt medical attention.

# Anatomy

The anatomy of the neural basis for visceral pain is more complex and less well understood than that of pain from superficial structures.

# Receptors

Visceral pain is caused by the activation of receptors in internal organs such as the intestines, the heart, the bladder, and sexual organs. Organs, such as the liver, lungs, kidneys, and the pancreas, have few receptors, but the pain from these organs comes mostly from the activation of receptors in the capsules of these organs.

There are only a few kinds of receptors in the internal organs; thus, less variations in visceral receptors than in somatic receptors (such as in the skin). If Robinson and Gebhart's definition of nociceptors is accepted, then 70-80 percent of receptors in the viscera may be classified as nociceptors [361].

Pain receptors in the viscera are mostly chemoreceptors that react to many kinds of chemicals including chemicals from inflammatory processes. Many of the receptors are free nerve endings. Receptors in the viscera also react to stretching of the organs, but burning and cutting do not activate these kinds of pain receptors. Ischemia also activates some visceral pain receptors, but ischemia of visceral organs can be painless, but produce other symptoms. The capsaicin receptor (TRPV1) is more common in visceral dorsal root ganglia (DRG) than in receptors in the skin and other superficial structures [361]. The functional, morphological, and biochemical differences between visceral and non-visceral (somatic) afferents has recently been reviewed by Robinson and Gebhart (2008) [361].

Mechanoreceptors (stretch receptors) in the viscera respond to innocuous stimulation of moderate strength, but strong stimulation of these receptors produces the sensation of pain. Pacinian corpuscles are other kinds of mechanoreceptors in visceral organs, but their exact functions are not fully known [50]. Activation of these receptors is probably perceived as deep touch.

Receptors in the viscera that respond to weak innocuous stimulation may cause a pain sensation in response to strong stimuli. Thus, these receptors have a dual way of responding.

# Afferent nerve fibers

Most organs in the abdomen are innervated by two different nerves, the pelvic and the splanchnic nerves, which innervate both the colon and the urinary bladder. The visceral organs also have a nervous system of their own, the enteric (associated with the intestines) nervous system of the gastrointestinal organs.

Spinal visceral afferent fibers project segmentally to lamina I and V and to deeper layers of the spinal dorsal horn. Pelvic afferent neurons also travel alongside parasympathetic efferent pathways, but their cell bodies are in the dorsal root ganglia (DRG) of the spinal cord. Other spinal nerves (e.g., greater splanchnic) travel alongside sympathetic efferent pathways, have cell bodies in the DRG, and pass through prevertebral ganglia (e.g., the celiac ganglion, CG).

Intestinofugal afferents synapse onto efferent sympathetic neurons in prevertebral ganglia, such as the inferior mesenteric ganglion (IMG) and have their cell bodies in the myenteric or submucosal plexus (M/SP).

Afferent fibers of the intrinsic (or enteric) nervous system, termed intrinsic primary afferent neurons (IPAN), synapse onto intestinofugal fibers, either directly or via interneurons. Rectospinal fibers have cell bodies in the myenteric plexus or muscle layers, with axons terminating in the spinal cord.

Innervation of the viscera is sparse compared to the innervation of superficial organs such as the skin. Visceral afferents are C-fibers and Aδ fibers; thus, similar to pain fibers in superficial structures. However, the proportion between C and Aδ fibers is different; in the viscera up to 80 percent of the fibers are C-fibers and fewer than 40 percent are Aδ fibers. There is an exception, however. Fibers from the perianal mucosa have been reported to be 23 percent C-fibers and 77 percent Aδ fibers [361].

Visceral afferents are of three main types: 1. Low-threshold mechanosensitive afferents responding to the distension of hollow organs, muscle contraction, and other stimuli; 2. Specific chemosensitive afferents; and 3. high-threshold mechanosensitive afferents.

The afferent sensory and pain fibers that innervate receptors of the viscera have their cell bodies in the dorsal root ganglia and they terminate on cells in the dorsal horn of the spinal cord. Nerve fibers from visceral receptors pass through autonomic ganglia where they give off collaterals that have secretory organs and muscles as their targets (the fibers are not interrupted for synaptic contacts) (see Figure 4.1) [33]. Nerve fibers that innervate receptors in the viscera terminate in the dorsal horn of the spinal cord or join other afferents in the vagus nerve.

Visceral C-fibers terminate in larger regions of the spinal horns than the C-fibers that mediate pain signals from the surface of the body. Some receptors are innervated by afferent vagus nerve fibers. Vagal afferent neurons have their cell bodies in the nodose ganglia (NG) bilaterally and travel alongside parasympathetic efferent pathways to organs in the thoracic and abdominal cavities. Vagal nerve fibers do not innervate the urinary bladder or the distal gut.

Afferent sensory nerves that innervate visceral organs follow sympathetic nerve fibers although they are not part of the autonomic system.

116   PAIN Its Anatomy, Physiology and Treatment

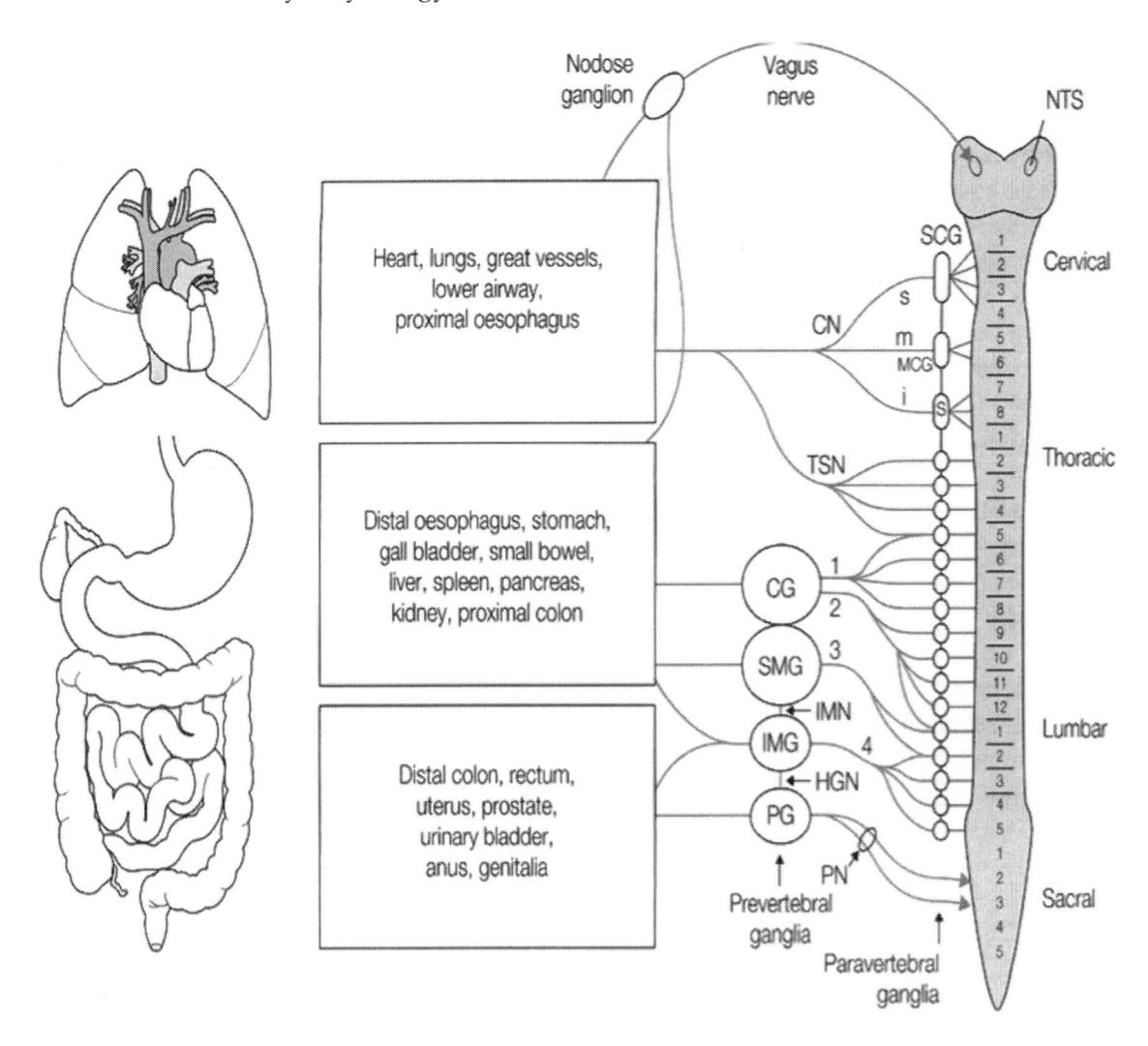

Figure 4.1. Innervation of the organs in the lower part of the abdomen. Nerve fibers from receptors in the viscera have their cell bodies in the superior and middle cervical ganglia and their target in cells in the dorsal horn of the spinal cord. For the vagus nerve, the targets are cells in the NTS nucleus.  CG: Coeliac ganglion; SMG and IMG: Superior and inferior mesenteric ganglia; PG: Pelvic ganglion; SCG and MCG: Superior and middle cervical ganglia; S: Stellate ganglion; PG: Prevertebral ganglia; CN: Cardiac nerves, s, m, i (superior, middle and inferior); TSN: Thoracic splanchnic nerves; IMN: Intermesenteric nerve; HGN: Hypogastric nerve; PN: Pelvic nerve. (Modified from Bielefeldt, K. and G.F. Gebhart, Visceral pain: basic mechanisms, in Textbook of Pain, S.B. McMahon and M. Koltzenburg, Editors. 2006, Elsevier: Amsterdam. p. 721-736 Reprinted with permission from Cambridge University Press [33].)

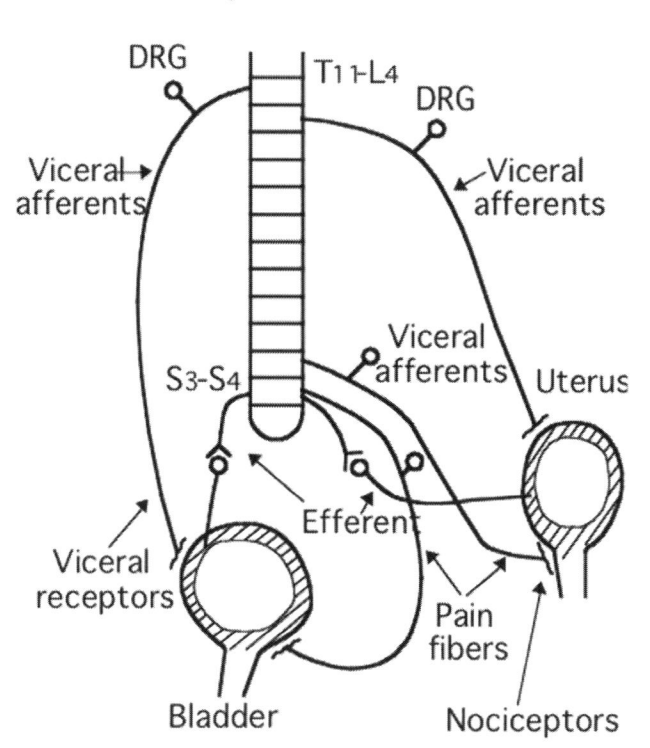

Figure 4.2 Visceral afferent innervation in the lower body and motor (efferent) innervation. The afferent pathways of visceral nociceptors in the bladder, and those of the neck of the bladder (including the prostate gland and the uterus) are shown together with motor innervation of the bladder and the uterus. (From Møller, A.R., Neuroplasticity and disorders of the nervous system. 2006, Cambridge: Cambridge University Press) Reprinted with permission from Cambridge University Press [288].

Once in the gut wall, vagal afferent fibers innervate neurons in the Auerbach's plexus of the intestinal wall or submucosal plexus (SP), circular and longitudinal muscle layers, and the mucosa (Figure 4.3). Most likely, specific chemosensitive afferents only contribute to the vagus nerve.

Pain elicited from receptors in some visceral organs is not only dependent on the activation of such receptors, but on the intensity of the stimulation. Thus, the discharge rate in spinal visceral afferents determines the kind of response (innocuous feelings or pain) [178]. Recordings of the electrical activity from afferent fibers in the pelvic nerve confirm that such afferents respond to distension of hollow visceral organs.

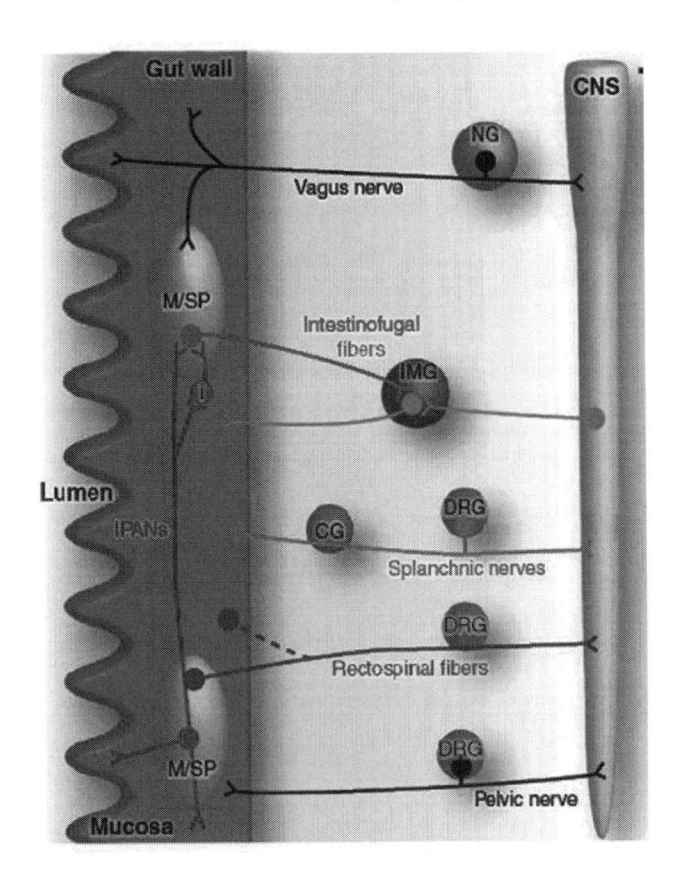

Figure 4.3 Simplified illustration of the functional neuroanatomy of the visceral sensory system. The gut is depicted here as an example of the sensory innervations of the visceral system. NG: Nodose ganglia; IMG: Inferior mesenteric ganglion; DRG: Dorsal root ganglion; IPAN: Intrinsic primary afferent neurons; M/SP: Myenteric or submucosal plexus, I: Interneurons. Note that not all of these nerves and fibers will terminate in the same areas of the gut, and inputs to the spinal cord may traverse a number of different levels; this figure has been simplified for clarity. (From Robinson, D., R. and G.F. Gebhart, Inside information: the unique features of visceral sensation. Mol Interv, 2008. 8(5): p. 242-53. [361].

Two systems of nerve cells and nerve fibers extend along the gastrointestinal tract. The myenteric (Auerbach's) plexus controls motility and the submucousal (Meissner's) plexus controls secretions. Five different types of afferent fibers have been reported in the colon: fibers that innervate cells that secrete, cells in the mesenteric (folds of the peritoneum), and muscular, mucosal, and muscular/mucosal sensory cells (Figure 4.4).

Each has a characteristic response to probing, stretching, and stroking the colonic wall, and each has a different putative functional role.

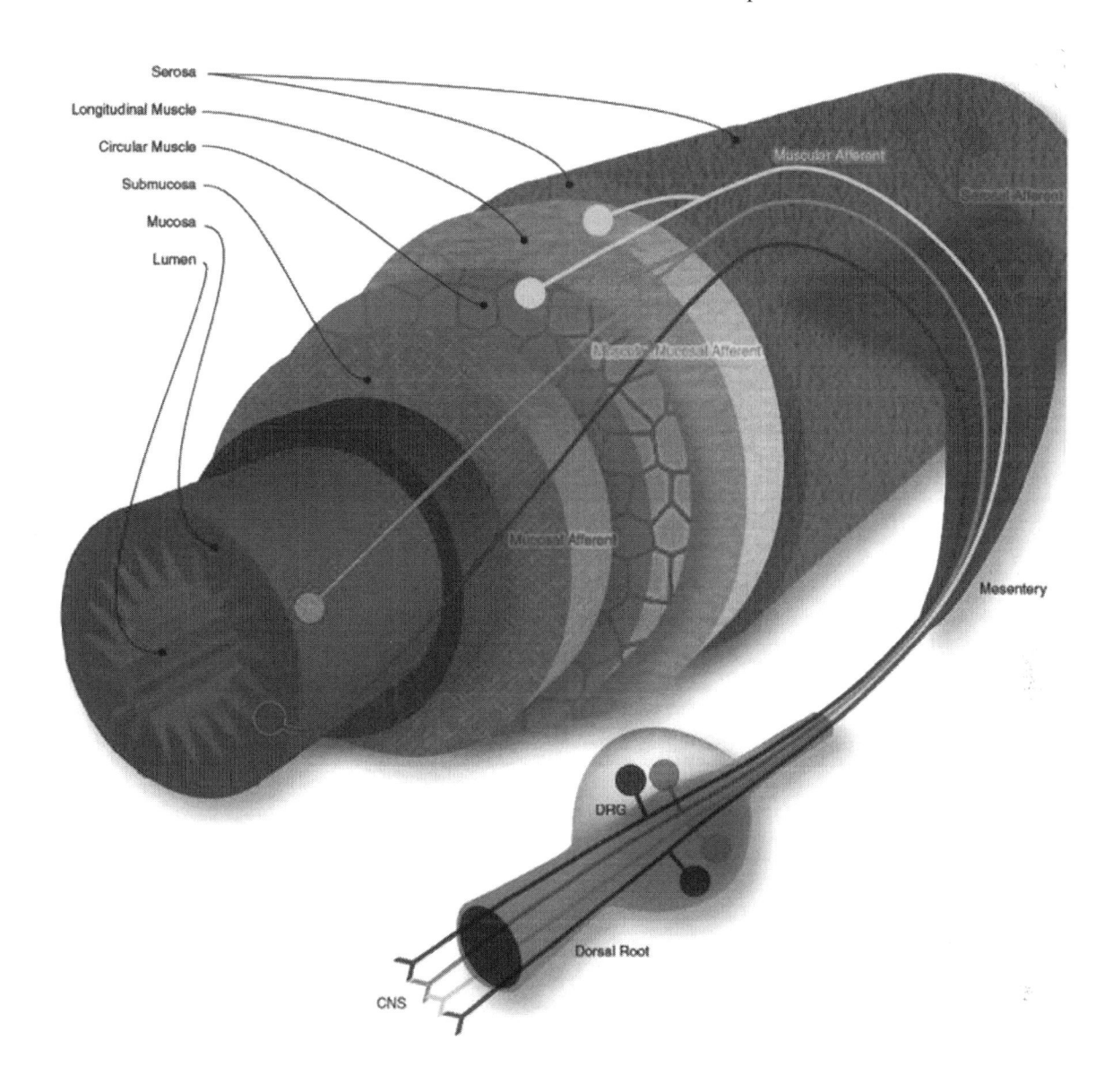

Figure 4.4 Illustration of the arrangement of the five different receptors in the colon. From Robinson, D.R. and G.F. Gebhart, Inside information: the unique features of visceral sensation. Mol Interv, 2008. 8(5): p. 242-53. [361]. After Brierley, S.M., R.C.R. Jones, G. Gebhart, F., and L.A. Blackshaw, Splanchnic and pelvic mechanosensory afferents signal different qualities of colonic stimuli in mice. Gastroenterology. 2004. 127(1): p. 166-78. [48]. Reprinted with permission from Gastroenterology.

Most serosal afferents are mechanosensitive and are thought to signal short, sharp events (e.g., muscle contraction). Mesenteric afferents are predominantly found near blood vessels and they respond to twisting of the colon wall and changes in mesenteric blood pressure, and they are possibly involved in inflammatory reactions. Muscular afferents of the gut respond directly to circumferential stretch with a low threshold of activation.

Muscular afferents generally are assumed to contribute to sustained filling, bloating, or distending sensations. Mucosal afferents respond to fine probing and stroking of the mucosal membrane. Thereby, they may provide feedback from physiological stimuli such as the normal passing of fecal material through the gastrointestinal tract. Muscular/mucosal afferents can detect both circular stretch and fine mucosal stroking, and they are a class of mechanoreceptors that are only found in pelvic innervation, at least in the mouse colon where they were studied. Innervation of deep structures by the vagus nerve is further illustrated in Figure 4.5.

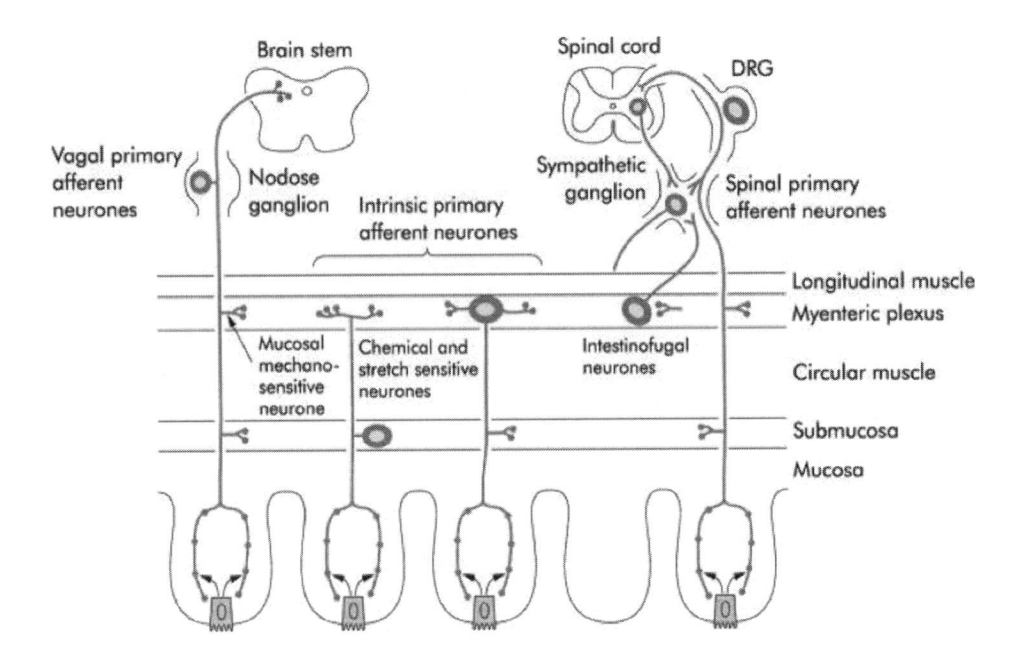

Figure 4.5 Innervation of receptors in the intestines by the vagus nerve (left part of the figure) and spinal afferent fibers (right side of the figure) and the arrangement of the primary afferent fibers and their targets. DRG: dorsal root ganglion. Grundy, D., Neuroanatomy of visceral nociception: vagal and splanchnic afferent. Gut, 2002. 51 (Suppl 1): p. 2-5. Adapted with the permission from Gut.

It has been learned from studies on the rat bladder that low-threshold mechanoreceptors can detect both non-noxious and noxious distension pressures, whereas high-threshold mechanoreceptors only respond to noxious distention pressures (A in Figure 4.6). Similar experiments have also revealed that mechanoreceptors (of either the high- or low-threshold type) that are innervated by the pelvic nerve can be sensitized by the addition of irritants (e.g., xylenes) into the bladder (B in Figure 4.6). In other studies, it was found that mice that were lacking the TRPV1 (capsaicin) receptor ("knock-out" mice) showed impaired visceral nociception.

A) Response from low-threshold mechanoreceptors (top curve) as a function of distension pressures of a rat bladder, and from high-threshold mechanoreceptors (lower curve) that only respond to noxious distention pressures. B) Effects of sensitization of high threshold mechanoreceptors (top graph) and low-threshold receptors (low graph) recorded from the pelvic nerve. C) Illustration of the effect of impaired visceral nociception in mice lacking the TRPV1 receptor. The visceromotor response (electrical activity recorded in the abdominal musculature) is shown as a function of distension of the colon to a noxious pressure (e.g., 60 mmHg) (lower curve). Top curve reflects control recordings in a wild-type mouse used as a control. Modified from Robinson, D., R. and G.F. Gebhart, Inside information: the unique features of visceral sensation. Mol Interv, 2008. 8(5): p. 242-53 [361]. (Panels A and B are adapted with permission from Su, X., Sengupta, J.N., and Gebhart, G.F. Effects of opioids on mechanosensitive pelvic nerve afferent fibers innervating the urinary bladder of the rat. J. Neurophysiol. 77, 1566–1580 (1997). Panel C is adapted with permission from Jones, R.C.W., III, Xu, L., and Gebhart, G.F.

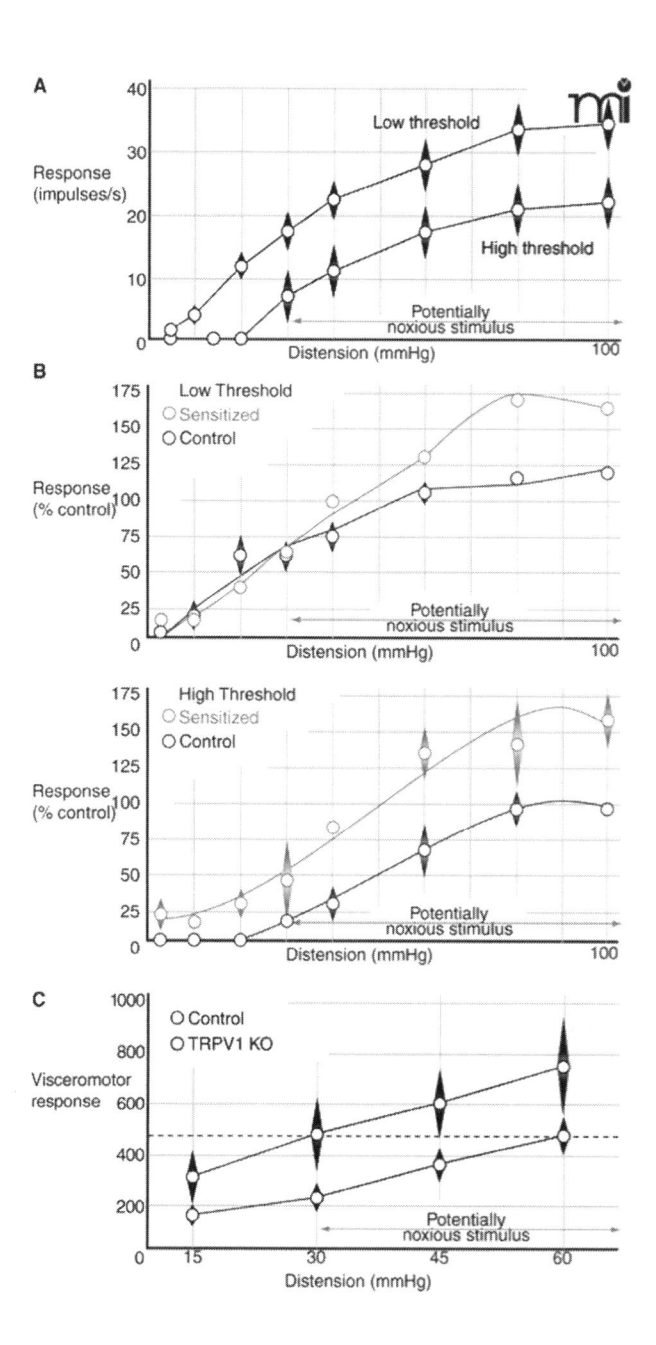

Figure 4.6. Responses from pelvic nerve afferent fibers (innervating visceral mechanoreceptors) during distension of a hollow visceral organ in animals.

The mechanosensitivity of mouse colon afferent fibers and their sensitization by inflammatory mediators require transient receptor potential vanilloid 1 and acid-sensing ion channel 3. J. Neurosci. 25, 10981–10989 (2005). [196]). There is evidence that some of the fibers that innervate visceral receptors and target cells in the spinal cord have redundant innervations from the vagus nerve. There is also evidence that indicates that the vagus nerve may substitute spinal pathways from genitalia in case of spinal cord injuries providing the possibility of tactile stimulation to evoke orgasms in females with spinal cord injuries [402, 403]. It is not known to what extent these "redundant" connections are also active in individuals who have intact spinal cords and whether they may furnish some pain information from that part of the body.

# Cardiac pain

Despite enormous importance of understanding the signs of cardiac problems, such as cardiac ischemia, it is still unclear which signs and symptoms are reliable indicators of cardiac muscle ischemia such as it occurs in the common heart attack. The ways heart attacks occur are often misunderstood.

Stents and bypass operations, which are often used to reduce the risk of further heart attacks, aim at opening arteries narrowed by atherosclerotic plaques. However, such narrowing of arteries is not what causes heart attacks; only the pain (angina) is caused by narrowing of cardiac (coronary) vessels. Instead, heart attacks are normally caused by pieces of arthrosclerosis plaque that come loose from the wall of an artery and travel by the blood stream to a narrow place where it blocks a vessel [469]. Thereby, the part of the muscle that losses its blood supply becomes ischemic and a long chain of events and processes begin. One of these is eliciting pain from nociceptors in the part of the heart muscle that has been deprived of blood.

The classical signs are chest pain and/or pain radiating out from the shoulder and neck, but studies have shown that these symptoms are only present in about half of the instances of cardiac ischemia [309]. Those who do not have these signs are sometimes known as "silent" heart attacks. More recent studies indicate that the symptoms are feeling sick such as occurs in severe influenza and perhaps shortness of breath. Thus, what is called a silent heart attack is not silent; it does indeed give signs, but different ones than a "normal" heart attack. The symptoms may be mediated by the vagus nerve. It is not uncommon in visceral systems to give such different symptoms for similar events, such as ischemia.

# Central pathways for visceral pain

The involvement of the central nervous system in deep pain is extensive and in many aspects, different from that of somatic pain [361]. Little is known, however, about the central connections of visceral afferents except that the spinal nerves from viscera essentially use the same pathways from the spinal cord to the brain (spinothalamic tract, STT). However, the vagus nerve that has a completely different central projection than spinal nerves may play a role. We have shown in other parts of this book that the nucleus of the solitary tract (NST) that is the target of the afferent fibers in the vagus nerve project to many different regions of the brain. Activation of the vagus nerve may, therefore, give different signs than similar activation of spinal nerves.

## The vagus nerve and visceral pain

The notion that visceral afferents only target spinal neurons is outdated and there is now considerable evidence that afferents in the vagus nerve communicate visceral sensory information including pain [32].

There is also evidence that there are two parallel targets of innervation to the organs in the thorax and the abdomen; one is the vagus nerve and the other source includes nerves that become dorsal roots of the spinal cord.

Approximately 80 percent of the fibers in the vagus nerve are afferent (ascending) fibers, but so far, most studies have concerned the efferent (descending) fibers of the vagus nerve (which supply internal organs in the abdomen with parasympathetic innervation). The afferent fibers terminate in the nucleus of the solitary tract (NST). The afferent parts of the vagus nerve can influence processing of pain signals in the brain, but little is known about the specifics of the neural circuits through which the vagus nerve can modulate pain impulses. Recent studies have found that the nucleus of the vagus nerve (NST) can influence many structures of the brain and the spinal cord, including pain circuits (including those involved in pathological pain) (see Figures 3.13B and 12.2B).

Vagal afferents from the small intestine have inhibitory influence on central input to the pre-ganglionic neurons that innervate the adrenal medulla and there is evidence that the vagus nerve provides a natural modulation (suppression) of pathological pain from neural activity in the intestine [181].

Activity in the preganglionic neurons innervating the adrenal medulla and thus, controlling the liberation of adrenalin into the blood stream, are modulated by vagus nerve fibers that innervate the small intestine, being inhibitory. Thus, interruption of vagal input from the small intestine increases adrenal secretion. It has been hypothesized that these reflex kinds of circuits in the lower brainstem are in turn controlled by the upper brainstem, the hypothalamus, and the forebrain (see Figure 12.2B).

There are indications that vagus nerve activity may contribute to more complex signs than just a sensation of pain. However, little is known about the role of the vagus nerve regarding communicating noxious information from internal organs involving affective symptoms. Feelings of illness may be one such complex sensation. There is also evidence that the vagus nerve may exert regulation of cerebral functions.

The axons of the NTS travel to several brain centers such as the paraventricular nucleus of the hypothalamus and the amygdala. The paraventricular nucleus connects to the pituitary gland, thus connecting to endocrine structures. The fact that electrical stimulation of the vagus nerve can suppress epileptic seizures also indicates that the vagus nerve has connections to many parts of the brain.

The left and right vagus nerves are different in several respects. For example, it is the right vagus nerve that slows the heart and this is why electrical stimulation of the left vagus nerve can be applied safely and is used clinically for various purposes such as controlling pain or epileptic seizures without affecting the function of the heart. It is not known if the afferent parts of the left and the right vagus nerves are different.

The fact that pain medication effective in alleviating pain from superficial structures is much less effective in treating visceral pain is an indication that the central targets of the ascending pain pathways that communicate visceral pain are different from those of pain from superficial structures (see Chapter 3).

Vagus nerve stimulation (VNS) is more potent than stimulation of spinal neurons in the $C_1$–$C_3$ segments of the dorsal horn of the spinal cord [100]. Vagal afferent fibers can modulate the processing of information of cells receiving afferent input from the heart of the thoracic spinothalamic tract by activating tracts in the brain and nuclei.

Vagus nerve stimulation is a potential treatment for essential tremor, cognitive deficits in Alzheimer's disease, anxiety disorders, and bulimia.

Finally, other studies explore the potential use of VNS in the treatment of resistant obesity, addictions, sleep disorders, narcolepsy, coma, and memory and learning deficits. These possibilities are now studied intensively [6, 209, 302] (see Chapters 7 and 12).

Pairing vagus nerve stimulation with a sensory stimulation seems to be a powerful method to activate neuroplasticity and this may be the most effective way to alleviate sensory hyperactivity such as that causing tinnitus [114]. Similar methods are under development for treating other plasticity disorders such as some forms of pain.

# The vagus nerve and the illness response

The illness response, in addition to hyperalgesia (lowered threshold for pain) and pain, may be elicited by the stimulation of receptors in the viscera such as by proinflammatory cytokines released from immune cells. These cytokines may activate afferent fibers in the vagus nerve and subsequently, activate cells in the nucleus of the solitary tract (NST). From there, illness responses may be elicited, including hyperalgesia and pain. This may be mediated through connections from the NTS neurons to the raphe magnus nucleus, which has both facilitating and inhibitory influence on spinal cord pain neurons.

It is possible that the hypothalamus-pituitary-adrenal system is also involved in lowering the pain threshold (hyperalgesia). The illness response may also be elicited through activation of the paraventricular nucleus of the hypothalamus and limbic structures such as the hippocampus (Figure 4.7).

## The vagus nerve and immune reactions

Afferents of the vagus nerve may serve as an important rapid signaling pathway for communicating immune changes from the periphery to the areas in the brain that respond to infection and inflammation. Infection and inflammation elicit the production of vasoactive and neurohumoral compounds [100, 142].

The release of inflammatory cytokines, such as interleukin (IL)-1, IL-6, IL-1$\beta$, and tumor necrosis factor $\alpha$, trigger several systemic responses depending on the integrity of the vagal afferent pathway.

Activity in the vagus nerve can change pain sensitivity and metabolism, cause hyperthermia, and can cause an increased release of adrenocorticotropin, glucocorticoids, and liver acute phase proteins that are all related to the immune responses. Stimulation of afferent vagal axons can also activate the hypothalamus–pituitary–adrenal axis. The hypothalamus and the amygdala may also be activated by vagus nerve activity.

It is possible that activity in afferent vagal axons that results from the release of cytokines might inhibit spinothalamic tract cells and spinal neurons in the thoracic segments. Thus, the vagal afferent pathway to structures in the brain might be important for eliciting the immune responses resulting from systemic infections and inflammation contributing to the perception of pain such as in angina pectoris [100]. Studies have shown that the cholinergic anti-inflammatory pathway can be activated through activity in the vagal afferents[441]. This means that events in the gut can influence the ability of the immune system to fight invasions of bacteria and viruses. It also implies that electrical stimulation of the vagus nerve can modulate immune reactions.

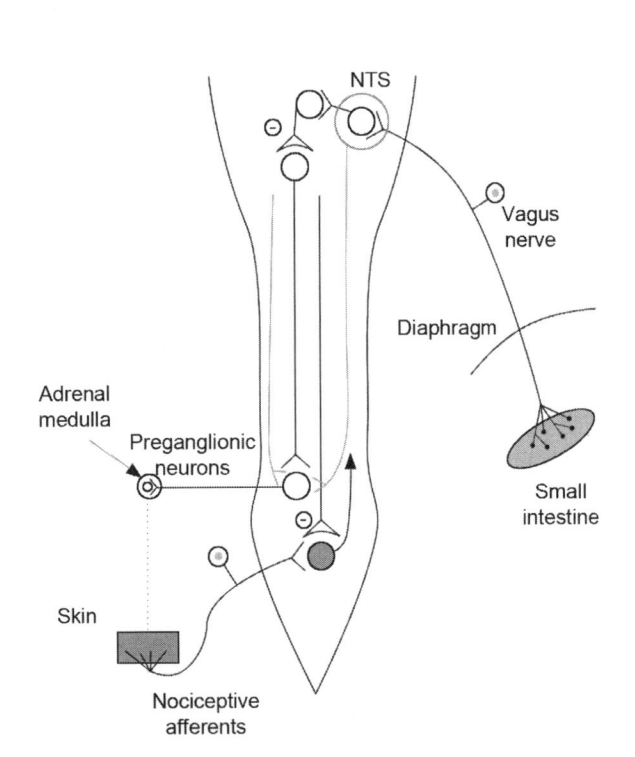

Figure 4.7 Illustration of how the illness response may be mediated by the vagus nerve through the nucleus of the solitary tract (NST) causing hyperalgesia and pain through descending pathways via nucleus raphe magnus, possibly involving the hypothalamus-pituitary-adrenal system (Modified from Jänig, W., & Levine, J. D. (2006.) Autonomic-endocrine-immune interactions in acute and chronic pain. In S. B. McMahon & M. Koltzenburg (Eds.), Wall and Melzack's Textbook of Pain (Vol. 5th). Amsterdam: Elsevier. and Goehler et al 2000 [142]) [183]. (Artwork by Monica Javidnia.)

This means that the vagus nerve is involved in protective mechanisms of the body of which the illness response is an important one (see Chapter 2, Figure 2.5).

# Visceral organ cross-sensitization

The interaction between pain from different internal organs has just began to attract attention [55]. There is recent behavioral, morphological, and physiological evidence of mechanisms underlying cross-organ sensitization.

Noxious input from different visceral organs converges on cells in the central nervous system and it has been assumed that cross-organ sensitization arises from a similar convergence-projection mechanism as the one that is involved in referral of pain in internal organs to locations on the surface of the body. This includes highly organized immune-sensory systems with pathways for activating host defenses against infection and other insults to the body [142].

# Referred pain

Pain from internal organs is localized to the surface of the body, but the location is not over the organs that cause the pain. This is known as referred pain. Figure 4.8 shows the general outline of the location of pain from internal organs, but there are considerable individual variations.

The visceral afferents that travel to the spinal cord terminate on cells in the dorsal horns, and they often share the same cells as fibers from somatic nociceptors. The axons of these cells travel in the anterior lateral tracts towards the thalamus and several other brain structures (see below).

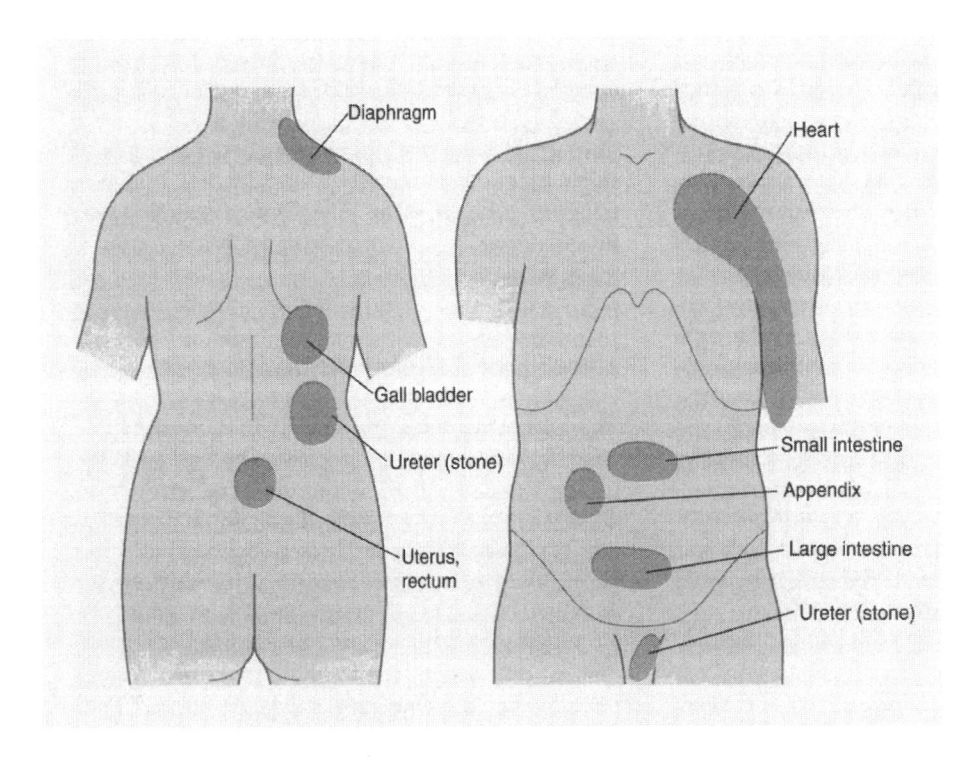

Figure 4.8. Referred pain (From Brodal, P., The central nervous system. 3rd ed. 2004, New York: Oxford Press.) [51]

Pain caused by stimulation of pain receptors in the heart, intestines, and other internal organs is not felt at the anatomical location from where it is elicited, but referred to locations on the surface of the body (known as referred pain) [81, 82, 336, 364] (Figure 4.8). The location to which the pain is referred is less specific than somatic pain and varies among individuals [81].

The anatomical basis for referred pain is not known in detail. Several hypotheses have been presented regarding the mechanisms [81, 83]. One hypothesis regarding referred pain from viscera assumes that the same cells in the dorsal horn receive input both from receptors in the viscera and from receptors in the skin [33] (see Figure 4.9). Referred pain has also been attributed to a change (extension) of the receptive fields of neurons by activating dormant synapses, thus, an expression of neuroplasticity. The regions of the body to which pain is referred often extend with time, thus a form of lateral spread of activation. It has been suggested that a peripheral nerve trunk is capable of sustaining a "flare" response similar to that observed in injured skin and other tissue[508] and thus cause an extension of the region from which pain sensation originates.

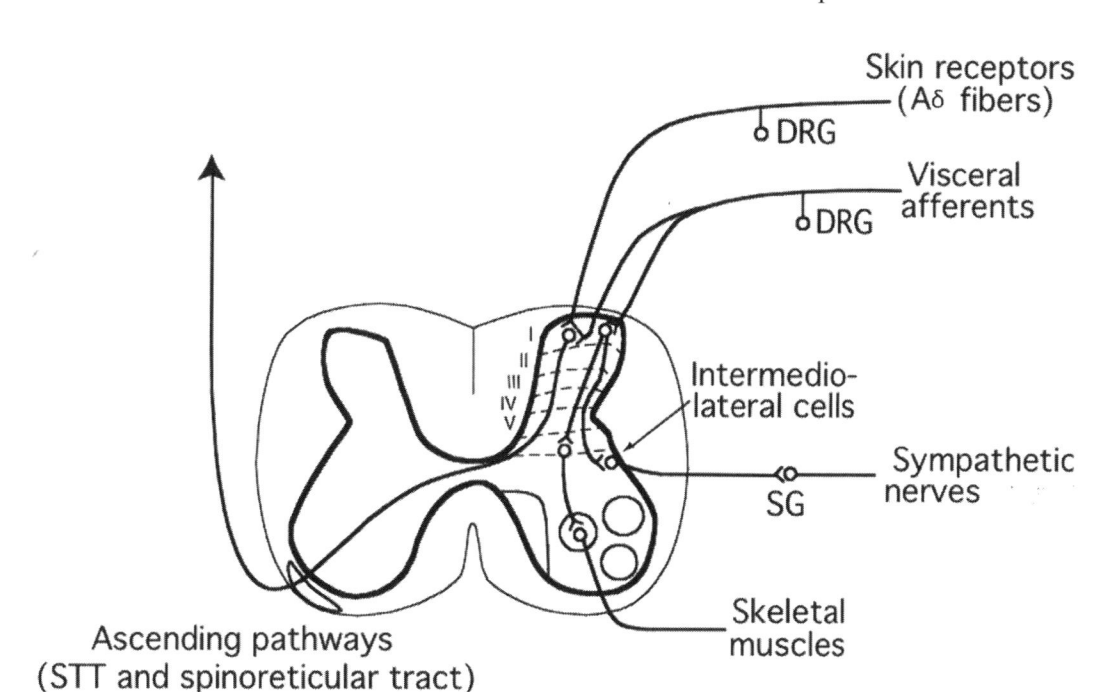

Figure 4.9. Schematic diagram of the anatomical basis for one hypothesis for referred pain. Sharing of target cells in lamina I (the axons of which form the anterior portion of the STT is shown). SG: Sympathetic ganglion. (From Møller, A.R., Neuroplasticity and disorders of the nervous system. 2006, Cambridge: Cambridge University Press [288], Adapted from [82] Reprinted with permission from Cambridge University Press).

The reason that pain from viscera is poorly localized could also be related to the fact that the cells in the spinal cord that receive signals from visceral structures are much fewer than those that receive input from superficial body structures (skin, etc.) [70]. The fact that the vagus nerve mediates pain from viscera may also contribute to the difference in the perception of such pain compared with other forms of physiological pain [32].

Pain from organs in the lower abdomen, including reproductive organs, are often referred to as $T_{12}$-$L_1$, dermatomes; thus, in accordance with the location where the afferent nerves enter the spinal cord [83]. However, as mentioned above, the receptors of some parts of pelvic organs are innervated by nerve fibers that follow the sympathetic-fibers and enter the spinal cord as parts of dorsal roots of the sacral spine. This means that some pain from pelvic organs may be referred to the distribution (dermatomes) of sacral somatic nerves.

Referred muscle pain may also occur as a result of the diffusion of substance P (SP) and calcitonin generated peptides in the dorsal horn of the spinal cord [267], which may explain the pathophysiology of trigger points that are associated in some forms of muscle pain [171]. (Trigger points are locations on the skin (or in the mouth) where sensory stimulation (touch, cold, or warmth) elicits an attack of pain.) Some forms of pain have distinct trigger points from which pain can be elicited or from which attacks of pain can be initiated.

# An odd manifestation of referred pain

Facial pain, in rare occasions, has been shown to present as a symptom of lung cancer [373]. These investigators described patients with lung cancer who had attacks of debilitating facial pain, presenting as cluster headaches. Moreover, 32 reported cases of lung cancer-related facial pain have been reported. The facial pain is almost always unilateral, and is most commonly localized to the ear, the jaw, and the temporal region. It was hypothesized that such pain is a form of referred pain caused by the invasion or compression of the vagus nerve, or secondary to the production of circulating humoral factors by the malignant tumor cells. Radiotherapy and tumor resection with severance of the vagus nerve has been effective in aborting the facial pain. The interval between the presentation with pain and the discovery of the lung cancer varied between 6 weeks and 4 years.

# The role of the sympathetic nervous system in visceral pain

The sympathetic nervous system may be involved in referred pain. The sympathetic nervous system plays an important role by increasing the sensitivity of skin receptors. Activation of α-motoneurons may occur causing contraction of skeletal muscles, which may cause pain. Referred pain may also be caused by the convergence of pain impulses at more central locations such as the thalamus.

Diagnosis of disorders on the basis of pain is more difficult for visceral pain than somatic pain because of the variability of the location of the pain. The fact that the location is not directly associated with the anatomical location of the organ that is affected contributes to the ambiguities of the symptoms and signs from internal organs.

# Involvement of the dorsal column in deep pain

The dorsal column-medial lemniscal system has earlier been regarded to only mediate innocuous sensation and not pain perception. Recent studies, however, seem to show that the dorsal column may be involved in relaying visceral nociceptive information [326]. Clinical studies have shown that small lesions made on the dorsal columns close to the midline of the spinal cord can relieve pain and decrease analgesic requirements in patients suffering from cancer originating in visceral organs [326]. Studies in animals have shown that lesions in the dorsal column can lead to decreased activation of cells in one of the dorsal column nuclei (gracilis) by visceral stimuli [326]. The fact that dorsal column stimulation can relieve pain [494] may have other reasons.

# The role of the insula lobe in visceral pain

The insular lobe is a little known structure of the brain that is located under the temporal lobe [316]. It may play an important role regarding visceral pain [306]. The insula is a complex structure that provides extensive functional connections to many parts of the brain, but little is known about the behavioral aspects in humans. Cells in the insula have connections to many parts of the brain, such as both the primary and secondary somatosensory areas, the anterior cingulate cortex, the amygdala, the prefrontal cortex, the superior temporal gyrus, the temporal pole, the orbitofrontal cortex, the frontal and parietal opercula, the primary and association auditory cortices, the visual association cortex, the olfactory bulb, the hippocampus, the entorhinal cortex, and the motor cortex [306].

There is anatomical and some functional evidence that the insula plays an important role in the integration of multimodal sensory input (including pain). It is also believed that the insula has an important role in some neuropsychiatric disorders [55].

There are signs of a close relationship between the insular cortex and neuropsychiatric diseases such as mood disorders, panic disorders, post traumatic stress disorders (PTSD), obsessive-compulsive disorders, eating disorders, and schizophrenia [306].

The activity from visceral organs arrives at the viscero-sensory cortex that is located in the middle part of the insula and also projects to the right anterior insula and orbitofrontal cortices [316, 389, 417]. The right anterior insula is involved in diverse tasks, one being the sympathetic arousal associated with mental tasks. This brain region also receives input from many other parts of the brain, including pain and painful stimuli.

There is evidence that the insular cortex is involved in the processing of sensory information, especially visceral sensations, but also in visceral motor, vestibular, attention, pain, and emotion, verbal, and motor information. The insula lobe is involved in functions related to eating such as taste and smell.

Studies using semi-permanently implanted electrodes (Figure 4.10) in humans undergoing treatment for intractable epilepsy have provided a wealth of information about the function of the insular lobe [416, 417]. These studies suggest that sensory information, including gustatory, olfactory, visual, auditory, and tactile inputs, converge on the insular cortex and may be coordinated there [416]. Electrical stimulation of various locations within the insular lobe in awake and alert individuals gave responses such as various forms of taste, a metallic sensation in the nose, odd feelings in the stomach, and pulsations in the foot [416, 417] (Figure 4.11).

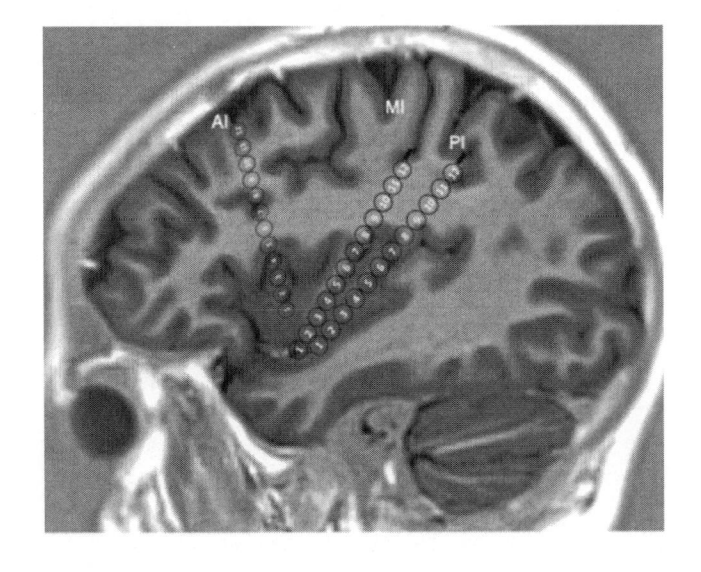

Figure 4.10. Electrode placements for stimulation and recording (123 electrodes) in the insula of a person undergoing diagnostic work-up for surgical treatment for epilepsy. From: Stephani, C., G. Fernandez Baca-Vaca, M. Koubeissi, R. Maciunas, et al. Stimulation of the insula. In Second Congress, International Society of Intraoperative Neurophysiology. 2009. Dubrovnik [416]. Reprinted by permission of the editor of the Proceedings and the author of the chapter).

It has been learned from studies of the rat bladder that low-threshold mechanoreceptors can detect both non-noxious and noxious distension pressures, whereas high-threshold mechanoreceptors only respond to noxious distension pressures (A in Figure 4.6). Similar experiments have also revealed that mechanoreceptors (of either the high- or low-threshold type) that are innervated by the pelvic nerve can be sensitized by the addition of irritants (e.g., xylenes) into the bladder (B in Figure 4.6). In other studies, it was found that mice that were lacking the TRPV1 (capsaicin) receptor ("knock-out" mice) showed impaired visceral nociception.

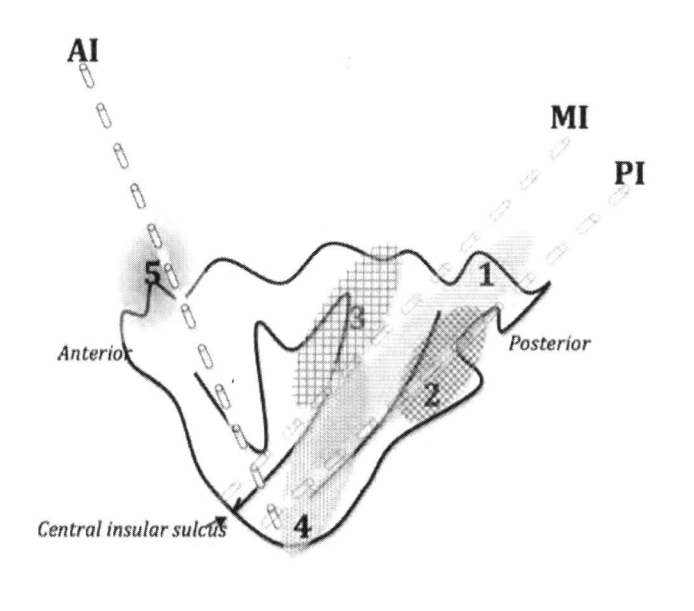

Figure 4.12 Electrode tracks in the insula of a person undergoing diagnostic work-up for surgical treatment for epilepsy. AI: Anterior insula, MI: Middle insula, PI: Posterior insula. 1. Somatosensation; 2. Temperature; 3. Taste; 4. Sensation from internal organs (viscera); 5. Perception of speech (From Stephani, C., G. Fernandez Baca-Vaca, M. Koubeissi, R. Maciunas, et al. Stimulation of the insula. In Second Congress, International Society of Intraoperative Neurophysiology. 2009. Dubrovnik) [416]. (Reprinted by permission of the editor of the Proceedings and the author).

There is evidence that the insula may provide convergence of different kinds of neural activity such as from different sensory systems. Studies have shown connections from the somatosensory system to limbic structures, from the insula to limbic structures, insula to orbital to temporal connections, and from the prefrontal cortex to the basal ganglia to the basal forebrain [389]. There is evidence that these same structures are involved in the processing of pain signals from viscera.

# Deep sensations

Sensations that are not painful can be elicited from mechanical stimulation of viscera. These sensations are probably evoked by the stimulation of Pacinian corpuscles and may occur by the activation of non-classical sensory pathways [287].

There is also evidence that painful stimuli activate cells in the basal ganglia [42]. The highly specialized organization of the parts of the central nervous system that concern pain may couple pain and its intensity and form with specific autonomic states.

The anterior cingulated cortex that plays a crucial role in pain perception is directly involved in the control of autonomic functions. Thus, the pain system and the autonomic nervous system closely interact in many processes such as in maintaining internal homeostasis.

# CHAPTER 5
# Pain from Peripheral and Cranial Nerves
## The role of inflammation

# Abstract

1. Neuralgias are characterized by sharp shooting pain that is felt in the radiation of one or more peripheral nerves.

2. Disorders of peripheral nerves are known as mononeuropathies when they affect a single nerve and as polyneuropathies when several nerves are affected.

3. Mononeuralgies may be caused by viral infection, trauma, or unknown causes. Polyneuralgies may occur in connection with diabetes or may be age related, but often no cause can be found.

4. Trigeminal neuralgia is often regarded as a model of neuralgias.

5. Compression of nerves such as spinal nerve roots have been blamed for causing pain, but compression of a normal nerve would only affect larger myelinated fibers with little or no effect on small myelinated fibers and unmyelinated fibers that are involved in pain.

6. Carpal tunnel syndrome and low back pain have been regarded as "nerve compression disorders", but recent evidence shows pain from nerve compression only occurs if the or nerve root is inflamed.

7. Peripheral nerves have receptors (nervi nervorum) in the nerve sheet. These may be involved in causing pain.

8. The location of the pathology that causes pain in "nerve compression disorders" can also be the central nervous system (spinal cord or brain) if plastic changes occur.

9. Nerve inflammation by the herpes virus is a common cause of mononeuropathies such as shingles.

10. Polyneuropathies typically affect mainly sensory nerve fibers of small diameters (Aδ and C-fibers), which explain the bilateral burning pain that is common for these disorders. Distal portions of the nerves are often affected first and more severely than proximal fibers and that explains that foot pain is often the first sign of polyneuropathy.

11. Trauma to nerves, including severance of nerves, promotes creation of neuromas, which are pain sensitive and, therefore, may contribute to trauma-induced pain.

12. Slightly injured nerves may fire in bursts and such bursts may be more powerful in exciting their central target cells than steady firing.

13. Neuropathy may promote activation of neuroplasticity that can shift pain from being physiological pain to becoming pathological pain.

# Introduction

Disorders of peripheral and cranial nerves are known as neuropathy. By definition, neuropathic pain is all pain caused by pathologies of the nervous system, but this is too broad a term to be practical. Neurologists use the term "neuropathy" to describe disorders of peripheral nerves and cranial nerves only. We will do the same in this book and use the term "central neuropathic pain" for pain caused by disorders (or changes in the function) of the spinal cord and the brain.

This chapter will discuss the various causes of pain from peripheral and cranial nerves, including viral infections and trauma (as well as surgically induced trauma). We will also discuss controversial issues such as the cause of low back pain.

# Different kinds of disorders of nerves

In this chapter, the term "mononeuropathies" [255] will be used for disorders that affect a single peripheral nerve and the term "polyneuropathies" will be used for disorders that affect several nerves [376]. Neuropathies may have symptoms other than pain such as numbness, tingling, or itching. The term "neuralgia" describes pain that may be caused by disorders of the nerve in question (neuropathy) or have other causes. Pain that follows a single nerve is known as mononeuralgia and pain that follows several nerves is polyneuralgia.

# Neuralgias

Neuralgias are pain conditions that are related to one or more nerves. Many neuralgias cause severe suffering in many people [453]. When only one nerve is affected, it is known as mononeuralgia (or mononeuropathy [255]) and when more than one nerve is involved, it is known as polyneuralgia (or polyneuropathy [376]). Neuralgias are characterized by pain that is related to the anatomical location of one or more of a nerve's anatomical location. Neuralgias are characterized by pain. The pain can have the form of shooting pain that comes in attacks, such as in trigeminal neuralgia, or it can be in the form of burning pain, such as in polyneuralgia in diabetes or age related neuropathy [341].

Neuralgia can be caused by minor injuries to any nerve, but it may start without any known cause. Post-herpetic neuralgia can affect any nerve after an infection with the herpes virus. Mononeuralgias may be caused by trauma or virus infections, or may have no known cause such as trigeminal neuralgia. Polyneuralgia typically occurs in connection with diabetes or vitamin deficiencies or it may be age-related, but in many cases, the cause is unknown.

These disorders, as so many other disorders, only manifest if more than one condition is present. This is one of the reasons for controversies where some investigators claim one cause whereas other investigators claim a different cause of a disease. The truth is probably that more than one abnormality must be present at the same time to produce symptoms.

If two causes are necessary to cause symptoms, removal of either one will relieve the symptoms. This makes it possible for investigators with different opinions regarding the cause of a disease to claim that their suggestion of cause is the correct one.

A specific neuralgia, trigeminal neuralgia, belongs to a group of diseases known as microvascular compression disorders. Trigeminal neuralgia (TGN) (or tic douleroux) [129, 477] is a typical mononeuralgia that occurs without any known cause. Individuals with TGN have sharp shooting pain that is perceived in the distribution of a branch of the trigeminal nerve. The pain comes in attacks, often triggered by a touch at specific places on the face or in the mouth. TGN is a rare disease with an incidence of 5.9 per 100,000 in women and 3.4 in 100,000 in men in a white population in the U.S.A. [202].

TGN is interesting in many ways. For example, it has the highest success in treatment of any of the neuralgias (about 85 percent of the patients get total freedom of pain [24]) and it can be treated equally successful by three different methods (see Chapter 7). TGN has a complex pathophysiology, involving the central nervous system. It is not a neuropathy because there is probably nothing wrong with the nerve itself; the pain is most likely caused by hyperactivity of the trigeminal nucleus.

TGN is similar to hemifacial spasm (HFS) in that both can be successfully treated by moving a blood vessel off the respective nerve root. For a long time, it was assumed that the symptoms were caused by ephaptic transmissions (direct transmission between nude axons along a nerve [352] that would occur in the facial and trigeminal nerve roots and cause the spasm in HFS and pain in TGN [132, 315]). This hypothesis had to be abandoned by studies of patients with HFS [283]. HFS that has lasted many years involves all mimic muscles including the platysma, but excluding the muscles of the forehead that have bilateral innervation. It was realized that to explain the extensive contractions of facial muscles in hemifacial spasm, it would be necessary that almost all axons in the nerve root had contact with each other. Naturally, this is not realistic [115]. Any amount of demyelination that would be necessary to satisfy the ephaptic hypothesis has not been detected either.

Evidence that the abnormal activity is caused by functional abnormalities in the facial motonucleus has been presented in studies in patients with HFS undergoing microvascular decompression (MVD) operations [284, 297, 298] . This means that these microvascular compression disorders are not peripheral nerve disorders, but disorders of functions of the central nervous system caused by activation of neuroplasticity (see Appendix A).

We know more about neuralgias from studies of trigeminal neuralgia than from any other neuralgia [128, 388]. Trigeminal neuralgia has been regarded as one of the most excruciating pains and before effective treatment was available, it was a cause of suicide. Glossopharyngeal and intermedius (geniculate) neuralgias have similar characteristics.

Other forms of face pain include atypical face pain, which is characterized by constant burning pain [145] and anesthesia dolorosa which is a burning pain with numbness. Anesthesia dolorosa is very rare and has been described as a sequel to surgical operations where the central portion of the trigeminal nerve has been injured [325, 425]. It is assumed to be caused by deprivation of input through large diameter nerve fibers to pain circuits in the brain [254].

In this book, we discuss neuralgias in Section II on physiological pain. There are, however, pain receptors in peripheral nerves that may cause physiological pain under some circumstances when mechanically or chemically stimulated.

# Painful neuropathies

Painful neuropathies are diseases where disorders of a peripheral or cranial nerve cause pain (Figure 5.1). Viral infection and trauma of various kinds are the common causes of painful neuropathies. Demyelination usually does not give pain.

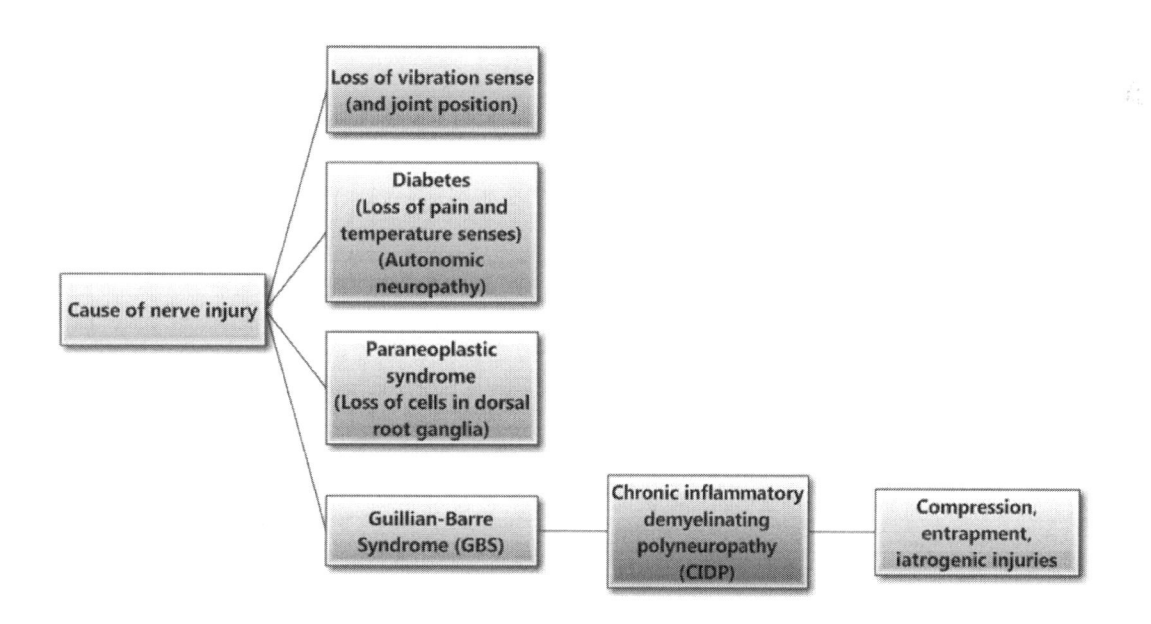

Figure 5.1. Causes of nerve injuries. (Artwork by Monica Javidnia).

Many studies have shown that nerve injury and axon degeneration can cause spontaneous discharges by axons proximal to the injury level [462]. When such nerve activity is interpreted in the same way as activity that is caused by stimulation of nociceptors, pain results, but it depends on which axons are affected. Injury induced activity in large, myelinated somatosensory fibers (A$\beta$ fibers) typically causes tingling or "pins and needles" sensations (paresthesia). Activating C-fibers is more likely to cause a burning sensation that is diffusely localized, while activating A$\delta$ fibers is more likely to cause stinging and well-localized pain. Mechanical stimulation of slightly injured nerves mostly affects larger myelinated nerve fibers.

The finding that the covering of peripheral nerves contains pain receptors (nervi nervorum) [421] may explain some forms of acute pain from mechanical stimulation of peripheral nerves. Whether or not the activation of the nociceptors in the sheaths of the nerve is regarded to be normal or pathological is a matter of opinion. Pain may also be caused when a nerve acts as a mechanoreceptor as it often does after injuries.

Many forms of peripheral neuropathies are associated with deficiencies of $B_1$ and $B_{12}$ vitamins. Administration of these two vitamins can often relieve pain in many forms of neuralgia, such as that caused by diabetes or alcohol and neuralgias associated with drugs used in cancer treatment such as Taxol (used in the treatment of breast cancers) and other cancer chemotherapy drugs [483]. Administration of B vitamins, especially vitamins $B_1$ and $B_{12}$, is specifically effective in the treatment of some forms of peripheral neuropathies such as painful diabetic neuropathy and alcohol-induced neuropathy.

As shown in Chapter 7, relief of the pain can often be achieved by administration of vitamin B supplements (in sufficient amounts).

# Mononeuropathies

Injuries to a single nerve can occur from trauma, including surgical manipulations. Trauma to cranial nerves can occur during various kinds of surgical operations. Tumors, strokes, and bleeding often cause injuries to more than one cranial nerve. Inflammation and vitamin deficiency are examples of other common causes of disorders of peripheral nerves and nerve roots that cause numbness, muscle weakness and pain, often in the form of burning, mostly in the peripheral regions of a nerve ("burning feet")

# Nerve compression

Mechanical compression of peripheral nerve affects nerves with axons of different diameter differently. Compression of nerves with axons of small diameter is little affected and healthy unmyelinated fibers are generally unaffected by mechanical compression. Mechanical compression such as from entrapment may change the ability of the respective nerve to conduct nerve impulses, which will affect the target nerve cells. A nerve may act as a mechanoreceptor when compressed generating nerve impulses (becomes an impulse generator). This may also occur from chemical stimulation [102].

Nerve compression may also affect the axonal transport (axoplasmatic flow). There are two kinds of transport, slow and fast. For a 1-meter long nerve the fast transport will take approximately 2.5 days from one end to the other, and the slow transport will take approximately 125 days [103].

Imaging studies often show that nerves are compressed, such as occurs in some forms of spinal stenosis that is common in elderly people. When such compression occurs in people with pain such as low back pain it is often regarded as being the cause of a person's pain. However, acute compression of a healthy mixed nerve mostly affects large diameter, myelinated nerve fibers while unmyelinated (C-fiber) nerve fibers are rather insensitive to compression. Most people have experienced the effect of nerve compression of their sciatic nerve when sitting on a seat with a hard edge or from crossing of the legs. The effects are tingling and numbness, which are assumed to be caused by interruption of the axoplasmatic flow in the large, myelinated axons and ischemia [220].

Recall from Chapter 3 that compression of a mixed nerve mainly affects large diameter myelinated nerve fibers causing numbness, tingling and muscle weakness rather than pain because unmyelinated fibers are unaffected. This is different when a nerve is inflamed or injured. C-fibers and small myelinated fibers of inflamed or injured nerves often become sensitive to stretching or compression. Axons of an injured nerve can become sensitive to deformation similar to what occurs normally in mechanoreceptors in the skin, joints, and tendons.

The compression of nerves as is evident from imaging studies of for example individuals with lower back pain is more to be regarded as a coincidence. There is evidence that injured nerves or inflamed nerve and nerve roots are sensitive to compression causing pain[146, 236, 420]. Anti-inflammatory drugs such as ibuprofen can often cure inflammation and injured nerves from trauma often heal by time without any treatment.

Clinically, mechanical sensitivity of peripheral nerves is known as the Tinel sign, which is a sensation of tingling or of "pins and needles" that is felt when a nerve is tapped. It is taken as an indication that the nerve in question is inflamed or injured or that it is in the process of regenerating after being injured.

The reason that a peripheral nerve becomes sensitive to mechanical stimulation is that the membrane of the axon has been changed so that it becomes sensitive to deformation; thus, similar to that of the common mechanoreceptors in the skin, joints, tendons, and muscles. Injured nerves may become impulse generators and, thereby, generate nerve impulses without any outside stimulation. Such nerve impulses are interpreted as pain signals by the brain.

Low back pain is often regarded to be caused by ruptured or herniated vertebral discs or by compression of nerve roots in people with spinal stenosis. While disc herniation (DH) may cause acute pain (such as in sciatica), it is usually not the cause of the aching pain that characterizes common low back pain, as indicated by the fact that many people have similar compressions of nerve roots, but no pain [168]. This means that root compression alone cannot cause pain, but another factor must also be present and this other factor (or factors) has (have) no verifiable signs. One of such two factors that must be present may be injury or inflammation of the nerve and compression of the nerve in order to cause pain. This is likely what causes the pain in such common disorders as lower back pain and in the carpal tunnel syndrome. This means that low back pain is an example of pain where two factors must be present at the same time to produce the symptoms (pain).

Many forms of pain that are referred to the extremities often occur coincident with different forms of compression of spinal nerves or nerve roots [239, 407] , but the causal relationship is not obvious [407]. On the contrary, it has been shown that similar nerve root structural changes occur in individuals who do not have pain [168]. Studies have shown that many people have similar compression without having any symptoms, including pain [168, 471] . Other studies found both false positive and false negative MRI findings in individuals with cervical radiculopathy (disorders of nerve roots) [221].

Compression of spinal roots has been regarded as the cause of low back pain because of the often-impressive abnormalities that are seen in MRI and other imaging studies. However, the causal relationship between the structural abnormalities and the symptoms are often lacking [471]. Nerve compression as seen on MRI occurs frequently in individuals who do not have pain [168, 239, 407, 471] . That the root compression seen on MRI is not a cause of many forms of back pain is supported by the poor results of surgical treatment that relieves the compression.

The fact that many forms of the common low back pain can be treated successfully anti-inflammatory drugs such as NSAIDs supports the hypothesis that inflammation of nerves or nerve roots plays an important role.

The pathology of chronic back pain is complex and poorly understood. The way it starts is not known. There are indications from different studies that inflammatory processes plays a role in the early stage of low back pain but there is less evidence that it plays a significant role in chronic low back pain. It is however, known that peripheral and cranial nerves may become sensitive to compression or stretching by activation of receptors in the nerve sheaths. Some of the acute pain from mechanical stimulation of nerves or nerve roots may be explained by the finding that nerves have pain receptors (nociceptors) in the nerve sheaths [421].

Evidence have been presented that inflammatory mediators such as phospholipase A2, prostaglandin E2, leukotriene, nitric oxide, immunoglobulin, pro-inflammatory cytokines such as interleukin (IL)-1α, IL-1β, IL-6, and tumor necrosis factor alpha (TNF-α) may be involved in creating some forms of low back pain[146]. These investigators also found evidence that autoimmune reaction mediated by macrophages expressing IL-1β, intercellular adhesion molecules played a role in creating pain in connection with disk herniation. They presented the hypothesis that the leakage of these substances could excite nociceptors or cause neural injury or inflammation and enhance sensitization to other pain-producing substances (such as bradykinin) and that that could lead to the nerve root pain. The role of these inflammatory mediators in the pathophysiology of lumbar radiculopathy has not been proven.

There may be several reasons that vertebral disk herniation is often present in persons with low back pain can cause pain. There is evidence that unmyelinated (pain) fibers may grow into damaged vertebral disks. A recent study [236] has shown that low pH favor such ingrowth. These investigators suggested that low pH may promote the production of the inflammatory mediators in a damaged intervertebral disk and that together with depletion of proteoglycan may cause an inflammatory response in the dorsal root ganglia, which changes the balance between molecules in the ganglia. These investigators suggested that such as sequence of events could result in the establishment of a vicious cycle that would lead to forms of chronic back pain.

A form of low back pain, known as sciatica is a shooting pain that is probably caused by an acute insult or injury to one or more spinal nerves. This form of pain is usually short lasting and resolves naturally through rest and pain medication. After some time of pain from such causes functional changes in the central nervous system may occur causing pathological pain (see Chapter 8).

Pain that is mediated by C-fibers is of another form, more like a burning and aching sensation, and that is not what is experienced in acute mechanical compression of (mixed) peripheral nerves. There are many reasons why surgical decompression of nerves and nerve roots has poor results[420]. All forms of surgery sever peripheral nerves in the skin and in other tissue that are cut. Severed nerve fibers sprout and these sprouts are mechanosensitive, causing pain from manipulations of the wound even after complete healing. Even without manipulations, sprouts often cause pain. This is one of the reasons that any kind of surgical operations are followed by pain that can last for months, thus yet another reason to act conservatively regarding choosing surgical treatment of low back pain.

The general lack of objective signs of back pain has suggested that the pain in some cases has psychiatric causes [239], a not uncommon conclusion when detectable abnormalities are absent. The innervation of the nerve sheet may play a role in pain caused by mechanical compression of nerve roots. Mechanical irritation (compression) of peripheral and cranial nerves can cause pain by stimulating nociceptors in the nervi nervorum [44].

The structures surrounding peripheral nerves (*nervi nervorum*) [44], which are small nerve filaments that innervate the sheath of a nerve. In fact, these structures were described more than 100 years ago (1884) by the neurosurgeon Sir Victor Horsley, but not recognized until much later [421]. These filaments of nerves may serve as receptors for mechanical stimulation of nerves. Thus, this is a sign that specific nociceptors can be directly involved in causing the pain that is experienced from mechanical compression of peripheral nerves or their roots.

Carpal tunnel syndrome is the second most common industrial injury in the U.S.A. [407]. It is believed to be caused by entrapment of the median nerve or pressure on the nerve [255, 407]. However, the pain (and tingling) is often treated surgically by decompressing the nerve in question, but the symptoms can be relieved by many other forms of treatment that do not relieve any nerve compression such as splinting, cortisone injections, massage, and immersion of the hand in water. The pain from carpal tunnel syndrome sometimes worsens with psychosocial factors such as boredom, stress, job dissatisfaction, monotonous routines, and insecurity; this all points to a central cause of at least some forms of carpal tunnel syndrome. It is unlikely that the pain in the carpal tunnel symptoms is caused by compression of a normal nerve, it is much more likely that the nerves in question are inflamed or injured in one way or another. It is also possible that the pain is caused by changes in the function of the central nervous system (central pain) (see Chapter 8).

Ulnar nerve entrapment has similar symptoms as carpal tunnel syndrome. It is the second most common entrapment neuropathy [255, 407] causing numbness and tingling in the distribution on the hand of the ulnar nerve (the fifth digit and the lateral aspect of the fourth). Similar symptoms occur from other peripheral nerves such as the sciatic and common peroneal nerves [255].

The hyperexcitability that often occurs in connection with low back pain is likely to be the cause of the often-observed muscle contractions (spasms) in individuals with low back pain. This can contribute to the pain because these muscle contractions are usually tonic. This also makes the muscle contractions difficult to be observed. The finding supports that muscle contractions contribute to the experienced pain that back pain is often reduced by administration of benzodiazepines such as Valium.

# Polyneuropathies

Polyneuropathies involve more than one peripheral nerve. Neurologists distinguish between axonal polyneuropathies (mainly as loss of axons or damage to axons) and demyelinating polyneuropathies (primarily pathology loss of myelin). Metabolic diseases, such as diabetic neuropathy, are the most common causes of axonal polyneuropathies and the incidence is increasing. Available data show prevalence of pain from 10 percent to 20 percent in individuals with diabetes and from 40 percent to 50 percent in people who have diabetic neuropathy [453].

There is evidence that hyperglycemia-induced pathways cause nerve damage and dysfunction leading to hyperexcitable peripheral and central pathways of pain.

Alcohol, diabetes, solvents, heavy metals, and many drugs, including chemotherapeutic agents such as Taxol, vincristine and cis-platinum, can also cause polyneuropathy. Vitamin $B_1$ and $B_{12}$ deficiency can lead to autoimmune processes such as lupus. The pain is regarded to be caused by peripheral and central sensitization.

A better understanding of the peripheral and central mechanisms resulting in the symptoms caused by neuralgias could promote the development of more targeted and effective treatments. Also, better awareness of the role of vitamin deficiency could promote the use of vitamin supplements, which often provides better results than sophisticated medication, without side effects.

Typically, the pain is bilateral and burning in nature, and affects mainly sensory nerve fibers of small diameters (Aδ and C-fibers). Distal fibers are often affected first and more severely than proximal fibers. Pain first occurs in the feet in many of these disorders. This can be explained by the fact that distal portions of peripheral nerves have a longer way to their supply of nutrients and that the axon diameter decreases with the distance to their cell body. Common diagnostic methods, such as electromyography (EMG) and nerve conduction studies, are not sensitive to injuries to the small fibers conducting pain impulses and which are involved in the burning pain that is often the actual kind of pain.

Inflammation of nerves or nerve root infections by strains of the herpes virus can cause pain that is felt in the radiation of single or multiple nerves (shingles, Ramsay-Hunt syndrome, etc.). Infection by the chickenpox virus (varicella zoster virus, VZV) can cause severe pain (shingles) in the areas of the skin that are innervated by spinal nerves (dermatomes).

Polyneuropathy is likely to involve activation of neuroplasticity and, over time, cause pathological pain (central neuropathic pain) that often persists long after healing of the initial pathology. When physiological pain has persisted over a long period of time, a component of central neuropathic pain often occurs as an addition to the physiological pain that is caused by stimulation of nociceptors.

Activation of neuroplasticity may occur over time as a sequel to acute somatic pain and it often persists long after healing of the initial pathology. Deafferentation pain and phantom limb pain are other examples of pathological pain (central neuropathic pain, see Chapter 8) that may be associated with pathologies of peripheral nerves. A component of central neuropathic pain that has persisted over a long period of time is often caused by stimulation of nociceptors.

Pain is rare in demyelinating neuropathies, such as the Guillain-Barré syndrome, because of the sparing of the unmyelinated C-fibers that are important for pain.

# Neuritis (inflammation of nerves)

Inflammation from various causes may affect a single nerve (mononeuritis) or several nerves may be affected. Inflammation may affect a nerve (or nerves) at different locations. Inflammation of blood vessels (vasculitis) may also affect the function of nerves.

# Viral infections

There are several viruses that can cause pain from infecting peripheral nerves. Members of the herpes virus family are the best-known causes of virus infections that cause pain from peripheral nerves. Viral infections may also affect single or multiple cranial nerves. Nerves may recover their function after the inflammation has resolved or the inflammatory processes may have caused permanent damage that leaves a nerve without function or with a changed function. Like other disorders of peripheral nerves, neuritis may also activate neuroplasticity and cause central pain.

# Herpes virus

The herpes zoster (HZ) or varicella zoster virus (VZV) has been associated with many forms of mononeuralgies. The virus lives in the ganglia of sensory nerves for a long time without producing any symptoms. Occasionally, it may travel outside the ganglia and cause pain and eruption of vesicles on the skin over some part of one, or more than one, dermatome (shingles). It is the same virus that causes chicken pox.

The herpes zoster virus can involve the seventh and eighth cranial nerves in a similar way as shingles and is known as the Ramsay-Hunt syndrome. This syndrome causes a painful rash and blisters around the ear and in the ear canal. It may also cause facial weakness and hearing loss.

Herpes simplex is the cause of painful blisters and sores most common to occur around the mouth, nose, and genitals.

# Shingles

The herpes zoster virus causes shingles in adults. Schmader et al, 2008 [380], showed that herpes zoster affects millions of people worldwide, particularly older adults. This virus, the chickenpox virus, is dormant in many people, but can become activated causing significant suffering by causing acute and chronic pain, known as post-herpetic neuralgia.

The pain is severe and may persist for a long time. The frequency of shingles increases with age. The incidence and severity of herpes zoster (HZ) and post-herpetic neuralgia (PHN) increase with age [380]. The lifetime risk of shingles is estimated to be 20-30 percent with the risk increasing rapidly with age and is estimated to be approximately 50 percent for people of 85 years of age. There is now a vaccination available that can decrease the risk of getting shingles by a factor of 2.

Between the age of 20 and 50, it occurs at a rate of 2.5 per 1,000 per year; the rate doubles between the age of 50 and 60 (to 5 per 1,000 per year). It then doubles again between the age of 80 and 90 (10 per 1,000 per year).

# Trauma to peripheral nerves

Surgical operations are probably the most frequent cause of trauma to nerves. Essentially, all operations cause severance of small nerves and larger branches may inadvertently be severed. Severed nerves cause sprouting of axons and these sprouts are pain sensitive and likely to cause pain without any known stimulation.

It has also been suggested that trauma to the spine (such as almost always occurs in operations for decompression of spinal nerves) may cause the outgrowth of unmyelinated thin filaments of nerves that are pain sensitive and which may cause pain without any known stimulation[49]. Surgical operations, such as those aimed at correcting spinal stenosis, traumatize bone and cause an outgrowth of unmyelinated, pain sensitive, thin nerve fibers. This may explain why pain can be worse after operations to correct what was thought of as the cause of a person's pain. Outgrowths of pain sensitive nerves occur in other operations and may explain why most people have pain after any form of surgical operation.

Even without any mechanical compression, degenerative vertebral discs may also have an outgrowth of unmyelinated nerve fibers that can cause pain [49].

# Formation of neuromas

Sprouting of axons and the formation of neuromas may occur whenever a peripheral nerve is severed or seriously injured. Neuromas are pain sensitive and may cause pain without any stimulation. Experimental studies have found that sprouts of axons can cause spontaneous discharges in nerve fibers proximal to the injury level [462]. Again, such abnormal neural activity is interpreted in the same way as activity that is caused by stimulation of nociceptors and thereby, causes pain.

Some forms of pain from mechanical stimulation of peripheral nerves may be explained by stimulation of the pain receptors in the nerve sheets (nervi nervorum) [421].

# How do nerves cause pain?

We have shown above that many of the seemingly clear causes of pain are questionable for several reasons. Compression of nerves is easy to detect, but many studies have shown that it does not cause the common aching pain that is associated with nerve compression.

Viral infections that affect the function of nerves are not easily observable, but it is a convenient explanation that is difficult to disprove. Thus, it seems odd that viral infections often only affect one nerve such as, for instance, the facial nerve on one side of the body as occurs in trigeminal neuralgia. Only one or a few spinal nerves are affected in shingles, which causes pain in only one or a few dermatomes.

Compressions of peripheral and cranial nerves are easily observable on commonly used imaging techniques, but these techniques do not show how different kinds of nerve fibers are affected and do not show the effect on the function of the nerves. Imaging signs of nerve or nerve root compression are often taken as indications for surgical treatment of low back pain, despite the fact that asymptomatic individuals have similar or identical signs and the well documented fact that surgical treatment rarely is beneficial, but often causes other, and lasting, pain and symptoms.

These are just examples that established knowledge is not true and may cause incorrect diagnosis and incorrect treatment to no benefit for the patients, occasionally causing serious side effects.

It is appropriate perhaps to cite Mark Twain (Samuel Clemens):

*"It ain't what you don't know that gets you into trouble. It's what you know for sure that just ain't so."*

# Slightly injured nerves

Slightly injured nerves are nerves that function, but do so differently from normal nerves. Any injury, be it stretching or compression, can cause the conduction velocity to decrease and, typically, the changes are different for the different nerve fibers of a peripheral or a cranial nerve.

There are always small differences in the conduction velocity of nerves and that causes the neural activity to arrive at the target neuron more or less temporally dispersed.

Slight injuries affect different nerve fibers differently and cause this temporal dispersion to increase. The effect of this may be a change in the way neural activity in a nerve excites the target neurons. Assuming that there is a certain degree of convergence at the target nerve cell, increased dispersion causes a decrease in the amplitude and a broadening of the resulting excitatory postsynaptic potential (EPSP) in the target neurons (Figure 5.2).

A decrease in amplitude of the EPSP decreases the ability of neural activity in the nerve to activate (fire) the target neuron. However, if the membrane potential is sufficiently low, it may still cause the target neuron to fire.

In such a situation, the increased dispersion may not have any effect, or the broadening may make it possible for the target neuron to fire twice because the EPSP, in response to a transient stimulus, may exceed the refractory period of the target neuron. This means that increased spatial dispersion causing temporal dispersion of the activity that arrives at a neuron may not influence the firing of the neuron, may prevent the neuron from firing, or it may increase the firing of the neuron.

Thus, slight injuries to a nerve may have three very different effects on the neural activity in the target neuron as illustrated in Figure 5.2.

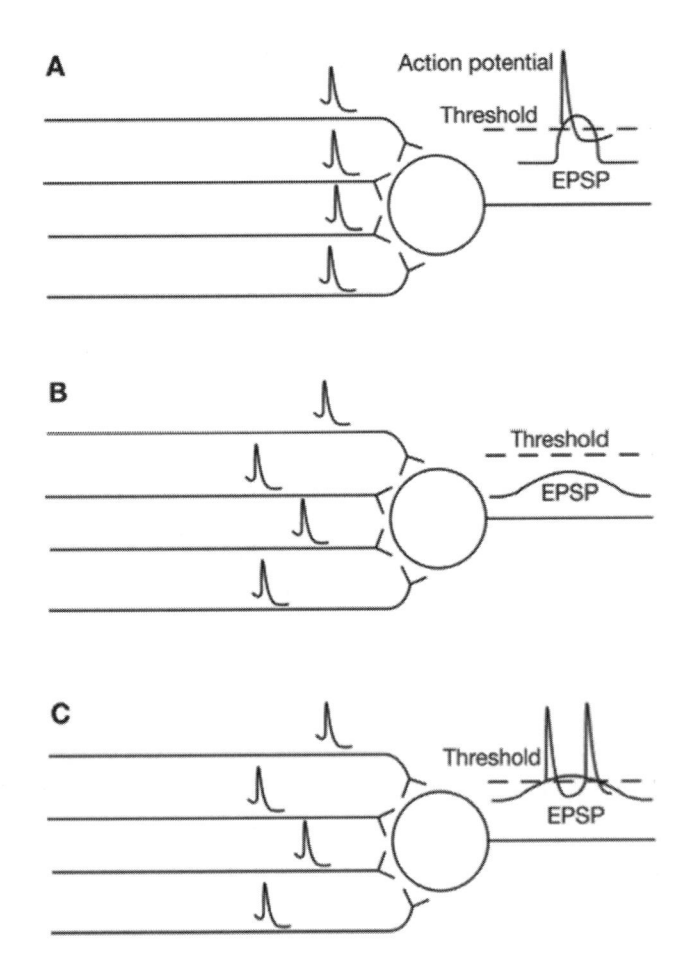

Figure 5.2 Hypothetical illustration of the effect of spatial integration by a cell on which many axons converge.
A: Little spatial dispersion
B: Increased spatial dispersion, but the high threshold of the neuron prevents it from firing.
C. Large degree of spatial dispersion and low threshold of the neuron. The prolonged EPSP makes the neuron fire twice. (From Møller, A.R., Neuroplasticity and disorders of the nervous system. 2006, Cambridge: Cambridge University Press [288], Adapted from [82] Reprinted with permission from Cambridge University Press.)

Injury to axons of a peripheral nerve may make them fire without stimulation. This means that they will act as impulse generators and their activity may be interpreted in the central nervous system in the same way as (normal) stimulation would do. This may be one way that an injury to a nerve can cause pain.

Thus, increased temporal dispersion of neural activity in a nerve can:
- Increase the duration of firing of the target neuron
- Prevent activation of the target cell
- Make it possible to activate neurons that are not normally activated.
- Degrade temporal information, which may be important in sensory systems such as in hearing.

Temporal and spatial dispersion also degrades temporal information, an effect that may have little importance in connection with pain.

More severe injuries to a nerve can also cause changes in the way the axons fire in response to stimulation or it may cause axons to fire without any stimulation. Such abnormal firing may include firing in bursts. Burst firing, instead of the normal continuous firing, can increase an axon's ability to excite its target neuron as illustrated in Figure 5.3. This means that burst activity may be able to activate neurons that are normally dormant and may re-route neural activity. Re-routing of neural activity plays a role in causing phenomena such as allodynia and burst firing that may result from injuries to peripheral nerves may, therefore, be a cause of abnormal functioning of structures in the central nervous system.

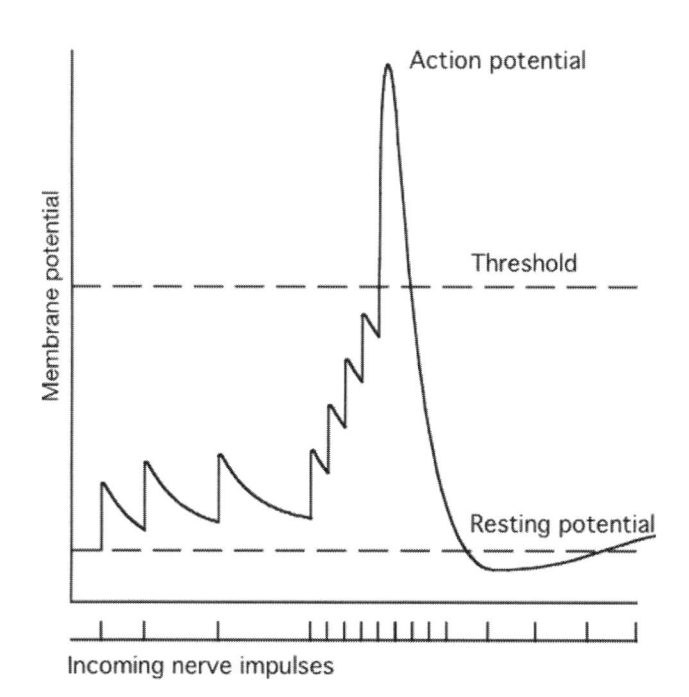

Figure 5.3 Hypothetical description of the effect of burst activity on the excitation of a cell. (From Møller, A.R., Neuroplasticity and disorders of the nervous system. 2006, Cambridge: Cambridge University Press [288], Adapted from [82] Reprinted with permission from Cambridge University Press).

Other forms of malfunction of peripheral nerves include the effect of demyelination. Much emphasis has been placed on the possibility of ephaptic transmission between demyelinated (denuded) axons, known as ephaptic transmission (direct transfer of impulse activity from one axon to another). While this phenomenon may indeed exist, it is much more rare than often given the impression of from the presentation of hypotheses of various effects of demyelination. Demyelinating diseases, such as multiple sclerosis, do not seem to be associated with pain. Demyelination is, therefore, not of interest in connection with pain.

With regard to pain, these abnormalities in the function of peripheral nerves may have their greatest importance in that they can induce plastic changes in the function of structures in the central nervous system that can cause pathological pain and, in addition, hyperpathia and allodynia.

# CHAPTER 6
# Modulation of Physiological Pain

## Abstract

1. The activity in neural circuits that are involved in pain can be modulated at many levels of the nervous system, including the receptors.

2. Peripheral sensitization may occur because sympathetic nerve fibers located close to pain receptors can modulate the receptors' sensitivity by liberating norepinephrine.

3. Since pain increases the activity of the sympathetic nervous system, causing an increase in the liberation of norepinephrine, a vicious circle can be created.

4. If the sensitivity of the receptors is increased enough, pain signals may be sent without external stimulations, thus causing constant pain.

5. Inflammatory processes may produce substances, such as prostaglandin $E_2$, which also can increase the sensitivity of pain receptors.

6. Trauma of various kinds may cause the release of chemicals, such as bradykinin, histamine, serotonin, cytokines, and excitatory amino acids, which can increase the sensitivity of pain receptors.

7. Injuries may cause the development of primary and secondary mechanical hyperalgesia.

8. Administration of pain medication of various kinds can modulate (decrease) pain by affecting neural transmission at different levels of the pain pathways.

9. Modulation of pain may occur in the dorsal horn of the spinal cord where $A\beta$ fibers can influence cells in lamina I and II that are the targets of pain fibers in peripheral nerves.

10. Circulating adrenalin in the blood increases pain by affecting pain transmission in the spinal cord and the (caudal) trigeminal nucleus.

11. Endogenous opioids can affect neural transmission and different levels of the pain pathways.

12. C-fibers can secrete chemicals that can increase the firing of cells in the spinothalamic pathways.

13. Mental activities, such as attention and distraction, can both increase and decrease pain sensations.

# Introduction

Pain can be modulated by affecting the sensitivity of pain receptors and by controlling neural transmission in the ascending pain pathways before reaching the part(s) of the brain where awareness of pain is achieved. Pain from stimulation of pain receptors can be affected by sensitization of pain receptors (peripheral sensitization) or neural circuits in the spinal cord and the brain can be sensitized or de-sensitized. Liberation of endogenous opioids in the central nervous system is another factor that can modulate pain sensations. Modulation of pain, peripherally and centrally, is the basis for most forms of treatment of pain. Understanding sensitization is important for understanding the mechanisms and causes of pain. Understanding de-sensitization is important for the treatment and management of pain (discussed in Chapter 7).

# Basis for modulation of physiological pain

Neural transmission and processing of pain signals elicited by stimulation of pain receptors can be modulated in the dorsal horn and in the caudal trigeminal nucleus by signals from receptors in the skin that respond to innocuous stimulations mediated by large diameter peripheral nerve fibers (Aβ).

Pain processing in the spinal cord and in the trigeminal nucleus can be modulated by neural activity generated in the brain. Pain can be modulated by external (artificial) factors such as medications. Electrical stimulation of the skin (transdermal electrical nerve stimulation, TENS) is a commonly used method for the treatment of pain. Other examples of induced modulation of pain signals include electrical stimulation of the dorsal column of the spinal cord, the somatosensory cortex, and the premotor cerebral cortex.

Now, the most obvious way to affect pain is by administration of medications, such as the common analgesics including aspirin, various kinds of non-steroid anti-inflammatory drugs (NSAID), morphine, and different kinds of opioids including modern synthetic or semi-synthetic opioids.

These medications can control many forms of pain, but not all, and they all have various forms of side effects, some serious ones in the form of fatal damage to organs such as the liver and the kidneys. However, little is known about their exact actions on the spinal cord and the brain, perhaps with the exception of opioids.

Emotional factors, mood, and factors, such as distraction, can also modulate (increase or decrease) the strength of pain. The belief that a certain treatment is beneficial can have a profound beneficial effect on symptoms such as pain (placebo effect). The placebo effect, where an inactive treatment can decrease the perception of pain, is a prime example of pain control from activity in regions of the brain that concern cognitive functions, such as expectation, and it is related to Pavlovian conditioning [30].

Hypnosis that induces an extreme state of relaxation can also reduce the perception of pain. It is especially used in the treatment of pathological pain, although sparsely (discussed in Chapter 12). Hypnosis is used in surgical operations, mainly in non-Western countries such as China.

# Peripheral sensitization

Peripheral sensitization refers to the increased sensitivity of nociceptors. It is based on the fact that the sensitivity of nociceptors is not fixed, but internal, and external factors of various kinds can affect the strength of the pain.

One major source of sensitization of receptors is the secretion of noradrenalin that occurs from sympathetic nerve fibers; thus, a reaction to the activation of the sympathetic nervous system. Such an increase in the sensitivity of pain receptors causes stronger activation of pain circuits when pain receptors are stimulated. Increased pain causes increased activity in the sympathetic nervous system.

This causes more norepinephrine to be secreted near pain receptors which causes a further increase in sensitivity and more activation of pain circuits in the central nervous system. This means that sympathetic induced sensitization of pain receptors can start a vicious circle.

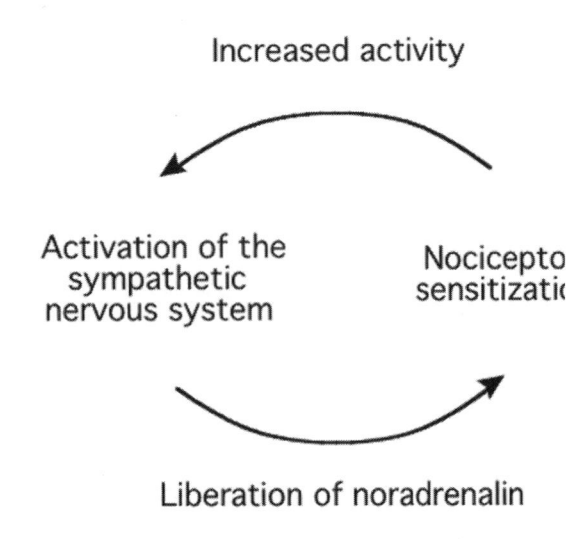

Figure 6.1 Vicious circle from activation of the sympathetic nervous system that increases the sensitivity of pain receptors. (Artwork by Monica Javidnia.)

This is an example of the few biological systems that are controlled by positive feedback. Positive feedback causes instability of systems, in this case, of the pain circuits in the nervous system. (Most biologic systems have negative feedback that promotes stability.) At some point in this process, pain stimulation is no longer necessary for keeping this vicious circle active and pain is caused even without any pain stimulation.

Trauma can initiate processes that result in a vicious circle involving the sympathetic nervous system. As shown in Figure 6.2, trauma to the skin or other structures that have pain receptors can activate these pain receptors. This activates the sympathetic nervous system causing liberation of noradrenaline near the receptors (A), increasing their sensitivity in such a way that they can be activated by light touch (B).

The pain further increases the activation of the sympathetic nervous system, which may reach a level where the pain receptors become active without any stimulation (C). This means that the vicious circle is now closed (Figure 6.1) and the pain is permanent without any external stimulation.

# The role of the sympathetic nervous system in modulation receptor sensitivity

As has been shown above, secretion of noradrenalin near pain receptors increases their sensitivity. The sympathetic nervous system can also affect neural processing of pain in the spinal cord and the brain. Sympathetic afferent fibers that enter the dorsal horn of the spinal cord can modulate neural transmission in pain circuits of the dorsal horn. Sprouting sympathetic nerve fibers that project to the dorsal root ganglia may also be involved in causing sympathetically maintained pain (see Chapter 11).

# The role of inflammation

Inflammatory processes can sensitize the pain system and cause hyperalgesia. Thus, the secretion of prostaglandins ($E_2$) near the receptors can sensitize the receptors which may occur as the result of an injury or inflammatory process [56].

Prostaglandin $E_2$ provides sensitization of dorsal horn cells causing inhibition of glycinergic transmission in cells in lamina I and II of the dorsal horn. This causes an enhanced transmission of pain signals from receptors; thus, strengthening the pain that is elicited by the stimulation of pain receptors. Prostaglandins can be blocked by aspirin, indomethacin, and the common non-steroidal anti-inflammatory drugs (NSAID) that can inhibit the enzymes cyclooxygenase 1 and 2 (COX-1 and COX-2).

This cannot explain all of the pain relieving effects; it is only one of the several pain relieving effects of these drugs. The other effects of these drugs on pain are complex and poorly understood. These drugs can probably influence pain circuits in the spinal cord and brain as well.

# Neural transmitters involved in peripheral sensitization

Chemicals released through an injury, such as bradykinin, histamine, serotonin, several cytokines, and excitatory amino acids (EAA) , are some of the best-known examples of substances that cause sensitization of cells in the pain pathways.

However, increased acidity (proton, $H^+$) can also cause sensitization. Activation of vanilloid receptors (TRPV1) by, for instance, capsaicin is also a powerful sensitizer of pain systems. Wallerian degeneration of nerves, such as the distal portion of peripheral nerves, can cause hyperalgesia (increased sensitivity to pain, thus a leftward shift of stimulus response curves) through the secretion of products from the breakdown of nerves [274].

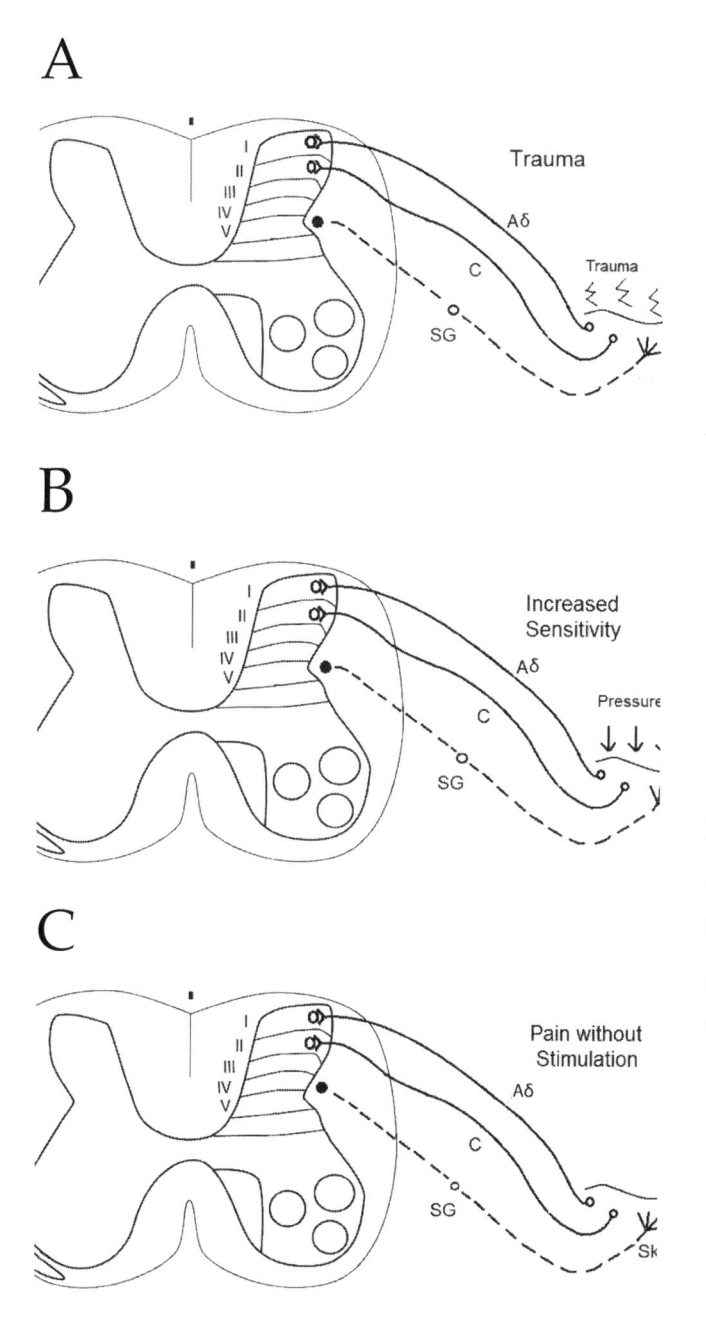

Figure 6.2 Illustrations of how trauma can start a vicious circle of sympathetic maintained pain.

A: Trauma causes activation of C-fibers producing pain.

B: After some time of pain activation, stimulation of receptors that are innervated by Aδ fibers can produce pain sensations (allodynia).

C: After more time, the sympathetic nervous system becomes activated and sympathetic C-fibers secrete noradrenalin near pain receptors causing pain without any stimulation. (Artwork by Irene Cunha.)

Many neural transmitters can modulate the neural activity in nerve cells in pain pathways (Figure 6.3).

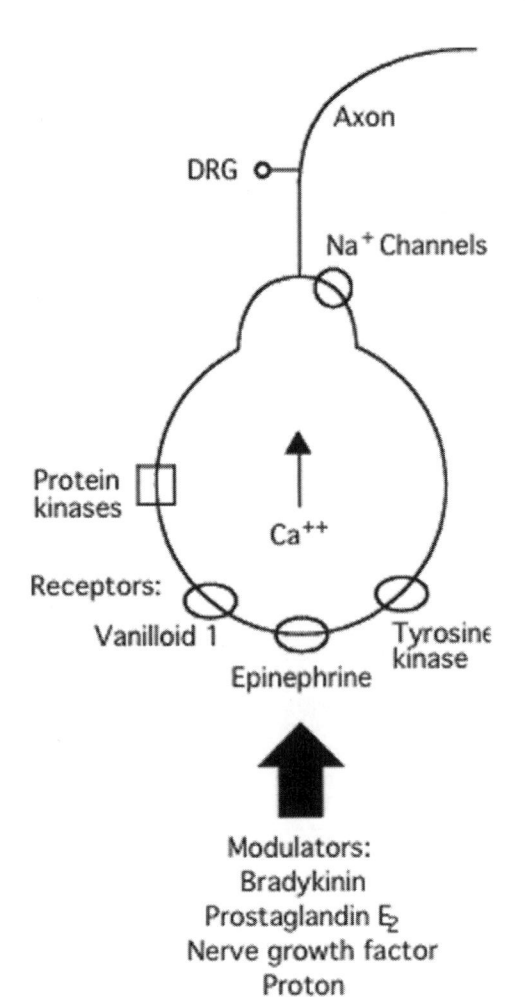

Figure 6.3 Molecular bases for peripheral sensitization. (Modified from Møller, A.R., Neuroplasticity and disorders of the nervous system. 2006, Cambridge: Cambridge University Press [288]. Based on Bolay, H. and M.A. Moskowitz, Mechanisms of pain modulation in chronic syndromes. Neurology, 2002. 59(5 Suppl. 2): p. S 2-7.) [39]. (Artwork by Irene Cunha.)

# Development of mechanical hyperalgesia after injury

A change in the sensitivity to mechanical stimulation (mechanical hyperalgesia) is present at the site of the skin that is burned (primary hyperalgesia) (Figure 6.4). Pain thresholds in adjacent uninjured skin areas are also lowered after burns (secondary hyperalgesia). Primary hyperalgesia is caused by inflammatory processes, thus involving the immune system [249]. The change in the function of receptors is induced by the platelet-activating factor (PAF).

Secondary hyperalgesia is caused by a descending influence from the brain; it is a protective mechanism that discourages from manipulating a region adjacent to an injured region. Thus, secondary hyperalgesia is a form of central sensitization.

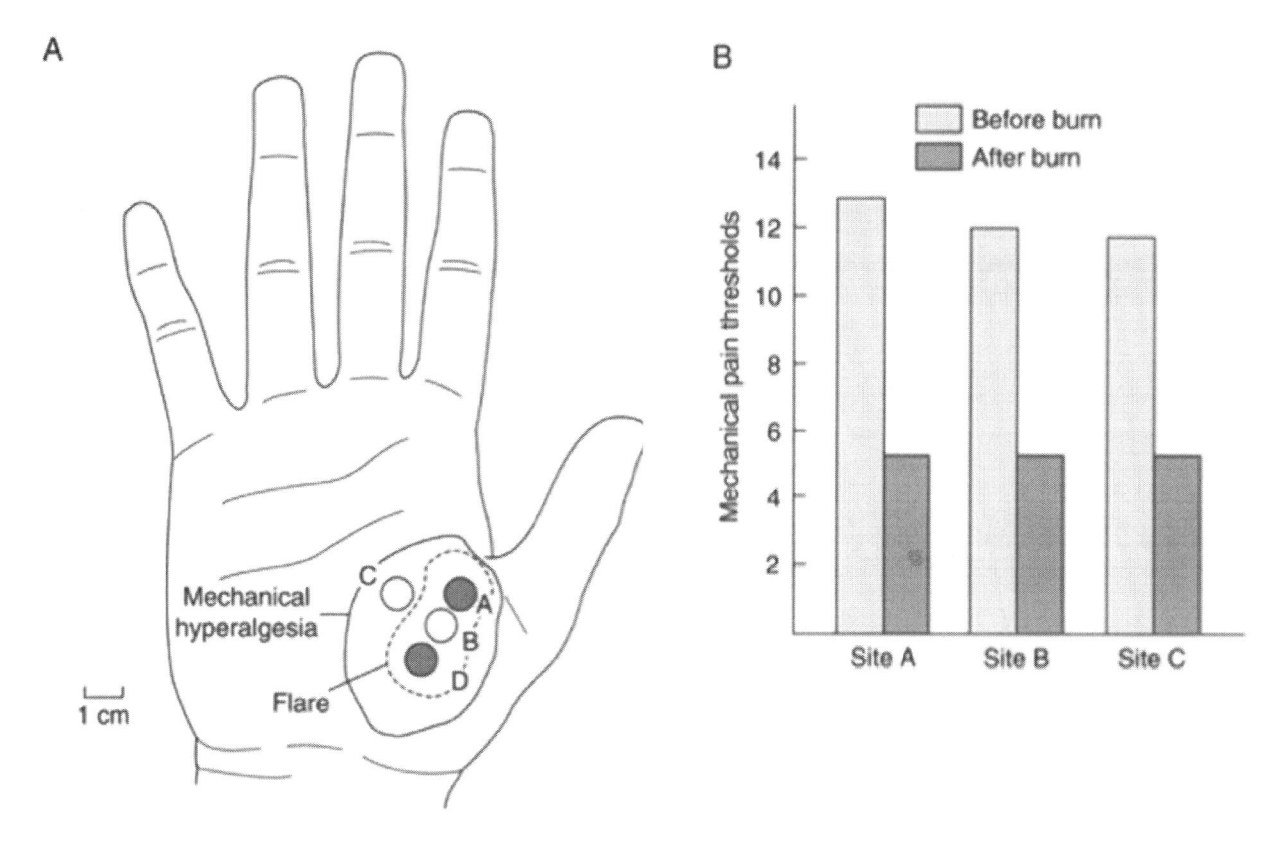

Figure 6.4 The effect of burns to skin (53 degree C for 30 sec) on hyperalgesia.
A: Mechanical hyperalgesia was recorded in sites A, B, and C.
B: Threshold to pain before and after burns at these three sites.
Based on Raja SN, Campbell JN and Meyer RA. Evidence for Different Mechanisms of Primary and Secondary Hyperalgesia Following Heat Injury to the Glabrous Skin. Brain 107: 1791-1188, 1984 [344]. (Artwork by Monica Javidnia.)

# The gate control hypothesis

The best known theory for peripheral control of pain is the gate control hypothesis published in 1965 by Wall and Melzack [264] (Figure 6.5). The hypothesis has undergone some changes since then, but the general principle is still valid. The hypothesis states that pain transmission in the spinal cord can be modulated by input from A$\beta$ fibers that innervate sensory receptors in the skin. The impulses that arrive from pain receptors activate cells in layers I and II of the dorsal horn and the excitability of these cells can be modulated by impulses from larger myelinated fibers (A$\beta$) through inhibitory interneurons that terminate on cells in layer II. The gate hypothesis has undergone some modifications since its publication in 1965 to take into account the descending influence on pain transmission in the spinal cord (see Chapter 8).

# The original gate hypothesis

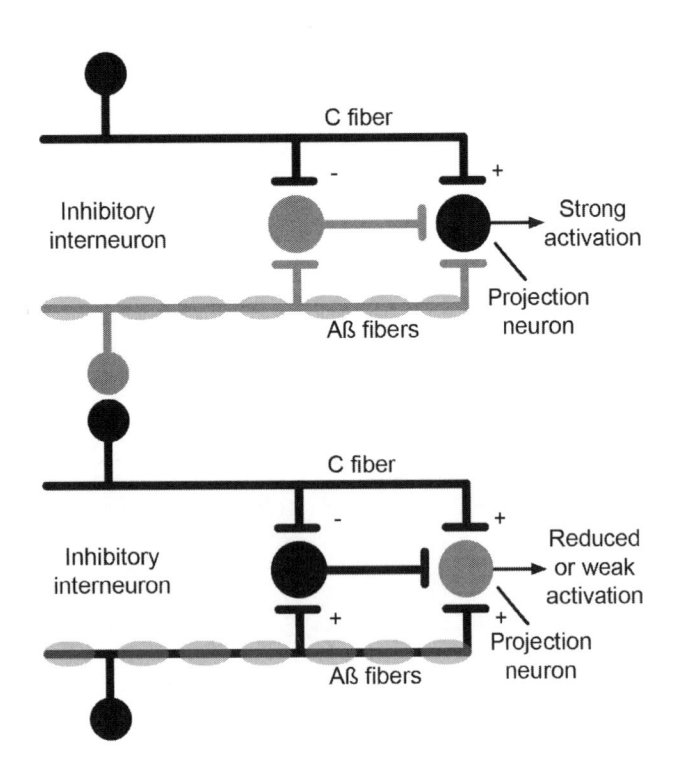

Figure 6.5 The original gate hypothesis. (Adapted from Melzack, R. and P.D. Wall, Pain mechanisms: A new theory. Science, 1965. 150: p. 971-979. [264]. (Art work by Monica Javidnia).

The original Melzack and Wall gating hypothesis as described in their 1965 paper [264] shows how pain impulses from pain receptors that arrive at the dorsal horn of the spinal cord in Aδ and C-fibers can be modified (decreased) by signals from larger (Aβ) nerve fibers before they reach the brain such as occurs normally through the spinothalamic tract (STT) (see Chapter 3,).

The hypothesis involves four different kinds of neurons: C-fibers, Aδ fibers, Aβ fibers, and nerve cells to which Aβ fibers project to through inhibitory interneurons. C-fibers terminate on neurons in lamina II and Aδ fibers terminate in lamina I of the dorsal horn. The cells in lamina I and II that receive input from pain receptors are conducted to cells in lamina V and these cells send axons to the brain in the STT. Large (Aβ) fibers connect to inhibitory interneurons in lamina II and, thereby, make it possible for Aβ fibers to inhibit pain impulses in neurons in lamina V before these are transmitted to the brain (in the STT). Further, C-fibers and Aδ fibers not only excite neurons in lamina V, but they also inhibit the inhibitory interneurons in lamina II, which are activated by Aβ fibers. This means that in addition to providing the normal excitation of STT fibers through neurons in lamina V, the C and Aδ fibers can also enhance this transmission; thus, opening a "gate" for noxious input to get to the brain.

It is believed that one of the beneficial effects of transdermal electrical nerve stimulation (TENS) on pain control is through mechanisms that can be explained by the Melzack-Wall gate control hypothesis as described in Chapter 7 (other effects of TENS are on the central nervous system, see Chapter 12).

# Endogenous opioids modulate acute pain

The neural basis for the action of opioids is not only important for the treatment of pain with opioids, but it is also important for normal functioning of the pain system because of the effect of endogenous opioids; thereby, providing a natural basis for the modulation of physiological pain.

Endogenous opioids (enkephalins and endorphins are morphine-like substances that are produced in the body) have an inhibitory influence on pain sensations. The endorphins and other opioids act on many parts of the nervous system in a similar way as the opioids that are administered for relieving pain.

The proof of the role of endogenous opioids in the normal modulation of pain is the observation that administration of an opioid receptor antagonist, Naloxone, causes increased pain (because the drug blocks opioid receptors).

This would explain why some studies have shown that administration of Naloxone worsens pain, such as postoperative pain. However, other studies have shown that administration of Naloxone reduces pain. The truth seems to be that Naloxone in low dosages has a (weak) pain relieving effect and in high doses, it increases pain because it blocks opioid receptors that have been activated by endogenous opioids [232]. It has been hypothesized that endogenous opioids are involved in the placebo effect in pain [374].

There are several endogenous opioids and different ones have the greatest affinity to specific opioid receptors. β-Endorphin is released from the pituitary gland and other structures including immune cells. It activates mainly $\mu_1$ receptors and with a lower affinity to $\mu_2$ and δ opioid receptors. Met-encephalin activates mostly the δ opioid receptor and it is produced widely in the central nervous system (in the dorsal horn of the gray matter of the spinal cord, the central part of the thalamus, the amygdala of the limbic system, and in other parts of the brain). It activates μ and δ opioid receptors. Dynorphine acts on κ-opioid receptors and is widely distributed in the brain. Endomorphine acts on μ receptors.

# The role of the vagus nerve in control of pain

The effect of vagal activity on pain is poorly understood. It may be mediated through the NA-serotonin descending system [428] as well as the endocrine system from the adrenal medullae [182]. As mentioned above, adrenalin and norepinephrine modulate the sensitivity of pain receptors. Since vagal afferents from the small intestine have inhibitory influence on the central input to the pre-ganglionic neurons that innervate the adrenal medulla, they may control the level of adrenalin in the blood and thereby, affect processing of pain signals. The vagus nerve can influence visceral pain as discussed in Chapter 7.

# CHAPTER 7

# Treatment of Physiological Pain

## Abstract

1. When the cause of pain cannot be treated to eliminate the pain or when the cause cannot be found, the pain itself must be treated.

2. There are many forms of pain and the optimal treatment is different for the different forms.

3. When selecting a treatment, side effects must be taken into account.

4. Most forms of minor to moderate pain can be treated by over the counter medications such as non-steroidal anti-inflammatory drugs (NSAID) that include such common pain relievers as ibuprofen, naproxen, and paracetamol.

5. These drugs inhibit enzymes such as cyclooxygenase type 1 and 2 that convert arachidonic acid into prostaglandins.

6. Paracetamol has a different action and acts mostly through its metabolites, which influence descending serotoninergic pathways to release serotonin (5-HT), which inhibits the release of several mediators of pain.

7. Side effects of ibuprofen and naproxen are mainly related to increased risks of stomach bleeding. The risk is greater for naproxen than ibuprofen; the risk of bleeding increases with age and the risk depends on a person's diseases.

8. There was evidence that these side effects were related to the reduction of the COX-1 enzyme. COX-1 enzymes are involved in "house keeping functions" and selective COX-2 inhibitors were developed.

9. The selective COX-2 inhibitors, known as Coxibs, however, turned out to be disappointing because of their many side serious effects, such as increased risk of cardiovascular events. Most Coxibs had to be taken off the market.

10. Paracetamol has side effects that do not exist for other drugs. Most serious is it hepatotoxicity, which can cause liver failure; a very high risk of irreversible liver failure when 4,000 mg or more of paracetamol are administered in one day.

11. Opioids (drugs that binds to opioid receptors) are powerful pain relievers.

12. The natural substances, such as heroin and morphine, are highly addictive and cause strong withdrawal symptoms. These adverse effects are considerably reduced in the commonly available synthetic, Fentanyl, or semisynthetic opioids (oxycodone, oxymorphone, and hydromorphone).

13. Opioids act through the rostral ventromedial medulla (RVM) system.

14. There are several other opioid-like pain reliving drugs (such as Tapentadol).

15. Long-term use of opioids can result in tolerance, which means that more must be administered to obtain the same effect.

16. Opioids can cause sensitization to pain (hyperalgesia).

17. The placebo effect is large regarding pain.

18. Peripheral neuropathy which causes burning feet and more wide spread pain is often caused by a deficiency of vitamins, especially vitamins $B_1$ and $B_{12}$, and the pain can be effectively treated by administrating these vitamins. This form of treatment has no known side effects but is often overlooked.

# Introduction

Pain is an important sign of disease and attempts to treat physiological pain should not be done before it is determined that the pain is not a sign of a treatable disease. When that has been ruled out, treatment of the pain can be initiated. To be successful in treating physiological pain (receptor pain), the abnormality that causes the pain must be identified. Many forms of physiological pain have no detectable signs from standard clinical tests such as imaging, chemical tests, or electrophysiological tests. Many people have various kinds of abnormalities, which may occur coincidentally to pain. The task of diagnosing is then to evaluate the results of such tests and to determine which abnormalities are related to the patient's pain and which are not. It is also important to distinguish coincidence of signs that occur in individuals who report that they have pain (two signs just occurring at the same time) from causality (one sign causing the other).

Pain can be referred to the anatomical location on the body where the abnormality (pathology) that causes the pain is located, or pain can be referred to a different location (referred pain). Referred pain occurs in disorders of internal organs (visceral pain, see Chapter 4). Often, it is not possible to find anything wrong in any location of the body. Such pain is known as idiopathic (cause unknown) pain.

Treatment of physiological pain can be directed to the pain itself, not attempting to find or correct the pathology that causes the pain, or treatment can be directed at correcting the pathology, thus attempting to cure the pain.

As discussed earlier in this book, pain often has two different expressions; one being the perception of the pain and the other being the adverse (negative) effect of the pain. The latter is more important to aim at in treatment because that is what reduces a person's quality of life. Many medications, such as opioids, have that aspect of pain as their target, and they may not change the perception much. A patient who is being treated for pain may say "I still have my pain, but it does not bother me anymore". This must be regarded as an effective treatment although the patient still has pain.

Some forms of physiological pain cannot be totally resolved with available treatments, but the condition can often be improved. Often, pain cannot be eliminated, but reduced. It is often possible to manage the pain, which means reducing the adverse effects of the pain as much as possible and to restore the person's quality of life to the greatest extent (discussed in Chapter 3).

Such management of pain can make life better for many patients. People often are searching for treatments that can completely solve their problems instead of just improve their situation. People believe in medicine, and often have a blind trust in the pharmaceutical industry and hospitals, but pay little attention to how they select their physician or surgeon and how they administer their medication. People often underestimade how side effects will affect their lives, and physicians and surgeons are not too eager to discuss side effects.

The armamentarium available for the treatment of pain has increased dramatically during the past few decades, but many of the treatments that are in use for common pain, such as low back pain, are ineffective. This chapter will discuss physiological pain; treatment of pathological pain will be discussed in Chapter 12.

# Diagnosis of pain and its cause

An incorrect diagnosis is worse than no diagnosis because it can cause treatment that is of no benefit, but still has side effects and costs money. Incorrect diagnoses occur, for example, when coincidence of a sign, such as an anomaly that appears on a MRI, is assumed to be the cause of a patient's pain. Coincidence of morphological changes occurs in common pain disorders, such as low back pain, where compression of spinal nerve roots is often taken as a cause of an individual's pain while it often is an independent occurrence that does not cause the pain. (Compression of nerves and nerve roots affect different kinds of nerve fibers differently, mainly affecting large fibers and having little effect on small diameter fibers that communicate pain, see Chapter 3) This is an example of imaging results (MRI or CT scan) that show changes that are unrelated to the patient's pain. Surgical correction of these changes, therefore, does not alleviate the pain, but may create pain in itself.

# Pain medication (analgesics)

There are many kinds of medications (analgesics) that are effective in the treatment of pain, some are best for one kind of pain and others are best suited for other kinds of pain. There are many different substances that have analgesic effects and many are used routinely. Pain medications of various kinds represent the most used pharmacological treatments.

Many different substances are commonly available and in common use without a prescription. They are, therefore, mostly administered without the guidance (and knowledge) of health care professionals. Medications for common pain are economically very important and the different kinds of medication compete heavily as evident from the extensive advertisings that emphasize their product's superior action, which is often exaggerated and mostly emphasizes the side effects of the competitor's drugs only. Rarely are the much less expensive generic versions of drugs mentioned, and patients are often reluctant to use a less expensive version of a drug in the belief that the expensive (and heavily advertised) version is better.

The different medications that are in common use have different efficacies in treating pain and the efficacy of each one may be slightly different for different kinds of pain. The duration of action of the different commonly used pain medications is mainly determined by the drugs' pharmacokinetics, which differs slightly although the advertising of certain kinds of pain medications is highly exaggerated. The effect of some pain relievers decreases with time of usage (tolerance) and some cause various forms of withdrawal symptoms when administration of the drugs is terminated. Some forms of pain are reduced for a longer period than indicated by the pharmacokinetics of the drug, especially if a sufficient amount is taken so that the pain is eliminated.

Pain medications can be divided into two main groups of drugs: non-steroidal anti-inflammatory drugs (NSAID) and opioids. The first group is by far the most commonly used, especially for acute physiological pain. Opioids have their main use in severe chronic pain, but are also used after trauma and surgical operations. Some commonly used analgesics, especially those belonging to the opioid family of drugs, can produce pleasure feelings that invite to misuse. Thus, laws to reduce misuse heavily regulate dispensing of opioids, but these laws are also obstacles in the legitimate use of effective painkillers.

Common for all pharmaceutical analgesics is that their side effects depend on the dosage and length of time they are used. There are great individual variations in both efficacy and side effects of commonly available pain medications. Disease processes, such as impaired liver or kidney functions, may affect the side effects.

# Non-steroidal anti-inflammatory drugs (NSAID)

This family of medications has pain-relieving effects, reduces swelling from inflammation (anti-inflammatory), and reduces fever (antipyretic). Drugs that suppress the synthesis of prostaglandins are in common use for the treatment of many kinds of pain and it is regarded that this effect is responsible for some, but not all, of the pain relieving effects of NSAID. Steroids (such as cortisone) have also been used for a long time in the treatment of some pain conditions. This is because such treatments dampen the reactions of the body's immune system. When it became evident that the central nervous system had its own immune system (see Chapter 10), it became clear that prostaglandins could also increase the immune reactions of the central nervous system [183, 249], which are involved in pathological pain (see Section III).

Some of these NSAID also have varying degrees of blood thinning effects by inhibiting thrombocyte aggregation. This can be an advantage, but also a disadvantage because it can promote bleeding. The different members of the family differ slightly in their side effects and the risks of severe complications differ considerably.

The most common NSAID are acetylsalicylic acid (Aspirin), ibuprofen (Advil, Motrin, see ibuprofen), naproxen (Aleve), and diclofenac (Voltaren). Indomethacin (Indocid) is another NSAID. Paracetamol (acetaminophen), (common brand name Tylenol) is in a class of its own with many similarities to NSAID. The difference is that it is not a blood thinner and that it has different kinds of side effects from that of the NSAID.

Also, tricyclic antidepressants have pain-relieving effects as well, but they are thought to do so by indirectly activating the endogenous opioid system. More recently, it has become evident that administration of omega-3 fatty acids have a pain relieving effect [250]. These fatty acids have no known side effects, thus, a marked difference from any of the conventional pain relievers.

## Actions of NSAID

The actions of NSAID are poorly understood, but there is evidence that the pain relieving action is related to inhibition of an enzyme, the cyclooxygenase 2 (COX-2) that facilitates synthesis of prostaglandins (especially $E_2$) that are involved in inflammatory reactions. This cannot account for the entire pain relieving effects of NSAID, nor can it explain the effect on reducing fevers (antipyretic).

Common NSAID also inhibit COX-1, which is believed to have a normal function in protecting the stomach lining among other "housekeeping" functions these substances have. The increased risk of stomach bleeding from administration of NSAID has been ascribed to their inhibition of COX-1 and this assumption initiated a search for drugs that were elective COX-2 inhibitors.

COX-1 and COX-2 enzymes convert arachidonic acid to prostaglandin, a substance that occurs naturally in the body and which is involved in causing pain and inflammation. The arachidonic acid pathway constitutes one of the main mechanisms for the production of pain and inflammation, as well as controlling homeostatic function. The different pathways produce different classes of end products: 1. Prostaglandins (PG) (from cyclooxygenase metabolism), especially PGE2, PGF2α, and PGD2; 2. Prostacyclines PGI2; 3. Thromboxane Tx A2; 4. Leukotrienes (from lipooxygenase metabolism).

Paracetamol exerts most of its therapeutic efficacy from the metabolite, AM404 (an endogenous cannabinoid re-uptake inhibitor), which enhances the release of serotonin and also interacts with the cannabinoid receptors. The effect of paracetamol, through its metabolite, is by activating descending serotoninergic pathways in order to increase the release of serotonin (5-HT), which inhibits the release of several mediators of pain. It also decreases cyclooxygenase (COX-1 and 2) activity.

## Side effects of NSAID

The best-known side effect from NSAID is stomach bleeding (Figure 7.1) and ulcers (Figure 7.2 and 7.3). The risk is different for the different members of the family of medications. The risk varies among individuals and it depends on a person's history of stomach ulcers from other causes and age.

Ibuprofen appears to have the lowest incidence of digestive adverse drug reactions (ADRs) of all the non-selective NSAID. However, this holds true only at lower doses of ibuprofen, so over-the-counter preparations of ibuprofen are, in general, labeled to advise a maximum daily dose of 1,200 mg.

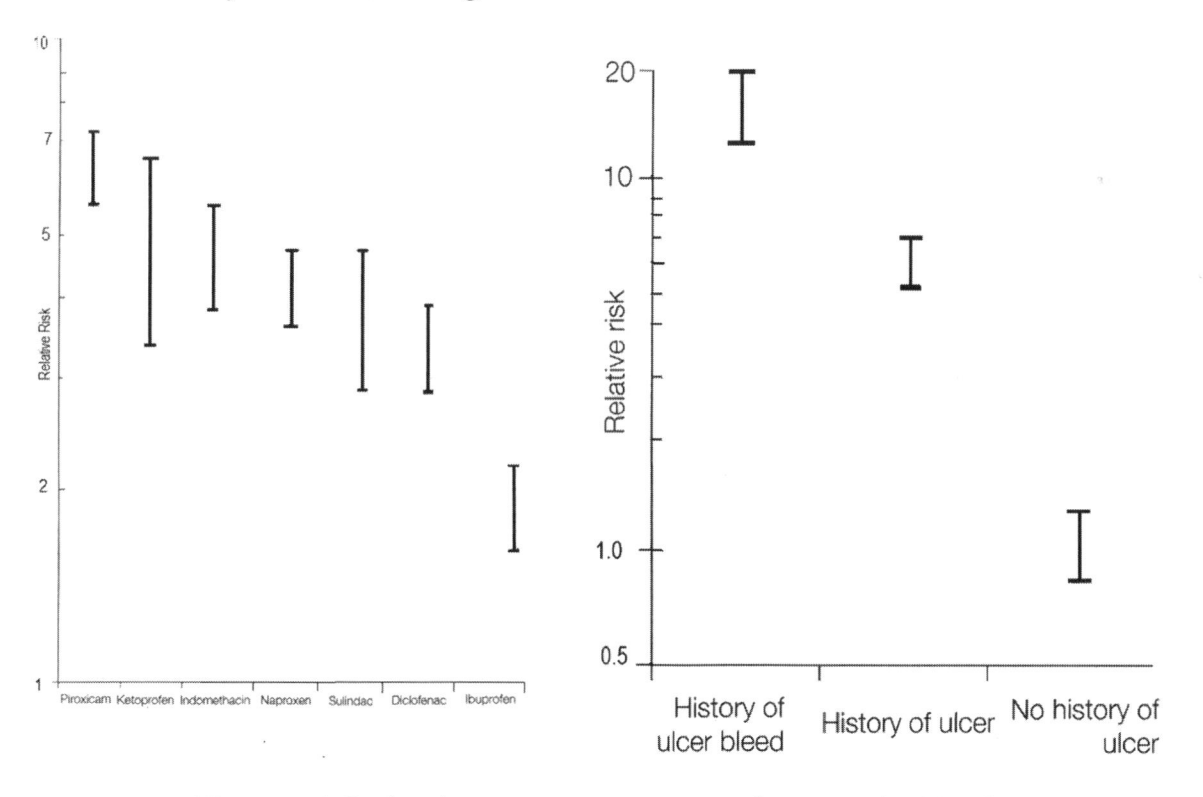

Figure 7.1 Risk of upper gastrointestinal (stomach) bleeding or perforation for different kinds of NSAID (Data from McQuay, H.J. and A. Moore, S and Coxibs: clinical use, in Wall and Melzack's Textbook of Pain, S.B. Mahon and M. Kolzenburg, Editors. 2006, Elsevier: Amsterdam. p. 471-480.) [262] (Artwork by Irene Cunha.)

172  PAIN Its Anatomy, Physiology and Treatment

Figure 7.2 Effect of history of ulcers (95 percent confidence of relative risk) (Data from McQuay, H.J. and A. Moore, S and Coxibs: clinical use, in Wall and Melzack's Textbook of Pain, S.B. Mahon and M. Kolzenburg, Editors. 2006, Elsevier: Amsterdam. p. 471-480.) [262].

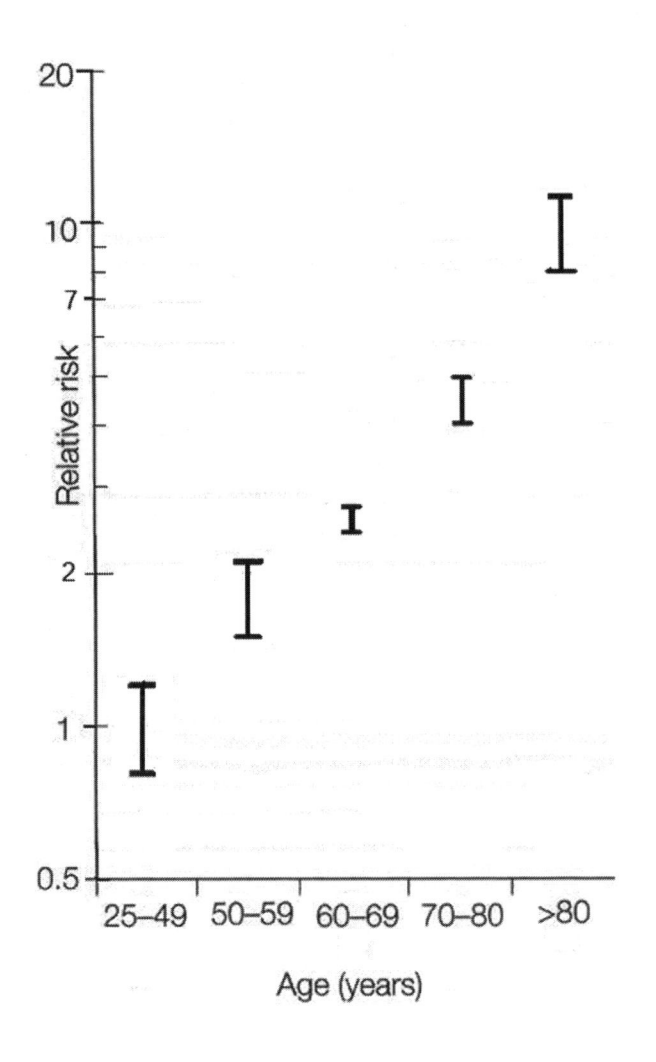

Figure 7.3 Effect of age in users of NSAID (95 percent confidence) on the risk of stomach problems. (Data from McQuay, H.J. and A. Moore, S and Coxibs: clinical use, in Wall and Melzack's Textbook of Pain, S.B. Mahon and M. Kolzenburg, Editors. 2006, Elsevier: Amsterdam. p. 471-480.) [262].

## Other side effects

Along with several other NSAID, ibuprofen has been implicated in elevating the risk of myocardial infarctions (heart attacks); in particular, among those who use high doses of the drug over a long time [166]. Aspirin, and Reye's syndrome should not be given to infants because of the increased risk of Reye's syndrome.

Paracetamol (acetaminophen) is in a class of its own because of its serious side effects at high dosages, but low risk of side effects when administrated in low dosages. Paracetamol may be regarded as a member of the NSAID family with similar analgesic effects as other members, but paracetamol stands out because of its side effects. While it has a lower risk of bleeding (it is not a blood thinner) than other NSAID, such as ibuprofen and naproxen, it has a very high risk of a particularly serious side effect (potentially fatal liver damage) when taken in high dosages.

People's belief that paracetamol is a safe drug is supported by the advertising that promotes Tylenol for its safety compared with other NSAID, such as acetylsalicylate (aspirin), ibuprofen, and Naproxen, which can cause bleedings such as of the stomach. When used correctly, paracetamol for pain control is indeed a safe medication.

The risk of liver damage is high when taking more than a certain amount; earlier regarded to be approximately 4,000 mg per day, up to 2,000 mg per day when drinking 3 or more alcoholic beverages per day (http://www.drugs.com/acetaminophen.html), but recently these limits have been regarded as too high. (There are tablets available (brand name in the UK is Paradote) that combine paracetamol with an antidote (methionine) to protect the liver in case of an overdose.) The biochemistry for liver toxicity from paracetamol is known (Figure 7.4).

## Biochemistry of liver damage from paracetamol

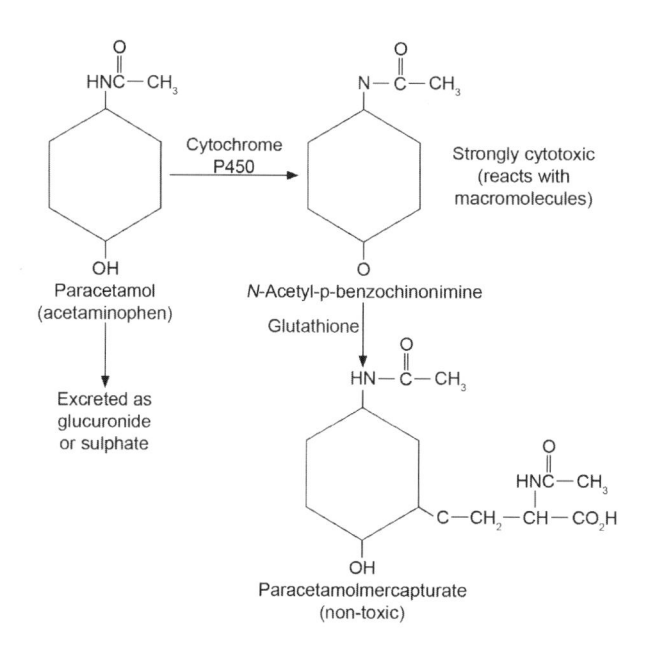

Figure 7.4. Schematic diagram of the metabolism of paracetamol (acetaminophen; Tylenol). Adapted from: Brune, K. and H.U. Zeilhofer, Antipyretic analgesics: basic aspects, in Wall and Melzack's Textbook of Pain, S.B. McMahon and M. Koltzenburg, Editors. 2006, Elsevier, Churchill, Livingstone: Amsterdam. p. 459-69. [56]. (Artwork by Monica Javidnia.)

Liver toxicity from an over dosage of paracetamol is by far the most common cause of acute liver failure in the United States. Taking paracetamol (acetaminophen, brand names such as Tylenol) causes many incidents of liver failure that may be fatal or require a liver transplant. In fact, a large percentage (30-50 percent) of liver transplants done in the USA are done for just that reason.

In a study of 662 individuals with acute liver failure over 6 years, 42 percent were from an overdose of paracetamol. The annual percentage of acetaminophen-related acute liver failure rose during the time of the study from 28 percent in 1998 to 51 percent in 2003. Unintentional overdosing accounted for 48 percent of those who had acute liver failure from paracetamol, 44 percent were from suicide attempts, and 8 percent were unknown intent. Eighty-one percent of unintentional patients reported taking acetaminophen and/or other analgesics for acute or chronic pain syndromes. The conclusion of the study was that paracetamol liver toxicity far exceeds other causes of acute liver failure in the United States [225].

Why does a person take too much of a medication? One reason is that the person does not know the safe limits of the medication. Some people trust the advertising that claims that paracetamol is safe and, therefore, do not watch how much they take of the drug. Another reason is that people do not know how much they are taking. This can occur because paracetamol is an ingredient in many products and it may cause people to take too much of the drug without realizing it. The advertisings for brand names, such as Tylenol, do not mention anything about the risks and how much is safe. Some causes may be attempted suicide just by taking any kind of pill without knowing what it is. Naturally, people with certain diseases, especially liver diseases, are more at risk of liver injury from paracetamol use.

While billions of doses of paracetamol are used every year by millions of people in many countries, its use has been reported to causes 56,000 emergency room visits, 26,000 hospitalizations, and 458 deaths annually in the United States, according to studies done between 1990 and 1998 [229]. In view of the enormous amounts of hydrocodone/paracetamol mixes, it is uncertain why there is not more liver damage, according to Richard DeNisco, MD, MPH, medical officer at the National Institute of Drug Abuse (NIDA) and a panel member (more information can be found in NIDA NOTES - Volume 16, Number 3. http://www.nida.nih.gov/NIDA_notes).

# Regulations to reduce the risk of side effects of paracetamol

An advisory committee voted that the single adult paracetamol dose should be no more than 650 milligrams, significantly less that the current 1,000 milligrams often contained in two tablets of certain over-the-counter pain products (why are people always recommended to take two tablets?). A panel of 37 doctors and other experts had arrived at a recommendation that the maximum total dose for 24 hours, which was 4,000 milligrams, should be decreased by July 1, 2009 and a person's medical condition should be taken into consideration:

(http://www.fda.gov/drugs/drugsafety/informationbydrugclass/ucm165107.htm).

The advisory committee also voted overwhelmingly to recommend that the FDA require a boxed warning -- often called a black box warning -- on the labels of prescription paracetamol combination products, with members noting this is considered the highest precaution the agency can give. They also called for limiting formulations of liquid over-the-counter paracetamol to only one concentration level in order to reduce confusion when people give the medicine to children. Such regulations usually meet heavy resistance from pharmaceutical companies.

Further, to reduce the risk of serious side effects, the Committee voted 20 to 17 that prescription products that combine paracetamol with other medications should be eliminated. It would affect billions of doses of products that are prescribed in which paracetamol is combined with narcotics (opioids), according to the American Food and Drug Administration (FDA). This recommendation would be a real change for the prescription industry and it would have serious economic implications for certain companies. Brand-name pain medications that would be involved would include Vicoden, Lortab, Maxidone, Norco, Zydone, and Tylenol with codeine, Percocet, Endocet, and Darvocet that all contain paracetamol. The combination of hydrocodone and paracetamol, for instance, has been the most frequently dispensed drug since 1997, according to the FDA.

# Action of non-steroidal anti-inflammatory drugs (NSAID)

The basic function of the commonly used non-steroidal anti-inflammatory drugs (NSAID), such as aspirin, ibuprofen, naproxen, and others, is related to the fact that they inhibit two enzymes (COX-1 and 2). It is believed that their effect in reducing swelling is related to their ability to block the synthesis of prostaglandins [162, 262].

Prostaglandins sensitize neurons in pain pathways, thereby increasing the response to painful stimuli. Reducing the sensitizing effect of prostaglandins can reduce pain (see Chapter 6, modulation of pain). Although it has been assumed that the effects of NSAID are (mainly) peripheral, this cannot explain all of the effects, such as the antipyretic effect. Peripheral neuromodulation cannot explain how these drugs can cause total absence of pain. This means that NSAID must also act on the central nervous system.

The effect on the periphery does not explain all of the effects such as pain relief in the absence of swelling and the effect on body temperature (antipyretic effect). Except for these functions, the mechanisms that are involved in the ability of NSAID in relieving pain is poorly understood; thus, less well understood than the mechanisms through which opioids exert their pain relieving action.

NSAID suppress both COX-1 and COX-2 enzymes. COX-1 is expressed normally while COX-2 is considered to be an induced enzyme that causes increased synthesis of prostaglandins. It is only COX-2 that is involved in pain and swelling from inflammation. COX-1 has other important functions such as protecting the stomach lining. It is, therefore, undesirable to also inhibit COX-1. COX-1 is necessary for the normal function of cells. Some studies have shown that the tendency to cause stomach bleeding was caused by the inhibition of the COX-1 enzyme and this was one of the reasons for the development of COX-2 selective drugs (coxibs). There are no reasons to inhibit COX-1 enzymes; on the contrary, such action may have undesirable effects.

A series of such selective COX-2 inhibitors known as Coxibs appeared on the market. However, when they came into practical use, these new drugs showed severe side effects, mainly in the form of increased risk for cardiovascular diseases. Many of these drugs were taken off the market after being in use for some time.

Coxibs were only available by prescription, which meant that the patients treated with these drugs were under the care of a physician. The patient reactions to drugs that can only be obtained by a prescription are monitored more extensively than that of drugs that can be obtained without a prescription.

The health professional who prescribes a pain killer for a patient will get to know if the patient has experienced side effects, whereas, the store that sells over-the-counter drugs will not have this feedback.

Therefore, side effects were detected promptly. Medications, such as aspirin, ibuprofen, and naproxen, that could be obtained without a prescription were not followed in the same way and their side effects, such as on the cardiovascular system, were probably not detected to the same extent as that of the new selective COX-2 inhibitors.

This means that the introduction of Coxibs has caused an increase in our understanding of the side effects of Coxibs, but also of old common NSAID.

Again, this is an example of how the enormous complexity of biological systems and our scant knowledge about their function brings unexpected effects. Manipulating biological systems that have been developed over millions of years is a daunting task.

# Opioids

Opioids have played a critical role in achieving pain relief in both modern and ancient medicine. They are still used extensively to control many forms of pain including acute and chronic physiological pain and for pathological pain. Postoperative pain is often treated by the administration of opioids. Yet, their clinical use is limited because of unwanted side effects such as tolerance and dependence (addiction). However, the risks of addiction, craving, and tolerance are side effects of opioids that are very different for the different synthetic and semisynthetic opioids and, in particular, for natural opioids (opiates). Thus, natural opioids, heroin, and morphine are highly addictive and produce euphoria when administered.

There is a wide confusion regarding the two terms, opioids and opiates. The term opioids is used for substances that bind to opioid receptors whereas the term opiate is used for the constituents or derivatives of constituents found in opium that come from the opium poppy. The synthetic opioids have much less risks of addiction and produce little or no euphoria, but are still powerful pain relievers. The name opiates should, therefore, not be used for synthetic opioids, which are substances that bind to opioid receptors, but are unrelated to opium. By far, most of the opioids used in medicine are synthetic substances or semi-synthetic.

## Action of opioids

Some of the complex action of opioids was discussed in Chapter 3 and the role of endogenous opioids in modulation of pain was discussed in Chapter 6. Opioids activate specific receptors that are found peripherally as well as centrally (spinal cord and brain). Three different receptors, $\mu$, $\kappa$, and $\delta$, respond to opioids. Most of the opioids activate all three receptors, but to a varying degree.

There are opioid receptors in many parts of the spinal cord and the brain. Animal experiments have shown that opioids can exert their pain relieving effects locally, such as in the skin, but the main effect is on the spinal cord and the brain [406].

Much of the pain relieving action of opioids is mediated by their action on cells in the periaqueductal gray (PAG), activating the descending pain pathways, mainly the rostral ventromedial medulla (RVM) as discussed in Chapter 3. Morphine and other opioids have opposite effects on the on and off cells of the RVM. They inhibit "on-cells" and excite "off-cells", thereby causing a decreased transmission in the pain pathways through both the RVM on and off pathways. Modulation of pain by administrating opioids, activating the RVM and PAG systems, involves several different opioid receptors ($\mu$, $\kappa$, and $\delta$ receptors) that all are found in many parts of the nervous system.

## Different kinds of opioids

The naturally occurring opioids, such as Morphine and codeine, synthetic opioids, such as Fentanyl and its variations (alfentanil, sufentanil, remifentnil), methadone, and semisynthetic opioids, such as oxycodone, oxymorphone, and hydromorphone, are widely used as pain relievers. Fentanyl is used in surgical operations and also as skin patches for the treatment of chronic pain.

The semisynthetic oxycodone and hydromorphone are the most used for relief of moderate to severe pain and they have very little risk of creating addiction; thus, very different from the natural opioids (opiates) such as morphine and, in particular, heroin. Even the commonly used semisynthetic opioids, such as oxycodone, may, however, produce withdrawal symptoms when administration is stopped abruptly. Adverse effects occur mainly when administration is terminated abruptly, but most individuals who use these drugs do not experience any withdrawal symptoms. In general, the risk of addiction to the modern synthetic opioids that are now in common use is very small. Most people do not like the side effects and are just waiting to no longer have to take these drugs.

The risk of death from overdosage of the extensively used semi-synthetic opioids used in general have had much less publicity than the risk of addiction. In fact a death from overdosage of the conventional semi-synthetic opioids (prescription pain medication) in the US occurs every 19 minutes [69]. It is the second leading cause of accidental death (after car accidents).

# Other side effects of administration of opioids

Suppression of respiration occurs in high dosages of opioids. This is not a problem with ordinary use of the medication such as with oxycodone that is administered in the forms of tablets; respiratory suppression would normally only occur in serious overdosing. Respiratory arrest has occurred by ingesting the substance in Fentanyl patches and from heroin when used as a recreational drug.

# Other analgesics

Tramadol activates opioid receptors, has a weak action on μ receptors, releases serotonin, and inhibits re-uptake of norepinephrine. Some drugs, such as Tramadol, do not bind to opioid receptors, but act as agonists to $\mu_1$ and $\mu_2$ opioid receptors, thus enhancing the effect of opioids. Tapentadol [64] (trade name Nucynta) is a centrally-acting analgesic with a dual mode of action as an agonist at the μ-opioid receptor and as a norepinephrine re-uptake inhibitor.

Tricyclic antidepressants, such as imipramine, amitriptyline, etc., have pain-relieving effects. The common selective serotonin re-uptake inhibitors (SSRIs) also have pain-relieving effects, but they are less effective. Some of these medications also have norepinephrine re-uptake inhibitor effects. The greatest effect of these drugs may be in enhancing the effect of opioids. In fact, they have been thought to have some of their pain relieving effects by indirectly activating the endogenous opioid system [470].

Alcohol has considerable pain relieving effects and it was the first commonly used analgesic for severe pain and for surgical procedures before anesthetics, like ether, became available. Alcohol is not used as an analgesic now except by self-administration.

When discussing analgesics, it is also worth mentioning that drugs that reduce muscle contractions, such as members of the benzodiazepine family, can have pain-relieving effects because many forms of pain are, in fact, caused by muscle contractions.

# Non-analgesics that can relieve pain

Recently, it has been shown that administration of several substances that are not traditional pain relievers can be effective in controlling many forms of pain. This is discussed in Chapter 12 in connection with managing of chronic neuropathic pain. Here we will discuss administration of substances that can help manage physiological pain and peripheral nerve pain.

## Omega-3

Omega 3 fatty acids have pain relieving effect without any known side effects [250]. Substances derived from omega 3, such as lipoxins and D and E series resolvins [409] that are specialized pro-resolving lipid mediators (SPM), prevent excessive inflammation and promote removal of microbes and apoptotic cells, thereby expediting resolution and return to tissue homeostasis. These substances [386] have the effect of reducing inflammation and these substances are candidates for becoming effective pain relievers in the future.

## Cannabis

We discuss in Chapter 12 the use of cannabis to treat chronic neuropathic pain and central neuropathic pain. It is especially one of the two main active substance (CBD) in cannabis that has pain relieving effect in chronic pain [482]. This component of cannabis is also effective in treating physiological pain [2, 331, 357].

## Benzodiazepines

Muscle contractions may contribute to some forms of pain such as low back pain. Some of the pain may, therefore, be relieved by the administration of a muscle relaxant and in that way muscle relaxants of various kinds can serve as pain relievers. Benzodiazepines, such as Valium, which is an effective central muscle relaxant, are effective in reducing pain in connection with low back pain and neck pain of various causes. However, GABAergic inhibition affects descending activity from the PAG that has inhibitory influence on pain mediating neurons in the dorsal horn (the RVM pathway). This means that enhancement of GABAergic inhibition from administration of benzodiazepines may in fact decrease the (natural) inhibitory influence on transmission of pain signals in the spinal cord (and the trigeminal nucleus).

## B-vitamins

Some forms of pain from peripheral neuropathy may be relieved by the administration of B vitamins. Administration of $B_1$, $B_6$, and especially $B_{12}$, has been shown to provide relief in some forms of pathological pain such as painful diabetes neuropathies (PDN) [427] and low back pain [256]. The common form of $B_{12}$, (cobalamin) must be converted in the liver. This step can be avoided by using methylcobalamin, which is available as a sublingual tablet. Treatment with $B_{12}$ is effective for in treatment of diabetes and alcohol induced peripheral neuropathy. Also pain from treatment of by some cancer drugs such as Tamoxifen that is known to cause peripheral nerve neuropathy that present with burning pain in feet.

## Relievers of sympathetic activity

Some kinds of pain are activated through increased sympathetic activity. Therefore, medications that reduce sympathetic activity, such as clonidine, may be effective in controlling pain.

## Anti-inflammatory drugs

Administration of drugs such as ibuprofen, naproxen and other NSAIDs that are COX-2 inhibitors have anti-inflammatory actions that helps reducing pain by inhibiting the synthesis of prostaglandin $E_2$.

## Electrical stimulation of the vagus nerve

Studies in cats and monkeys have shown that electrical stimulation of the vagus nerve attenuate the response from neurons in the dorsal horn to many different type types of noxious and innocuous stimuli[72]. Vagal activity elicited by endocrine stimulation from the adrenal medullae has similar effect[182]. The effect seems to be related to anatomical connections between the vagus nerve and the dorsal horn neurons that mediate pain[137, 182].

The beneficial effect of vagal nerve stimulation (VNS) depends on the stimulation parameters [6]. The difference in the reported results of VNS for controlling pain may, to some extent, be explained by the fact that different investigators have used different stimulus parameters.

Several studies report that electrical stimulation of vagal afferents inhibits spinal pain reflexes and transmission. However, results are partly contradictory. As mentioned above, adrenalin and norepinephrine modulate the sensitivity of pain receptors. Since vagal afferents from the small intestine have inhibitory influence on the central input to the pre-ganglionic neurons that innervate the adrenal medulla, they may control the level of adrenalin in the blood and thereby, affect processing of pain signals.

The left and right vagus nerves are different. The right vagus nerve slows the heart (cholinergic influence on the sinoatrial node), counteracting sympathetic influence (adrenergic) that increases heart rate. The left vagus nerve innervates the AV node and strong stimulation of the left vagus nerve can promote atrioventricular blocks. The left vagus nerve, however, can be safely stimulated electrically (may give hoarseness) for treatment at low to moderate stimulus intensities.

Other studies have shown that stimulation of the vagus nerve reduces the pain from controlled stimulation of nociceptors and it reduces the temporal integration of pain elicited by 5 consecutive impulses ("wind-up") and pain from tonic pressure[209]. However, the same study showed that pain associated with single impulses of heat was not affected[209]. This indicates that activity in the vagus nerve mainly affect the central processing of pain (central inhibition). Yet other studies have indicated that the effect of vagal activity on pain is mediated through the NA-serotonin descending system [428].

The vagus nerve seems to be involved in the opioid induced analgesia as studies in rats have shown that vagotomy decreases the analgesic effect of morphine administered intravenously in rats[137]. This means that intact function of the vagus nerve is necessary for the analgesic effect of morphine.

# Administration of pain medication

Perhaps the greatest obstacle in successful treatment of physiological pain by medications is the administration of the medication. Treatment of physiological pain often fails to provide complete relief from the pain despite the choice of excellent medications. The reason is often that the medications are administrated incorrectly.

While there are endless descriptions of the beneficial effects of many medications when administrated under ideal conditons, little attention is devoted to the importance of correct administration; teaching patients how to administer their medications.

Drug treatments for acute pain of moderate intensity, such as common headaches, should always be administered in such a way that the pain disappears. Often, less than optimal amounts of medication are chosen. Many people are afraid of taking pain medication and will only take so much that they can tolerate the pain. This will often prolong the pain compared to treating it so that it is eliminated.

Treatment of chronic pain especially is often much more efficient when the medication is administered on a regular basis using a scheme where the medication is given before the pain re-appears. For chronic pain, medications should not be taken just when the pain reoccurs. A person with chronic pain knows the length of time the medication he/she takes keeps the pain away and can plan to take the medication before the pain occurs. It is usually difficult, however, to convince patients about administrating pain medication in such a way because most people believe that medication should (only) be taken when the pain appears.

The description of how to administer medication is often given by a physician who is in a hurry (does not want to take the necessary time) or by a nurse who does not have sufficient qualifications for the task. Patients at an office visit are often only left with oral instructions from their physician about how to take their medications and without written instructions. This is despite the fact that most patients have a limited recall of what the physician said and many do not understand the instructions that were given.

It is a mystery why people do not get written instructions from their physicians. One cannot buy any gadget, simple or complex, that does not have detailed written instructions. Pharmacies are beginning to provide written instructions on how to take the medication and information regarding the side effects. These instructions are general instructions that would apply to the average individual. It would seem to be better if the physician would provide instructions that were tailored to the individual patient, taking into account the patient's age, gender, body weight, diseases, and which medications the person currently takes. Such a simple reform would increase the efficacy of many treatments and reduce the side effects.

In general, people would rather hear about new and sophisticated experimental treatments than trivial matters such as how to administer pain medication. People believe in medicine and have blind trust in the pharmaceutical industry and hospitals, but pay little attention to how they administer their own medication. The same is applicable to other suggestions that physicians may give to their patients. Often, changes in lifestyle can improve a patient's condition.

However, suggestions about how to change that lifestyle (exercise, control their weight, etc.) are also given in the same way as instructions about how to administer medications. Often, such simple treatment as taking vitamins can relieve some forms of pain, but physicians rarely recommend that form of treatment.

# Tolerance and addiction

Tolerance means that after some time of use, the amount of an analgesic drug that is administered must be increased to get the same effect. Addiction to a drug means that withdrawal symptoms are experienced when administration of a drug is terminated. Tolerance is especially pronounced for opioids and it often occurs after months of use.

## Tolerance to opioids

Opioid receptor desensitization and down-regulation of opioid receptors are believed to be major mechanisms underlying opioid tolerance. Facilitation of pain circuits in the spinal cord and the brain that occurs after some time of use of opioids also contributes to opioid-induced hyperalgesia. Tolerance is an obstacle in long term use of opioids [112].

There are 3 different receptors for opioids: μ, κ, and δ. The synthetic opioids that are in common use for pain management activate both μ and κ receptors. A change in the type of opioid from mainly μ receptor blockage to κ receptor agonist will help.

## Addiction to opioids

The focus of addiction from pain relievers has been on opioids. It is unfortunate that the same terms, opioid or opiates, are used both for such highly addictive drugs, such as heroin and morphine, and at the same time, are used for synthetic analgesics, such as oxycodone, a modern opioid used as a pain reliever.

It is the addiction to synthetic and semisynthetic opioids of various kinds that is of interest regarding treatment of pain. The risk of addiction has caused legal restrictions regarding dispensing and use of opioids that now affect their legitimate use in the treatment of pain. The matter is complicated by the fact that the different opioids have very different risks of causing addiction and there is also some confusion regarding the definition of addiction.

Often, all opioids, including the naturally occurring opiates, are regarded in the same way as the synthetic and semisynthetic opioids, despite that they have very different risks of causing addiction. There are many different definitions of addiction. Craving or an eager desire in general may be regarded as a form of addiction, for example, a craving for specific foods.

Stedman's Electronic Dictionary defines addiction as: habitual psychological or physiologic dependence on a substance or practice that is beyond voluntary control. Other medical definitions are: addiction is a persistent, compulsive dependence on a behavior or substance.

Diagnostic and Statistical Manual of Mental Disorders (DSM-IV) defines substance dependence in this way:

"When an individual persists in use of alcohol or other drugs despite problems related to use of the substance, substance dependence may be diagnosed. Compulsive and repetitive use may result in tolerance to the effect of the drug and withdrawal symptoms when use is reduced or stopped. This, along with Substance Abuse, are considered Substance Use Disorders...."

The terms abuse and addiction have been defined and re-defined over the years. The 1957 World Health Organization (WHO) Expert Committee on Addiction-Producing Drugs defined addiction and habituation as components of drug abuse:

Drug addiction is a state of periodic or chronic intoxication produced by the repeated consumption of a drug (natural or synthetic). Its characteristics include: (i) an overpowering desire or need (compulsion) to continue taking the drug and to obtain it by any means; (ii) a tendency to increase the dose; (iii) a psychic (psychological) and generally a physical dependence on the effects of the drug; and (iv) detrimental effects on the individual and on society.

Drug habituation (habit) is a condition resulting from the repeated consumption of a drug. Its characteristics include (i) a desire (but not a compulsion) to continue taking the drug for the sense of improved well-being which it engenders; (ii) little or no tendency to increase the dose; (iii) some degree of psychic dependence on the effect of the drug, but absence of physical dependence and hence of an abstinence syndrome (withdrawal), and (iv) detrimental effects, if any, primarily on the individual.

In 1964, a new WHO committee found these definitions to be inadequate, and suggested using the blanket term "drug dependence":

The definition of addiction gained some acceptance, but confusion in the use of the terms addiction and habituation and misuse of the former continued. Further, the list of drugs abused increased in number and diversity. These difficulties have become increasingly apparent and various attempts have been made to find a term that could be applied to drug abuse generally. The component in common appears to be dependence, whether psychic or physical or both. Hence, use of the term 'drug dependence', with a modifying phase linking it to a particular drug type in order to differentiate one class of drugs from another, had been given most careful consideration.

An Expert Committee recommends substitution of the term 'drug dependence' for the terms 'drug addiction' and 'drug habituation'. Since dispensing of opioids is controlled by laws in many countries, it is interesting to consider what the legal terms of (substance) addiction would be.

186 PAIN Its Anatomy, Physiology and Treatment

An authoritative definition of drug addiction is that propounded by the World Health Organization (WHO): Drug addiction is a state of periodic and chronic intoxication detrimental to the individual and to society, produced by the repeated consumption of a drug (natural or synthetic). Its characteristics include: (1) An overpowering desire or need (compulsion) to continue taking the drug and to obtain it by any means; (2) A tendency to increase the dose; (3) A psychic (psychological) and sometimes a physical dependence on the effects of the drug. This definition of drug addiction includes many drugs, which are not pain relievers, such as hypnotic and sedative drugs (barbiturates, etc.), alcohol, amphetamine, and mescaline (peyote).

The legal restrictions regarding dispensing of substances that are thought to cause addiction are supposed to have been created for the purpose of protecting individuals from harm. Like many other similar actions, they have considerable side effects. The obstacles in and limitations of the justifiable use of analgesics is one side effect. This means that the legal restrictions that are aimed at protecting people from harm (from addiction) in fact cause harm because they are obstacles to legitimate use of these powerful pain relievers that have minimal side effects.

# Sensitization from opioids

It may be surprising to find that opioids can sensitize the pain system. We have discussed in other chapters how different forms of sensitization can increase the sensitivity to painful stimulation causing hyperalgesia. Sensitization can occur as a result of administration of pain relievers such as opioids. Sensitization is a form of pain modulation that is discussed in Chapter 6. Sensitization can occur at the receptor level (peripheral sensitization) or in the spinal cord and in the brain (central sensitization).

Long term use of opioids can have a paradoxical effect on pain in that it can cause an increase in pain sensitivity (hyperalgesia) [438] caused by central sensitization. This paradoxical effect of treatment for pain is a little known effect of opioids and possibly other pain relievers.

Glia cells seem to be involved in some opioid side effects including those mediated by cytokine receptors, κ-opioid receptors, N-methyl-D-aspartate (NMDA) receptors, and the recently elucidated Toll-like receptors. Newer agents targeting these receptors, such as AV411, MK-801, AV333, SLC022, and older agents used outside the United States for other disease conditions, such as minocycline, pentoxifylline, and UV50488H, all seem promising for providing significant relief from opioid side effects while simultaneously potentiating the pain relieving effect of opioids [154].

# Misconceptions of side effects of pain medications

The side effects of common pain medications should not be ignored, but people often focus on the wrong side effects. Some people often regard certain pain medications that have severe side effects as being safe, while the same people are afraid of other medications that, in fact, have fewer side effects. Many people are afraid of taking the modern synthetic and semi-synthetic opioids in the belief that the risk of addiction is similar to those of the natural opiates such as morphine and heroin.

In fact, modern synthetic and semi-synthetic opioids have a very low risk of addiction. Thus, for example, paracetamol is usually regarded as being a safe medication compared with NSAID such as ibuprofen, although paracetamol has severe side effects. In fact, a large proportion of people have liver transplants because they have lost normal liver function due to paracetamol intake. Many who lose liver function from paracetamol intake die before they can get a liver transplant.

The side effects of conventional NSAID that inhibit COX-1 and COX-2 enzymes and Coxibs that only inhibit the COX-2 enzyme are similar, namely increased risk of stomach bleeding, renal failure, and congestive heart failure at therapeutic dosages. The risks depend on the length of time the drugs are taken, the age of the individuals who take the medication, and on renal status.

Thus, diseases of various kinds can increase the risks of side effects from administration of these medications. The effects of a person's age, gender, or body weight on the risks of side effects are often ignored and so is the effect of diseases and medications taken.

# The placebo effect

The placebo effect is the beneficial effect of treatment with inactive means, which can be any treatment including medications. Treatment that people believe will be beneficial is often beneficial and the placebo effect is real.

The placebo effect is probably best known from testing of treatments, especially drugs, where the effect of the administration of a substance that is to be tested is compared with the results of an inactive substance that was administered in a similar way and where the participants (and the person who administrates the test) do not know which of the substances is the active one.

The placebo effect of treatment for pain is a result of an expectation of pain relief from what a person presumes to be an effective substance, but which, in fact, is an inactive substance. Thus, the placebo effect is a product of a positive expectation. (The word placebo is Latin and means, "I shall please".)

The placebo effect in the treatment of pain is real pain [173] and it may be regarded as a form of modulating neural activity in structures of the spinal cord and brain that transmit pain information [149, 233]. Again, this is a reminder that pain is far more complex than normally assumed, involving high brain functions. Many other symptoms are subject to placebo effects.

The neural mechanisms behind the placebo effect on pain are not well understood. One hypothesis states that it is caused by the action of endogenous opioids that are liberated because of the expectation of a beneficial effect from a treatment. This hypothesis was supported by a study of postoperative patients that showed that those who responded positively to a placebo experienced increased pain after the administration of naloxone (naloxone blocks the effect of opioids). Those who did not respond positively to the placebo did not experience any effect after administration of naloxone [233].

Other hypotheses ascribe the effect to emotional factors, which are known to be involved in many forms of pain [149, 182]. The involvement of limbic structures and descending pathways from the prefrontal cortex has also been implicated in the placebo effect. It seems likely that several mechanisms may be involved in the placebo effect [292].

# Treatment of the cause of pain

Pain is traditionally treated by pain medication as discussed above. There are, however other means that are effective in treating certain kinds of pain. Naturally, the most effective is to treat the disorders that cause the pain. Peripheral neuropathy is a common cause of pain. The term peripheral neuropathy means, "sick peripheral nerves" and it can have many causes. Peripheral neuropathies are examples of diseases that often can be treated successfully so that pain relief is achieved without pain medication.

## Peripheral nerve neuropathy

The symptoms of peripheral nerve neuropathy are burning pain and sometimes numbness. Peripheral neuropathies are common in elderly individuals and in individuals with diabetes.

It is also a typical symptom of excessive use of alcohol, but it may appear without any known causes. Normally, peripheral nerve neuropathies first manifest with pain in the feet and perhaps also in the hands. This is because distal parts of a peripheral nerve are more vulnerable than more proximal parts that are closer to the axons' cell bodies. This is because of the longer distance to the cell body of the axon and it is, therefore, more difficult to supply distal portions of an axon with nutrients than more proximal portions. The diameters of axons decrease with the distance from the cell body, which may also contribute to the higher likelihood of pain in distal locations such as the feet.

Pain from peripheral neuropathies is often caused by a deficiency in vitamin $B_1$, $B_6$, and $B_{12}$, more pronounced for $B_{12}$ [256, 427]. The reason is due to poor absorption that often occurs in elderly individuals. Pain from peripheral nerve neuropathy can, therefore, often be reduced almost instantaneously by the administration of vitamin B, most importantly $B_1$ and $B_{12}$ [427].

In a randomized, single-blind clinical trial, the efficacy of parenteral vitamin $B_{12}$ and nortriptyline were compared in a group of 100 individuals with painful diabetes neuropathy (50 in each group) [427]. Pain scores based on a visual analogue scale decreased 3.66 units in the vitamin $B_{12}$ group and 0.84 units in the nortriptylin group ($P < 0.001$). The scores for paresthesia decreased 2.98 units in the $B_{12}$ group compared with 1.06 units ($P < 0.001$) in the nortriptylin group.

The tingling sensation decreased 3.48 units in the $B_{12}$ group and only 1.02 units in the nortriptylin group ($P < 0.001$). Changes in perception of vibration, position, pinprick, and nerve conduction parameters were not significant in either of the two groups. Absorption of $B_{12}$ may be impaired when the form that is commonly available in pharmacies is used. That form, cyanocobalamin, must be converted in the liver to methylcobalamin. Therefore, it is better to use methylcobalamin that can be obtained from many health stores. This form of $B_{12}$ vitamin must be dissolved in the mouth not swallowed.

Naturally, painful alcohol neuropathy can be treated by reducing alcohol intake, which is no doubt the best form of treatment. However, that is often not possible. The fact is that alcohol induced peripheral nerve neuropathy is not caused by a toxic effect from alcohol, but rather because persons with a large intake of alcohol eat poorly because they get a large amount of their calories needed from alcohol. A deficiency of thiamin (vitamin $B_1$) is probably the main cause of the pain symptoms associated with excessive alcohol intake [401]. This means that supplements of B vitamins can often reduce the effect of alcohol intake on painful peripheral nerve neuropathy.

Low back pain is a common disorder that is treated in many different ways. One severe symptom is pain and pain treatments vary. Some forms of pain from common low back pain may have similarities with peripheral neuropathy. Treatments using $B_{12}$ vitamins have been shown to be beneficial [256], indicating a similar etiology of this kind of pain as other forms of peripheral neuropathy.

Other B vitamins are possibly also involved such as vitamin $B_3$ (Niacin). Vitamin $D_3$ has also been shown to be beneficial in various ways. Administration of α-tocopherol and tocotrienol, E vitamins, may have a beneficial effect as well. Taking vitamins has no noticeable side effects except for large amounts of vitamin A.

Since modern healthcare is test-driven, a person with painful neuropathy may be recommended by his/her physician to have an expensive test for vitamin B deficiency. However, a much easier, less expensive, and more efficient way is to try a vitamin B supplement. If it does not help, it has not caused any damage or side effects. These tests typically show "normal" values at levels that are far below that needed to affect neuropathy. This is because these tests often use the "recommended daily allowance" (RDA) as a guide for how much to take. These RDA values are based on avoiding getting sick from deficit in young healthy individuals. Elderly individuals must take larger dosages than the RDA indicates because of decreased resorption.

Far larger intake is necessary to treat disorders such as various forms of painful neuropathy. Since none of the B vitamins have any known adverse side effects, even in very large dosages, they can be taken so that even people who have poor absorption of the vitamins can get sufficient amounts to avoid such unpleasant disorders as pain from peripheral neuropathy. The common form of $B_{12}$ vitamins must be converted in the liver and people with reduced liver function may experience reduced effect of such forms of $B_{12}$. As mentioned above a form of $B_{12}$, methylcyanobalamin, does not need to be converted and may therefore be more effective in some people.

While the role of vitamins in these common pain conditions is confirmed in several studies, many physicians are unaware of the role of vitamin deficiency as a cause of pain from peripheral neuropathy. Instead, many physicians prescribe other more sophisticated and often less effective treatments that are likely to have adverse side effects; one side effect being high costs.

Electrical nerve stimulation, special (expensive) socks, etc. are frequently advertised for the treatment of pain from peripheral neuropathy. These treatments may alleviate the pain, but do not remedy the cause of the pain as vitamins would do. People often shun simple remedies for complex and expensive ones, which are heavily advertised and in the belief that expensive remedies are better than inexpensive ones.

## Neuropathy as a side effect of medical treatment

Some medical treatments can cause painful peripheral nerve neuropathy. For example, treatment of breast cancers with taxol and other cancer chemotherapy drugs [483] often causes painful neuropathy. Prophylactic treatment with acetyl-l-carnitine (ALC) has been reported to have beneficial effects [493], but relief of the pain can also often be achieved by administration of vitamin B supplements (especially $B_{12}$).

# Electrical stimulation (Neuromodulation)

Acute pain can be modulated by activity of $A\beta$ nerve fibers as discussed in Chapter 6. Electrical stimulation of peripheral nerves in the skin (transderm electrical nerve stimulation, TENS) is a proven method that can relieve some forms of pain as is discussed in Chapter 6 in connection with Melzack and Wall's gating hypothesis.

More recently, stimulation of the different parts of the cerebral cortex has been introduced. These methods are mostly used for treating pathological pain and will be described in Chapter 12.

# Surgical treatment of pain

Few incidences of physiological pain are helped by surgical treatment. Surgical treatment of low back pain and carpal tunnel syndrome is often done. These disorders may, at a glance, appear to be physiological pain, but while physiological pain may be a component of the pain, the pain in these disorders is mainly pathological pain. The surgical treatment of these disorders will, therefore, be discussed in detail in Chapter 12, which also will discuss surgical treatment of vascular compression disorders such as trigeminal and glossopharyngeal neural neuralgia.

Mistaking correlation from causal relations can have serious consequences because it can lead to surgical operations and other treatments that are of no benefit to a patient, but which have risks of serious side effects and complications. As pointed out in other places in this book, almost all forms of surgical operations involve severance of many small nerves.

The severed axons sprout and these sprouts are pain sensitive [49]. This is the reason that almost all forms of operations cause pain in the wounds that may last a very long time. Therefore, treatment of pain using surgical operations must be carefully considered.

# Reducing the risk of pain

Our medical system and the sentiment of people in general is directed to treatment although it has been documented over and over again that prevention is often far more efficient and, in particular, has far less side effects. Pain is not an exception.

There are many possibilities of reducing the risk of pain, but available ways to reduce the risk of severe pain are not used to the extent that they could.

Viral infections can cause excruciating pain that may last a long time. An example is shingles, which affects older people more frequently than younger. A vaccine has recently become available, but it has not been promoted extensively. The efficacy for the vaccine is reported to be approximately 50 percent and should be compared with the findings that individuals in their 70s have an estimated risk for shingles of approximately 1 percent during the next year (or 10 percent during the next 10 years).

Given the central nervous system damage caused by herpes zoster infection, the difficulty of adequately treating herpes zoster infections to prevent postherpetic neuralgia (PHN), and the intractability of postherpetic neuralgia, the advent of the herpes zoster vaccine appears to be a crucial innovation.

## Reducing the risk of postoperative pain

The pain caused by medical and surgical treatments can be serious and it affects many people, often for a long time. There are techniques that are in general use which have proven to reduce neural deficits from surgical operations that affect the nervous system. These techniques, known as intraoperative neurophysiological monitoring (IONM) [294], can also reduce the risks of complications that are in the form of pain.

For example, it is known that in orthopedic operations, the prevalence of complex regional pain syndrome, phantom limb pain, chronic donor-site pain, and persistent pain following total joint arthroplasty (joint replacement surgery) is alarmingly high [355].

Pain occurs frequently after amputations. As mentioned in Chapter 8, there are two kinds of pain that occur often, sprouting of axons from severed nerves and phantom limb pain that occurs frequently after amputations together with other phantom limb symptoms. Splitting the nerve after it is cut and then joining the ends of the two parts and making an anastomosis can reduce the risk of pain from sprouting axons. This reduces the risk of sprouting and thus, the risk of pain from neuroma formation [22].

Developing phantom limb pain depends on several factors, some that have to do with conditions before the operation, some that occur during an operation, and some that occur after the operation. The pain that an individual has before the amputation plays a role as does the neural activity caused during the operation, which ascends to the spinal cord and the brain. This is discussed in more detail in Chapter 12.

As we have discussed in several places in this book, activation of neuroplasticity can cause the development of central neuropathic pain. Manipulations of nerves in the anesthetized patient result in massive and abnormal neural activity, which arrives at the spinal cord and the brain before it becomes blocked by the anesthesia. This abnormal neural activity has a large potential to cause activation of bad neuroplasticity that can cause persistent pain after the operation.

The remedy would be to block the neural activity that is caused by the surgical manipulations before it reaches the spinal cord. This can be done easily by local anesthetics applied to the nerves before the surgical manipulations begin.

The use of such preemptive or preventive multimodal analgesic techniques is limited though, probably because surgeons are unaware of it, but also because limited attention is directed to postoperative pain as a complication. Other methods would be to use an anesthetic regimen that is aimed at more peripheral structures of the nervous system.

Multimodal analgesia that allows a reduction in the doses of individual drugs for postoperative pain and thus, a lower prevalence of opioid-related adverse events, may also be beneficial [355]. Effective multimodal analgesic techniques include the use of non-steroidal anti-inflammatory drugs, local anesthetics, $\alpha$-2 agonists, ketamine, $\alpha(2)$-$\delta$ ligands, and opioids.

# New avenues for treatment of physiological pain

Perhaps the most effective future development would be to provide factual information about the difference in the efficacy and side effects of common pain relievers. Since much of the information that is generally available is provided by advertisings of various kinds there are great risks that product information is biased.

Pharmacies are beginning to provide written instructions on how to take the medication and information regarding the side effects. These instructions are general instructions that would apply to the average individual. I, for example, noticed that my pharmacist was not allowed to mention the differences in the risks of bleeding from administrations of the different NSAID that are available over the counter. It would seem to be better if the physician would provide instructions that were unbiased regarding commercial interests and which tailored to the individual patient, taking into account the patient's age, gender, body weight, all diseases, and which medications the person takes. Such a simple reform would increase the efficacy of many treatments and reduce the side effects.

There are hopes that the effect of tolerance to opioids can be reduced by new approaches involving the immune system of the spinal cord and the brain. A basis for that is the finding that tolerance may be related to the function of microglia (the brain's immune system) and thus, related to the immune system in the brain [120, 412, 478]. Glia cells seem to be involved in some opioid side effects including those mediated by cytokine receptors, κ-opioid receptors, N-methyl-D-aspartate (NMDA receptors) receptors, and the recently elucidated Toll-like receptors. Newer agents targeting these receptors, such as AV411, MK-801, AV333, SLC022, and older agents used outside the United States for other disease conditions, such as minocycline, pentoxifylline, and UV50488H, all seem promising for providing significant relief from opioid side effects while simultaneously potentiating the pain relieving effect of opioids [154].

It has been indicated that tolerance to the analgesic effect of morphine is associated with apoptosis in the central nervous system [159]. Studies in rats showed that administration of minocycline, an antibiotic that influences immune reactions in the central nervous system, together with opioids, decreased the number of apoptotic cells in both the cerebral cortex and lumbar spinal cord [159] (see Chapter 10).

The results of these studies point to the importance of the brain immune system in pain and in pain medications. More recently, tolerance has been related to glia cells, especially to microglia [412]. Administration of valproate (an anticonvulsant used to treat epilepsy and bipolar disorder) has been tried for reducing tolerance to opioids. A study showed that it may reduce the tolerance effect [107]. Use of NMDA antagonists (Ketamine and MK801) has been suggested as a way to reduce the effect of tolerance. There are indications that administration of Valporate can reduce $\mu$ receptor tolerance.

# SECTION III
# PATHOLOGICAL PAIN

Pain that occurs without activation of nociceptors is called pathological pain. This type of pain is comprised of central neuropathic pain, muscle pain, and other forms of pain including fibromyalgia, myofascial pain, stroke pain, pain from amputations (phantom limb syndrome), and pain from injuries to the central nervous system including pain from head injuries and spinal cord injuries. Thalamic pain syndrome that includes pain and changed sensitivity to painful stimulation is a form of pathological pain that is caused by damage to the thalamus. Many pain conditions are caused by a combination of physiological and pathological pain.

Devor, 1999, and Bovie, 1999 [38, 103], have defined three main types of pain, namely: 1. Physiologic, 2. Inflammatory, 3. Neuropathic (pathological). Physiologic pain (also known as nociceptive pain) is the result of normal stimulation of nociceptors. Inflammatory pain is caused by varying kinds of inflammation and by tissue damage. Inflammatory pain overlaps with physiological and with pathological pain, in that nociceptive pain includes both the normal condition of stimulation of nociceptors and inflammatory pain that involves abnormal stimulation of pain receptors (Figure III.1).

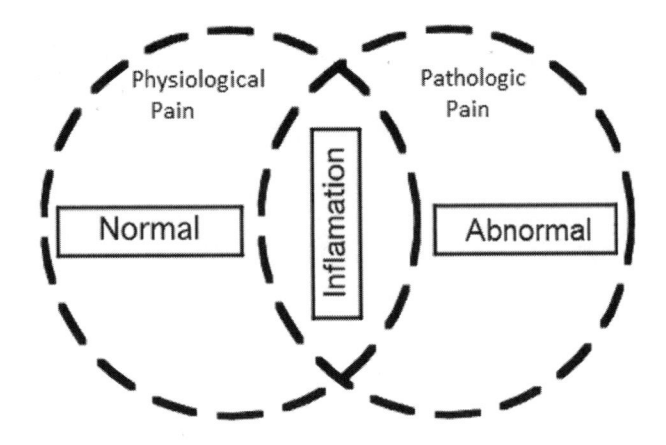

Figure III.1: A classification of pain that defines two main overlapping groups of pain, namely inflammatory pain that shares properties from both physiological pain and pathological pain. Physiological pain that can occur as a normal condition and as a result of inflammatory processes and pathological pain that also includes pain caused by inflammatory processes [103]. (Artwork by Irene Cunha.)

Inflammatory pain may be classified as a type of physiological pain (discussed in Section II) because it involves stimulation of pain receptors (nociceptors), but it can also be regarded as a form of pathological pain because it is not caused by the activation of pain receptors in normal tissue [103]. We will discuss inflammatory pain in Chapter 10.

In this section of Chapter 8, we will discuss central neuropathic pain; Chapter 9 will describe muscle pain. Inflammatory pain and the immune system in the central nervous system and its role in pathological pain will be discussed in Chapter 10. As is the case for physiological pain, pathological pain can also be modulated through activity in many parts of the brain. This is discussed in Chapter 11. Chapter 12 will discuss treatment for pathological pain, including ways to reduce the risk of developing pathological pain.

# CHAPTER 8
# Chronic Neuropathic Pain

# Abstract

1. Pathological pain that is caused by altered functions of specific parts of the central nervous system (central neuropathic pain) often lasts a long time; it is, therefore known as chronic neuropathic pain.

2. Chronic neuropathic pain causes enormous sufferings and it is a challenge to treat successfully.

3. Chronic neuropathic pain occurs without stimulation of pain receptors (nociceptors), but it may occur together with other forms of pain that are caused by stimulation of pain receptors.

4. Activation of (maladaptive) neuroplasticity plays an important role in creating and maintaining functional changes in the central nervous system that cause chronic neuropathic pain.

5. The functional changes that cause chronic neuropathic pain include changes in excitability, changes in routing of information, and changes in functional mapping of the body on many neural structures in the spinal cord and the brain. Changes in the mapping of the body on structures of the brain may change the perception of "self".

6. Therefore, chronic neuropathic pain is a plasticity disorder.

7. Absence of signals from the periphery can activate neuroplasticity causing deafferentation pain. Abnormal signals such as those of acute pain can also activate neuroplasticity, which creates central pain.

8. Many different parts of the brain are involved in central pain such the insular lobe, the premotor and supplemental motor areas, and the thalamo-cortical loop.

9. Also, the basal ganglia and parts of the "emotional brain", such as the amygdala, the anterior cingulate, the hippocampus, and the prefrontal cortex, are often involved.

10. Central pain occurs as one of several symptoms of many disorders such phantom limb syndrome, multiple sclerosis, strokes, and Parkinson's disease.

11. Chronic neuropathic pain has no apparent objective signs and it is, therefore, a phantom sensation.

12. Central neuropathic pain often has a strong emotional component such as depression indicating that the amygdala and the reward system of the brain are involved, as are the anterior cingulate gyrus and the hippocampus.

13. Pain from amputations is a part of phantom limb syndrome, which may include abnormal perception of "self" due to incorrect mapping on the brain of the amputated body part that can no longer be updated.

14. Spinal cord injuries may create pain as a part of the symptoms of spasticity.

15. The periaqueductal gray (PAG) plays a central role in modulation of pain.

16. Specific nerve cells, so-called wide dynamic range (WDR) neurons involved in generating the signals that cause the sensation of pain, are also involved in the modulation of pain. .

17. The sympathetic nervous system is heavily involved in many forms of central pain such as CRPS 1 and 2 and sympathetically maintained pain.

18. It has recently become evident that the immune system of the spinal cord and the brain can modulate pain.

# Introduction

Central neuropathic pain is a common form of pathological pain. The symptoms of central neuropathic pain are caused by abnormal functions of certain structures in the central nervous system (spinal cord and brain) without stimulation of pain receptors. Different authors have used different definitions of central neuropathic pain. Some [359][359][359] have used the (general) term neuropathic pain for pain caused by functional abnormalities and from structural lesions in the peripheral or central nervous system, which occurs without peripheral pain receptor stimulation. The term neuropathic pain, however, is now used to describe pain caused by pathologies of peripheral nerves and cranial nerves.

Central neuropathic pain causes enormous suffering and managing such disorders and other plasticity disorders is a challenge to the physician in regards to both its diagnosis and its treatment, which is generally unsatisfactory. Pain conditions that have lasted a long time often include a component of central neuropathic pain. However, central neuropathic pain may also occur alone and without any known cause.

The changes in function of the nervous system that cause pain without stimulation of pain receptors involve changes in the neural activity in different parts of the spinal cord and the brain. These changes may cause re-routing of information and alterations in the maps of the body that exist in the cerebral cortex and other parts of the brain. Naturally, that makes it difficult to diagnose these forms of pain and to choose the best treatment.

The change in function of the spinal cord and brain that causes central neuropathic pain is caused by activation of neuroplasticity. While plastic changes in function are often beneficial (good plasticity), are harmful (bad plasticity), causing symptoms of disorders ("plasticity disorders") [292][292][291](see Appendix A). Central neuropathic pain is an example of a plasticity disorder. Other types of plasticity disorders include some forms of tinnitus, spasticity, and synkinesis. Activation of neuroplasticity is suspected to play roles in causing the symptoms of diseases such as fibromyalgia (FM), chronic wide spread pain (CWP), low back pain, and carpal tunnel syndrome (CTS).

Central neuropathic pain often starts by physiological pain such as from trauma and that over time activate neuroplasticity and after some time the pain becomes permanent because of these changes while the initial cause of the pain has subsided or totally abolished.

# What is chronic neuropathic pain?

Chronic neuropathic pain (also known as central pain, CP) is a form of pathological pain that is a neurologic disorder caused by functional changes in the pain circuits in the spinal cord, the caudal trigeminal nucleus, and in several other parts of the brain. Chronic neuropathic pain occurs without signals from the peripheral part of the nervous system. CP often occurs together with other forms of pain including pain caused by stimulation of pain receptors (physiological pain). Chronic neuropathic pain causes more suffering than acute pain that is caused by stimulation of nociceptors, and it is more difficult to diagnose and treat this form of pain.

Chronic neuropathic pain is caused by abnormal neural activity generated by neural circuits in the spinal cord and the brain. Activation of neuroplasticity plays an important role in creating the functional changes that cause the pain. Central neuropathic pain is, therefore, a plasticity disorder [292]. The pathology of central neuropathic pain is a change in the function and in the organization of the dorsal horns of the spinal cord and in structures in the brain that normally process pain signals from the periphery of the nervous system. At the cellular level, neuroplasticity involves changes in synaptic efficacy, changes in protein synthesis, sprouting of axons and dendrites, and creation and elimination of synapses (see Appendix A).

These processes may be controlled by inherent (genetic and epigenetic factors) and environmental factors. Loss or reduction of normal inhibition in the spinal cord is assumed to contribute to the abnormal function that causes pain [214, 300].

Central pain occurs in many common disorders. Bonica (1991) [40] have estimated the prevalence of central neuropathic pain in spinal injuries, multiple sclerosis, epilepsy, Parkinson's disease, and after strokes (Table 8.1).

## TABLE 8.1

| DISEASE | TOTAL PERSONS | PEOPLE WITH CP | PEOPLE WITH CP |
|---|---|---|---|
| Spinal Cord Injury | 225,000 | 68,000 | 30 percent |
| Multiple Sclerosis | 150,000 | 42,000 | 28 percent |
| Stroke | 2,000,000 | 168,000 | 8.4 percent |
| Epilepsy | 1,600,000 | 44,800 | 2.8 percent |
| Parkinson's Disease | 500,000 | 50,000 | 10 percent |

Table 8.1 Estimated Prevalence of Major Disorders with Central Pain (CP) in the USA 1989 (population approximately 250 million). Data from Bonica, J. J. (1991). Introduction: semantic, epidemiologic, and educational issues. Pain and central nervous system disease: the central pain syndromes. K. L. Casey. New York, Raven Press: 13-29 [40]; and Rubinstein, B., T. Österberg, et al. (1992). "Longitudinal fluctuations in tinnitus reported by an elderly population." J. Audiol Med., 1: 149-155. [40]

# Symptoms and signs of pathological pain

Central neuropathic pain presents as pain of varying intensity and it may be referred to specific body parts. The pain is often accompanied by an abnormal perception of pain such as hyperpathia [371]. Hyperpathia is an abnormal reaction to pain caused by the stimulation of pain receptors, such as a needle prick. When hyperpathia is present, such light to moderately painful stimulation causes an exaggerated and prolonged pain sensation. Other abnormalities that often accompany central neuropathic pain are allodynia, which is pain from a light touch.

Individuals who have central neuropathic pain often have lowered thresholds to pain elicited by the stimulation of pain receptors (hyperalgesia). Also, temporal integration of painful stimuli is abnormal [300], often described as the "wind-up" phenomenon [105].

# Perception of pain

Pain has two components, namely, the perception (the strength and character) of the pain and its effect on a person causing emotional distress and affecting a person's entire life (quality of life). The effect that pain has on a person is not directly related to its strength and its character. It is often the strength of pain that is measured (for example, on an analog scale from 1 to 10) and that does not accurately describe the effect of the pain on a person. Thus, the way pain affects a person is not directly related to the intensity of the pain as it is assessed on an analog scale.

The same strength of pain may cause suffering in one person while another person may say, "I have pain, but pain does not have me". The way pain affects a person is closely related to the person's ability to cope with the pain. The opposite is catastrophizing where a person worries in an extreme way.

# Coping

Since pain often causes suffering, it is important to be able to cope with pain, especially chronic pathological pain. Coping has to do with how a person perceives his/her pain and deals with it; thus, a matter of quality of life. Coping is a learned skill and it is important that those who treat patients with chronic pain can help their patients learn the technique of coping. People have learned to live with their pain, by understanding their pain and by remembering that escapable and inescapable pain is different. Some of the structures of the brain that are involved in coping are known. It may be important that some of the neural structures, such as the nucleus accumbens, that are involved in pain are the same as those involved in rewards [74].

Severe tinnitus and pathological pain have many similarities and it has been shown that knowing about the auditory system and tinnitus is beneficial in the treatment of tinnitus. Tinnitus retraining therapy, TRT, is used as a common treatment and was developed by Pawel Jastreboff [190].

# Catastrophizing

Catastrophizing may be regarded as the opposite of coping (Figure 8.1) [422]. It has to do with increased worrying and fearing the worst. It is irrational thoughts that a bad situation will turn worse. Catastrophizing decreases the quality of life without actual causes. Studies have shown that catastrophizing painful stimulation contributes to more intense pain experiences and increased emotional distress.

The opposite of catastrophizing is confrontation with the problem and a positive attitude that involves expecting matters to improve and become better. Confrontation is beneficial in that it may in itself reduce the cause of matters such as pain. Many people are afraid of repeating a fall, for example. Confrontation of the problem would mean to examine and attempt to correct the causes of the fall. A person who catastrophizing will instead avoid situations with risk of falling.

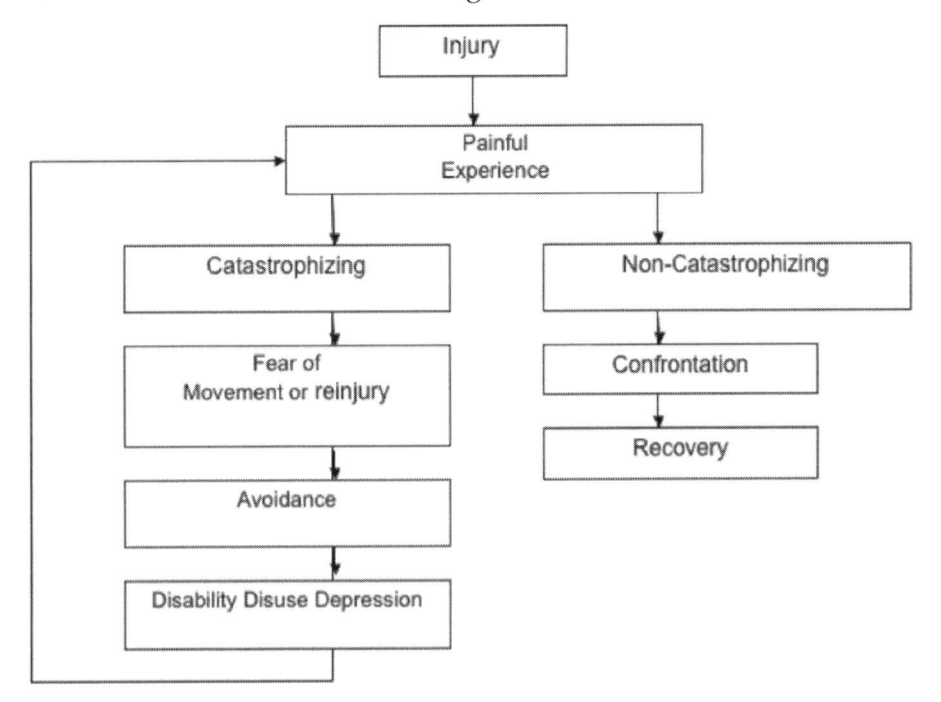

Figure 8.1 Cognitive-behavioral model of fear of movement and injury (Fear-avoidance belief). (Data from Fear of movement/(re) injury in chronic low back pain and its relation to behavioral performance. Vlaeyen JW, Kole-Snijders AM, Boeren RG, van Eek H. Pain. 1995 Sep, 62 (3):363-72 [455] Chpt. 20. Textbook of Pain, 2006.) (Artwork by Monica Javidnia.)

Studies of the effect of catastrophizing painful experiences are few, but the findings have been consistent in showing a relation between catastrophizing and the severity of the effect of pain. A review of the literature on the relationship between catastrophizing and pain shows several different theoretical models and suggests that catastrophizing might best be viewed from the perspective of hierarchical levels of analysis, where social factors and social goals may play a role in the development and maintenance of catastrophizing [422].

# Phantom sensations

Central neuropathic pain is a phantom sensation [291, 296]. Many forms of tinnitus are also phantom sensations [291, 296]. Phantom sensations are sensations that have no physical cause. Other phantom sensations include tingling, parenthesis, and other abnormal sensations including central neuropathic pain that may occur after the amputation of a limb (phantom limb syndrome).

The name phantom pain refers to sensations that are not caused by the stimulation of receptors, but created in the central nervous system [188]. Phantom sensations that often occur after amputations of a body part, such as a limb (phantom limb syndrome), are some of the clearest signs that changes of the function of the central nervous system (spinal cord and brain) can cause symptoms such as pain without any structural changes detected with the methods commonly available. Phantom limb symptoms, in addition to pain, include tingling and other abnormal somatic sensations (paresthesia) such as itching.

The anatomical and physiological bases for phantom sensations are tied to hyperexcitability and reorganization of neural structures in the spinal cord and the brain, especially in the brain stem, thalamus, and cortical sensory and motor regions. Activation of the autonomic nervous system also occurs in connection with central pain.

The functional changes may also include re-routing of information, which may explain symptoms that often accompany pathological pain such as allodynia, hyperpathia [371], and changes in temporal integration.

Phantom limb syndrome also often includes altered body perception (altered "self"). These changes in perception of the "self" that occur after amputations, such as of a limb, are assumed to be caused by changes in the maps of the body that are in the brain and which were created before the amputation and not updated as they used to be.

# Hyperpathia

Hyperpathia is the term used to describe the prolongation and exaggeration of the sensation from mild to moderate painful stimulations that often occur in connection with chronic neuropathic pain. Hyperpathia is a sign of central sensitization such as occurs in state 3 of Doubell's classification of different states in which the dorsal horn can operate[109]. Hyperpathia may be regarded as a pathology in itself that adds to the suffering of neuropathic pain. The pathophysiology of hyperpathia is unknown but clinical experience show that it can be alleviated by antidepressive drugs that affect serotonin receptors and that indicate that serotonin may play a role in causing hyperpathia (clinically amitriptyline and nortriptylin have been found to be the most effective antidepressive drugs in treating hyperpathia).

# "Wind-up" phenomenon

The "wind-up" phenomenon describes the increased pain sensations that are experienced when transient painful stimuli are repeated with short intervals. The pain sensation is stronger to a stimulus that follows immediately after another pain stimulation; thus, a sign of temporal integration. Temporal integration means that a response to stimulation is affected (increased) when it follows after a stimulus compared with when presented alone (see Figure 8.2).

Changes in temporal integration are signs that occur in pathological pain along with allodynia and hyperpathia that were mentioned above. A change in the temporal integration of painful stimuli has been demonstrated to occur for stimulations above threshold (known as the "wind-up" phenomenon) and at threshold.

Temporal integration (summation) is the opposite of adaptation. Individuals with central neuropathic pain often have exaggerated signs of this "wind-up" phenomenon. Studies have shown that the "wind-up" phenomenon is associated with a (glutamate) receptor, the N-Methyl-D-aspartate (NMDA) receptor. Administration of an antagonist to the NMDA receptor (5-aminophosphnovaleric acid) abolished the wind-up effect as shown by the change of the responses from cells in the dorsal horn (of anesthetized rats) (Figure 8.2). The results show signs that the "wind-up" phenomenon is NMDA mediated. Similar results were obtained using MK801 or 7-chlorokynurenic acid.

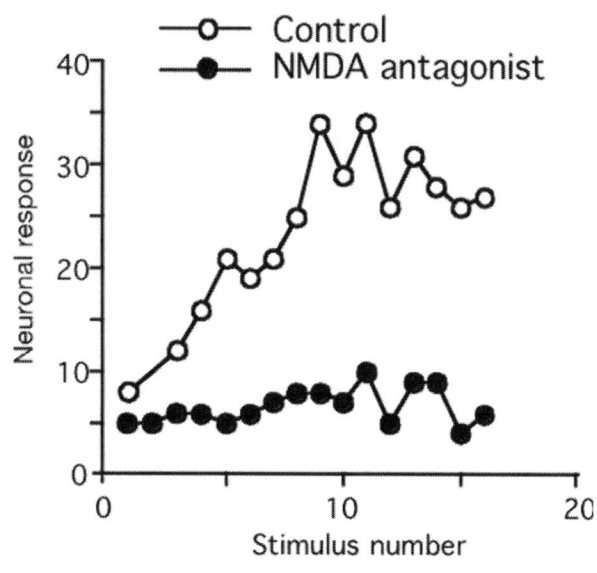

Figure 8.2 Neuronal responses from cells in the dorsal horn of the spinal cord in anesthetized rats to repeated pain stimuli before and after administration of a NMDA receptor antagonist. The responses without the receptor antagonist Increase after each stimulus, up to 8 stimuli, has been presented, indicating temporal summation (the "wind-up" phenomenon).

Response with and without a NMDA antagonist is shown. The open circles show control responses elicited by 16 consecutive, constant peripheral stimulation at three times the C-fiber threshold, applied at 0.5 pulses per second (pps).

Filled circles show the response after administration of a NMDA receptor antagonist, 5-aminophosphnovaleric acid. (Data from Dickenson, A.H., NMDA receptors antagonists as an analgesic. Prog. in Pain Res. and Management, 1994. 1: p. 173-187 [105].)

## Temporal integration at threshold

The "wind-up" phenomenon regards pain well above threshold. Temporal integration can also be demonstrated at threshold of pain. This can be done by applying electrical impulses to the skin at different rates. When obtained in persons with signs of central neuropathic pain, the results were different from results obtained in individuals who did not have pain [300] (Figure 8.3). The expression of temporal integration is different when assessed at threshold compared with the "wind-up" phenomenon, which reflects temporal integration for stimuli above threshold.

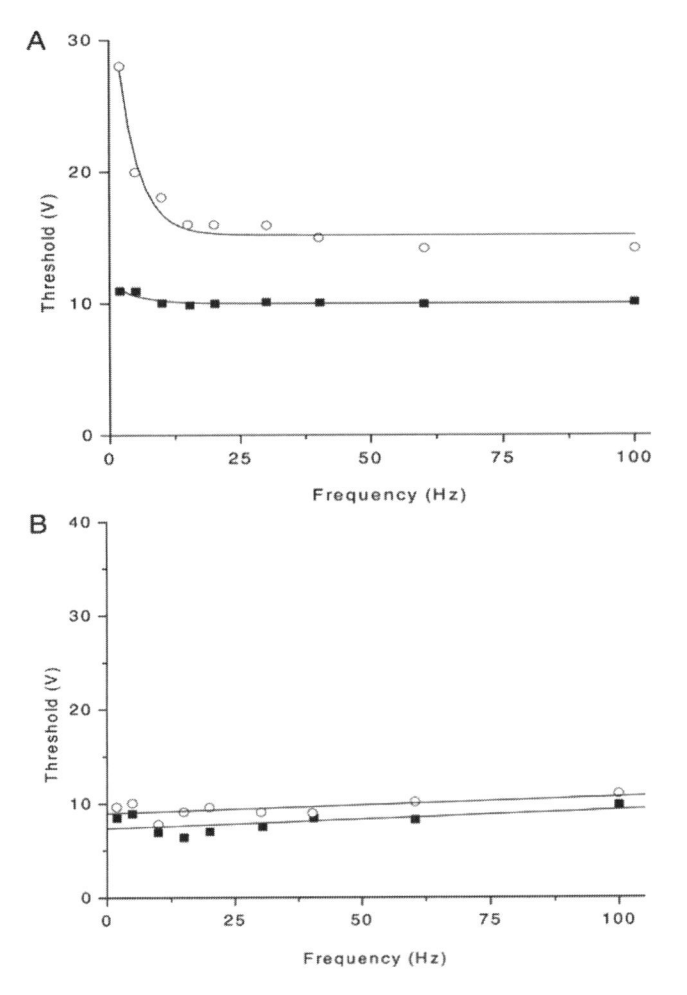

Figure 8.3 Temporal integration in an individual without pain (A) and in an individual with signs of central neuropathic pain (B). The threshold of sensation (filled squares) and pain (open circles) in response to electrical stimulation with impulses applied to the skin of the forearm are shown as a function of the frequency of the impulses. The threshold for just noticeable tingling (filled squares) and the threshold for a pain sensation (open circles) are shown to illustrate temporal integration in an individual without pain (From Møller, A.R. and T. Pinkerton, Temporal integration of pain from electrical stimulation of the skin. Neurol. Res., 1997. 19: p. 481-488, [300].)

In this study, electrical impulses, presented at different rates, were applied to the skin of the arm. When the strength was increased, the first sensation that was noted was a weak tingling sensation. When the strength of the electrical impulses was increased further, at certain strength, the sensation changes distinctly from a strong tingling to a painful sensation.

The study showed that in individuals who did not have pain, the threshold to painful stimulations decreased when the rate with which the stimuli were presented was increased (shorter intervals between individual impulses). This means that stimulation at a high rate was more effective in eliciting a sensation pain than impulses presented at a slow rate, thus with long intervals between the impulses. In other words, the threshold to an electrical stimulation is lowered by the presence of a preceding stimulus. This is a sign of temporal integration.

On the other hand, the threshold to innocuous stimulations that caused tingling only depended little on the rate with which the impulses were presented; thus, indicating an absence of temporal integration in the range of the frequency of the impulses that were tested. This means that transient painful stimulation, such as electrical stimulation, is normally subjected to temporal integration whereas the innocuous sensation from electrical stimulation has few or no signs of temporal integration (Figure 8.3).

The situation is different in an individual with signs of central neuropathic pain as shown in Figure 8.3B, which shows results obtained in a person who had developed central pain from trauma to an arm. In this individual, there is little difference between the threshold for tingling and the threshold for pain and the threshold is not noticeably dependent on the rate with which the stimuli are presented; thus, indicating that there were no noticeable signs of temporal integration for pain in this individual [300].

Also, the pain threshold was lowered and it became close to that of sensation (tingling).

# Emotional components of pain

There is considerable evidence that severe persistent pain can have negative effects on a person. Pain can cause or interact with affective (mood related) symptoms, such as fear, anxiety, and depression [312]. The nuclei of the amygdala play an important role in such interactions. Evidence from anatomical, neuroimaging, behavioral, electrophysiological, pharmacological, and biochemical data all implicate the amygdala in pain modulation and emotional responses to pain.

The amygdala is involved in memory functions, especially regarding memories of fearful events. A certain part of the amygdala is now defined as the "nociceptive amygdala" [312]. There is evidence that this part integrates nociceptive information with poly-modal information about the internal and external bodily environment. The amygdala seems both to have a facilitatory and an inhibitory role in the modulation of nociceptive processing at different levels of the pain neuroaxis. It is also known that the function of the amygdala is plastic and its function can change as a result of external and internal factors. This may explain the variations in affective components of severe pain [312].

# Depression

Depression often occurs as a part of the symptoms in chronic pain disorders [9]. It is known that many of the anatomical structures in the brain that are also activated by pain are activated in individuals who have depression. The structures include the insular cortex, the prefrontal cortex, the anterior cingulate cortex, the amygdala, and the hippocampus. Also, neural circuits that are associated with addictions (reward system) in the brain are also involved in some forms of pain [74]. The hypothalamic-pituitary-adrenal axis, limbic structures, and structures adjacent to the limbic structures are involved in addition to the ascending and descending pain tracts. Also, common neurochemicals, such as monoamines (epinephrine, norepinephrine), cytokines, and neurotrophic factors, are active in both pain and depression.

Cytokines are small regulatory proteins that are produced by white blood cells and a variety of other cells including those in the nervous system. The molecular structure of cytokines is quite diverse. Some of them form long-chain 4-helix bundles (e.g. interleukin (IL)-6); others form jelly rolls (e.g. tumor necrosis factor-alpha (TNF-$\alpha$)), or $\beta$-trefoils (e.g. IL-1b). Cytokines act at hormonal concentrations through high-affinity receptors [411].

Many psychological signs of pain and depression are similar. One explanation for the interaction and potentiation of the disease burden experienced by patients affected by both pain and depression is provided by the concept of allostasis (stability or balance, homeostasis) [362].

The secondary somatosensory cortex is also involved in the recollection of remote (not recent) memories of fearful events (not memories that were not associated with emotional charge) [368]. This further supports the hypothesis that suffering, such as from pain, may be related to memories, as has been suggested for severe tinnitus that has similarities with pain [189].

# Causes of chronic neuropathic pain

Changes in the central nervous system (spinal cord and brain) with pathological pain are extensive. The changes may be initiated by injuries to peripheral nerves that cause a cascade at the molecular and cellular levels that initiate neuroplasticity, resulting in widespread changes in function and morphology. Injuries to nerves together with inflammation are now believed to be conditions that can initiate processes that can cause pathological pain through expression of neuroplasticity.

Learning is assumed to underlie the mechanisms that makes pain become chronic[8, 117] and many forms of neuropathic pain may start with physiological pain (pain caused by activation of pain receptors), which, after some time, activate harmful plasticity resulting in activity in central nervous system structures that are perceived as pain sensations. This harmful neural activity may be maintained without input from pain receptors. Chronic neuropathic pain thereby becomes an example of how harmful plasticity can create dysfunctional neural networks in the brain by disrupting default-mode network dynamics (DMND).

The induced changes in function include altered synaptic efficacy, changes in protein synthesis, elimination and creation of synapses, dendrites and axons, and reduced synaptic inhibition in the dorsal horn of the spinal cord and in different parts of the brain (see Appendix A). Changes in excitability can occur by changes in the balance between inhibition and excitation (most cells have both inhibitory and excitatory input) and by changing the cell's threshold. The subsequent changes in function are increased excitability and re-routing of information. The plastic changes often occur in steps where different kinds of changes follow each other in a sequence.

Pathological pain may occur together with physiological pain caused by stimulation of pain receptors in normal or in pathological tissue. Sensitization, peripherally or centrally, plays an important role in the development of central pain. In fact, central sensitization is a fundamental component of the events that cause pathological pain. Central sensitization manifests as pain hypersensitivity, particularly dynamic tactile allodynia, secondary punctuate or pressure hyperalgesia, after sensations, and enhanced temporal summation that causes altered processing in the spinal cord [487].

Changes in pain sensitivity from central sensitization to pain is an important component of many different kinds of pain including fibromyalgia, osteoarthritis, musculoskeletal disorders, headaches, temporo-mandibular joint disorders, dental pain, neuropathic pain, visceral pain hypersensitivity disorders, and post-surgical pain [487].

Schwann cell and/or *nervi nervorum* activation could be an additional mechanism of pain generation. In the peripheral nervous system, Schwann cell activation in response to infection and trauma releases many neuroexcitatory substances [28]. Activation of the nervi nervorum in the peripheral nervous system also leads to the release of calcitonin gene related peptides, substance P, and nitric oxide. Such activation plays a role in initiating the plastic changes that cause central neuropathic pain.

The roles of glia cells (microglia and astrocytes) in these processes that cause central neuropathic pain are extensive, but have only relatively recently become apparent. Interestingly, microglia does not seem to be involved in physiological pain. There is a two-way involvement of microglia in that neuronal activity affects microglia though neuronal secretion of adenosine triphosphate (ATP) and microglia affect neuronal activity by secretion of many different cytokines, chemokines, neurotrophines, and tumor necrosis factor alpha (TGN-$\alpha$) [147, 278].

Identifying the cause of central pain is less important for the management of the pain (see Chapter 12) than what is the case for pain that is evoked by stimulation of pain receptors (physiological pain, see Chapter 3).

The start of a person's central neuropathic pain can rarely be found. There are, however, some factors that are believed to contribute to the development of central neuropathic pain. Post-herpetic neuralgia, trigeminal neuralgia, bodily trauma, diabetic neuropathy, spinal cord injuries, cancer, strokes, and degenerative neurological diseases may lead to central neuropathic pain [359]. Trauma naturally causes pain, but when the pain persists beyond healing of the wounds, the pain normally becomes central neuropathic pain, thus pathological pain rather than physiologic pain. It, therefore, becomes a different form of pain than the original trauma pain and any intervention at the anatomical location of the original lesion has little success in relieving the pain.

Trigeminal neuralgia and glossopharyngeal neuralgia were discussed in the chapter on peripheral and cranial nerves. However, it has become evident that these disorders are not directly disorders of the respective cranial nerves, but rather forms of plasticity changes in the function of their respective cranial nerve nuclei that are caused by activation of neuroplasticity. These disorders may, therefore, be regarded to be plasticity diseases.

# Pathology of chronic neuropathic pain

Despite much research, the pathophysiology of chronic neuropathic pain is incompletely understood. The process of developing chronic pain is complex and may be different for different forms of chronic neuropathic pain and different processes may be involved. It is generally assumed that activation of harmful (maladaptive) neuroplasticity plays an important role in initiation and maintenance of central neuropathic pain[339].

The pathways that are involved in severe central neuropathic pain are complex and poorly understood. At least parts of these pathways are probably the same as those mediating pain from stimulation of nociceptors. The organization of these pathways is dynamic and involves a high degree of parallel processing, including connections with autonomic systems and limbic structures.

While plastic changes (expression of neuroplasticity) in the nervous system undoubtedly play some role in most pain conditions, it plays a dominating role in chronic (central) neuropathic pain[8, 248, 488, 489].

Affective symptoms such as depression often accompany severe pain, and these symptoms may be explained by the establishment of new connections in the pain pathways in the brain or spinal cord or by amplifying existing pathways. The medial portion of the thalamus is likely to be involved providing subcortical connections to limbic structures such as the amygdala nuclei[227], the SMA, and prefrontal cortex. In these respects, central neuropathic pain has many similarities with other hyperactive sensory disorders such as tinnitus[62, 285, 299].

Studies have also found that structures of the hippocampus, the insula and amygdala are involved in many forms of pain. The insula is a complex structure that is poorly known. It has recently been associated with such complex functions as identification of one's own body - the "self". The techniques used have been resting state functional connectivity[20, 117, 273] . The thalamus and the corticothalamic loop has been suggested to play an important role in chronic neuropathic pain[237, 465].

Lesions in the cingulate gyrus have been made to treat severe chronic pain with some success[160, 329]. Although lesions in other limbic structures are effective in treating psychiatric disorders, their efficacy in treating pain has not been established[151]. This is another sign that many different anatomical structures are involved in the different forms of chronic neuropathic pain.

Chronic neuropathic pain is associated with several forms of changes in neural processing of pain. One such change is the abnormal processing causing allodynia and hyperpathia. Hyperpathia is a sign of changes in the processing of painful stimuli, whereas allodynia is a sign of re-routing of information (cross modal interaction).

Imaging studies such as MRI and conventional neurophysiologic tests usually do not reveal any noticeable abnormalities in persons with chronic neuropathic pain. The patient's description of the symptoms is the only assessable measure of central neuropathic pain.

The use of an analog scale of the patient' perception of the pain may be of some help but the fact that the suffering from pain is poorly correlated with the perception of the pain makes such measures of limited value in assessing the severity of and individual person's pain.

There is recent evidence that the neural activity in the brain that is related to chronic neuropathic pain is different from that of acute pain. Hashmi et al 2013 [158] described the transition between acute pain and chronic neuropathic pain using back pain as a model. They showed that brain activity in the acute or subacute stages of back pain back pain is limited to the same regions as involved in acute pain but in the chronic stage neural activity has shifted to circuits that are usually active in emotions. These investigators also found that reward circuitry was active both in the acute stage and in the chronic stage.

The results of these studies have thus demonstrated that areas of the brain that are active for the same percept of pain, can shift when pain changes from acute to chronic pain. These observations are another example of revised understanding of how different brain regions are activated and they confirm the contemporary understanding that connections in the brain are dynamic and that many different regions may be involved in a specific task.

During the development of chronic neuropathic pain, several changes in brain anatomy have been observed. There are morphological changes associated with chronic pain [18]. For example, gray matter density decreased and functional connectivity between nucleus accumbens with parts of the prefrontal cortex could predict the persistence of the pain Some investigators took this observation as a confirmation that corticostrial circuits are causally involved in the transition between acute pain and chronic pain [17].

Apkarian and his co-investigators found that the structure of the brain's white matter can predict how a person with low back pain would recover from the pain [247]. These abnormalities encompass emotional, autonomic, and pain perception regions of the brain, implying that they likely play a critical role in the global clinical picture of complex regional pain syndromes (CRPS). Members of the Apkarian laboratory have shown that the volume of grey matter in the brains of the same persons who had persistent pain decreased over a years time [158]. They showed that brain activity could be used to predict whether a subject would recover or would experience persistent pain.

There is thus evidence that many structures in the brain are involved in chronic pain including the hippocampus[305] and that changes in the connections between different structures may explain the emotional reactions to chronic pain [101].

# Reorganization of central pain pathways

It has been shown recently that there are many connections between different parts of the brain and the a specific task is not carried out only in a certain region of the brain but many parts are connected and involved in processing of information and generating commands. As an example it has been shown that much larger cortical regions are involved in simple tasks such as interpretation of a spoken word [440].

It was assumed earlier that diseases were caused by malfunction of a specific of the brain. That is not correct either and evidence has been presented that malfunction of many parts of the brain is involved in generating symptoms of disease. It has also been shown that these connections are dynamic, meaning that they can change. It is now believed that altered connections are in many cases signs of pathologies. There are recent studies that indicate that changes in connections between different parts of the brain are involved in age related changes [21, 377, 378] and in causing symptoms of disease [17, 379]

Recent studies have shown evidence of strong involvement of the state of the motivational and emotional mesolimbic-prefrontal circuitry of the brain. Nociceptive inputs elicit plastic changes within this circuitry are involved in shifting the pattern of brain involvement from acute pain to chronic pain thereby making the pain less somatic and more affective in nature [248].

# The role of the dorsal horn (and the trigeminal nucleus) in causing chronic neuropathic pain

Altered processing at the segmental and at supraspinal levels was discussed above in connection with physiological pain. Similar changes may be involved in chronic neuropathic pain[488, 489] and both peripheral and central sensitization are most likely play important roles in creating the symptoms of many forms of chronic neuropathic pain[39, 243]. Deprivation of input or overstimulation can cause such plastic changes of the nervous system.

Central sensitization and peripheral sensitization of pain receptors play important roles in creating chronic neuropathic pain [39, 489, 491]. Central sensitization of pain circuits may occur in the dorsal horn of the spinal cord (and of the CN V nucleus) and at supraspinal levels.

Changes in the function of specific parts of the spinal cord and the brain that are associated with central neuropathic pain are complex and poorly understood. At least parts of the structures that are involved are probably the same as those that are activated by stimulation of nociceptors. The pathways for physiological pain that were described in Chapter 3 have connections to many parts of the brain.

This may be viewed as a form of parallel processing that makes it possible for pain signals to reach many parts of the brain, including the autonomic systems and limbic structures. Since the connections between nerve cells depend on synapses being active, changes in synaptic efficacy that occur when neuroplasticity is activated can alter the routes that are used. Opening (unmasking) dormant synapses can establish new routes from connections that normally connect to their target cells through dormant synapses. Closing (masking) active synapses that connect axons to their target cells can inactivate (block) routes that have been active. This makes the organization of pain pathways dynamic.

The changes that may occur in the central nervous system causing central neuropathic pain may have several stages that may be executed sequentially or in parallel. Similar sequential processes are known from other pathologies such as, for example, the creation of diabetes neuropathy.

There is recent evidence that the neural activity in the brain that is related to chronic (central) pain is different from that of acute pain. Hashmi et al 2013 [158] described the transition between acute pain and chronic neuropathic pain and showed that using back pain as a model.

Hashmi et al showed that brain activity in the acute or subacute stages of back pain back pain group is limited to the same regions as involved in acute pain but in the chronic stage neural activity has shifted to circuits that are usually active in emotions. These investigators also found that reward circuitry was active both in the acute stage and in the chronic stage. The results these studies have thus demonstrate that areas of the brain that are active for the same percept, pain, can shift when pain changes from acute to chronic pain. These observations are another example of revised understanding of how different brain regions are activated and confirm the contemporary understanding that connections in the brain are dynamic and that many different regions may be involved in a specific task.

The organization of pain pathways is dynamic and involves a high degree of parallel processing, including connections with autonomic systems and limbic structures. Affective symptoms such as depression often accompany severe pain, and these symptoms may be explained by the establishment of new connections in the pain pathways in the brain or spinal cord or by amplifying existing pathways.

The medial-dorsal portion of the thalamus is likely to be involved providing subcortical connections to limbic structures such as the amygdala nuclei [227], the PMA, SMA, and prefrontal cortex. In these respects, central neuropathic pain has many similarities with other hyperactive sensory disorders such as tinnitus[62, 285, 299].

It has been shown recently that there are many connections between different parts of the brain and the a specific task is not carried out only in a certain region of the brain but many parts are connected and involved in processing of information and generating commands. As an example it has been shown that much larger cortical regions are involved in simple tasks such as interpretation of a spoken word [440].

There are many signs that chronic neuropathic pain is associated with changes routing of signals and in neural processing of pain. The abnormal processing causing allodynia and hyperpathia are examples of sign of changes in the processing of painful stimuli, whereas allodynia is a signs of re-routing of information (cross modal interaction). Studies have found that structures of the hippocampus, the insula and amygdala are involved in many forms of pain. The insula is a complex structure that is poorly known.

Chronic neuropathic pain has recently been associated with such complex functions as identification of one's own body - the "self". Reorganization of the thalamus and particularly the cortico-thalamic circuits shave been implicated in chronic neuropathic pain[54, 57].

Recent studies of functional connectivity in the brain have also provided valuable insight in the pathology of chronic neuropathic pain. The techniques used in studies of connectivity have been resting state functional connectivity[20, 67, 117, 273] . The thalamus and the corticothalamic loop have been suggested to play an important role in chronic neuropathic pain[54, 237, 465]. Such recent studies have shown evidence of strong involvement of the state of the motivational and emotional mesolimbic-prefrontal circuitry of the brain. Nociceptive inputs elicit plastic changes within this circuitry are involved in shifting the pattern of brain involvement from acute pain to chronic pain thereby making the pain less somatic and more affective in nature [248].

Learning is assumed to underlie the mechanisms that makes pain become chronic[8, 117] and many forms of neuropathic pain may start with physiological pain (pain caused by activation of pain receptors), which, after some time, activate harmful (maladaptive) neuroplasticity resulting in activity in central nervous system structures that are perceived as pain sensations. This harmful neural activity may be maintained without input from pain receptors. Chronic neuropathic pain thereby becomes an example of how harmful plasticity can create dysfunctional neural networks in the brain by disrupting default-mode network dynamics (DMND). Such studies have brought evidence that many connections in the brain are dynamic, meaning that they can change. It is now believed that altered connections are in many cases signs of pathologies.

Recent studies have indicated that changes in connections between different parts of the brain are involved in age related changes[21, 377, 378] and in causing symptoms of disease such as pain[54, 67] and tinnitus[17, 379]. It was assumed earlier that diseases were caused by malfunction of a specific part of the brain but such recent evidence indicate that malfunction of many parts of the brain is involved in generating symptoms of many kinds of diseases.

Altered processing of nociceptive information at the segmental and at supraspinal levels are also involved in chronic neuropathic pain[488, 489] and both peripheral and central sensitization most likely play important roles in creating the symptoms of many forms of central neuropathic pain[39, 243]. Deprivation of input or overstimulation can cause such plastic changes of the nervous system.

# Cortical representation of the body is dynamic

The sensory representation in the somatosensory cortex is well known (Figure 8.4). The surface of the body is mapped onto the surface of different regions of the cerebral somatosensory cortex.

Mapping of the body surface on the somatosensory cortices (mainly regarding primary cortices) has been described in detail. The map of the body on the primary somatosensory cortex is illustrated by the familiar homunculus by Penfield and Rasmussen [328] (Figure 8.4).

It deserves to be emphasized that the other cortical areas also have maps of the body, but more complex ones and these maps are less well known. Other brain regions that are activated in connection with pain probably also have maps of the body and these maps may be equally important to those of the primary cerebral cortices.

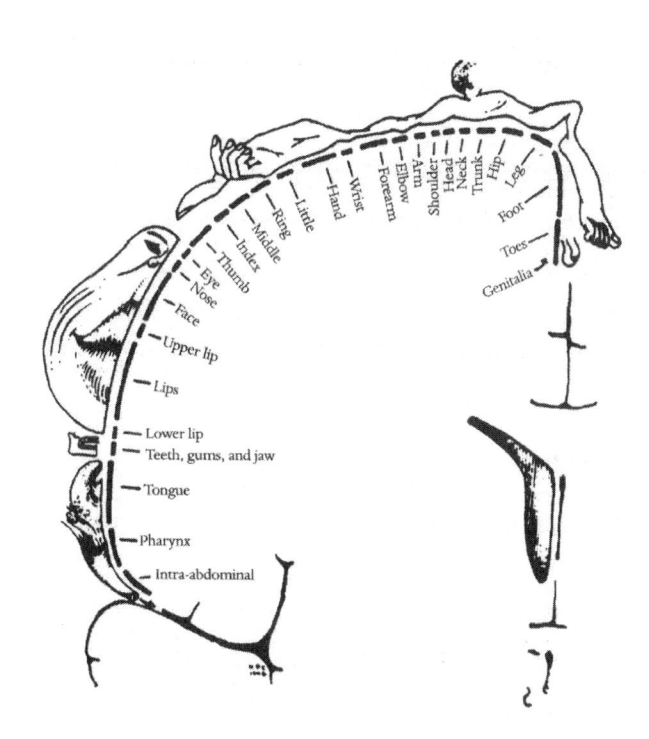

Figure 8.4 The representation of the body on the somatosensory cortex. Notice that the fingers are represented on the cerebral cortex close to the representation of the face (forehead). (Based on Penfield, W. and T. Rasmussen, The cerebral cortex of man: a clinical study of localization of function. 1950, New York: Macmillan. [328])

Cortical maps, however, are not stable, but subject to change as a result of the brain not being hard wired, but plastic (it is malleable). Many factors can activate neuroplasticity so that the representations of specific body parts change. Extensive use of, for example, one or more fingers causes the area of the sensory cerebral cortex that represents the finger in question to expand on the expense of neighboring cortical areas [113]. A decrease in use may cause shrinkage of the cortical areas that represent the function in question.

Amputations of limbs deprive large areas of the somatosensory cortex from sensory input, leaving areas unused. This promotes ingrowths of sprouts from cells in other neighboring somatosensory areas so that the unused areas may become taken over by other areas of the cerebral cortex.

Changes in cortical maps mainly occur because of changes in the efficacy of synapses. There is a morphological basis for extensive overlaps of cortical areas, but functionally, such overlap is limited by the fact that many synapses are non-conducting (dormant). These non-conducting (dormant) synapses can be made to conduct (unmasked) by activation of neuroplasticity [460], thereby extending cortical areas of representation of the body surface. Closing of synapses that are normally conducting can likewise change cortical maps in the opposite direction, shrinking the areas of the cortex that represent certain areas of the body or certain functions.

With regard to pain, there is evidence that its cortical representation is less pronounced than often assumed. Some studies have found evidence that the secondary somatosensory cortex may have a greater involvement than the primary cortices. This also agrees with the fact that the dorsal and medial thalamus, which are much involved with pain, project to secondary and association cortices, and to different other structures such as the anterior cingulate and the amygdala.

# Phantom limb syndrome

Phantom limb syndrome is sensations of pain, tingling and other somatosensory sensations that are felt as coming from a limb that has been amputated. These sensations are felt as if they come from specific parts of an amputated body part such as a limb. The phantom (ghost) limb symptoms are therefore a clear example of somatosensory sensations that are created in the central nervous system without input from receptors in the body. Phantom pain is a clear example of pain and other sensations that are felt at a different location of the body than that where the neural activity that causes the pain is generated. It is obvious that the neural activity that causes the phantom limb sensations is not evoked by physical stimulation at the location where the sensations are felt. Instead, the abnormal neural activity that causes the sensations must be generated in the spinal cord or the brain without any signals from outside reaching the central nervous system.

The cause is re-organization and changes in function of specific parts of the central nervous system. The abnormal functions that produce phantom limb symptoms are caused by maladaptive neuroplasticity [123] elicited by the absence of normal sensory input from the periphery or by excessive stimulation. Deprivation of input is the strongest promoter of plastic changes in the spinal cord and the brain.

The abnormal sensations associated with phantom limb syndrome, pain, tingling and itching, are referred to specific anatomical locations on an amputated limb. Phantom limb syndrome occurs frequently. In a study of amputees of war veterans where over sixty percent responded, 85 percent of these individuals who had had an amputation reported that they experience phantom sensations in their amputated limb, and the majority of the sensations are painful [390].

The existence of phantom limb syndrome confirms that neural circuits in the central nervous system (spinal cord and brain) can produce sensations that are referred to specific anatomical locations on the body without any physical stimulus being applied to that location.

Phantom sensations are some of the clearest signs of harmful plastic changes in the nervous system [293]. Other forms of deafferentation can also cause phantom pain sensations. Symptoms of harmful plastic changes include tinnitus, tingling, pain, parenthesis, and other abnormal sensations.

# Causes of pain after amputations

The anatomical and physiological basis for phantom sensations can be tied to hyper-excitability and reorganization of neural structures in the spinal cord and the brain. Activation of the autonomic nervous system plays an important role in the generation of phantom limb symptoms. It has been suggested that the risk of developing phantom limb pain depends on the pain that an individual has before the amputation and the neural activity caused during the operation (Figure 8.5). People who had a limb amputated, but did not have pain in the limb before the amputation, may still get phantom pain.

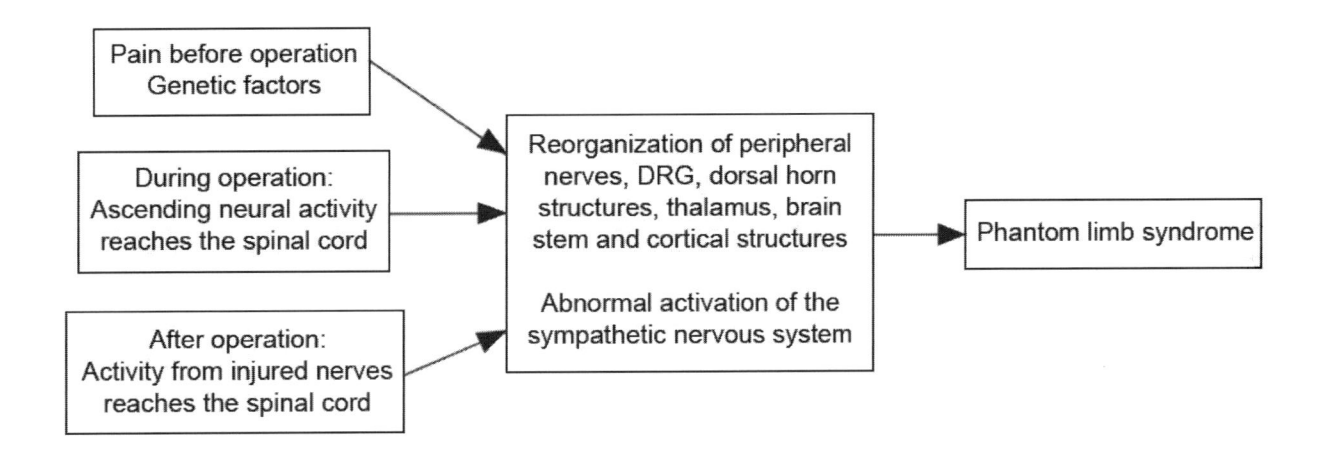

Figure 8.5 Proposed model of the development of phantom pain. (Information from Nikolajsen, L. and T.S. Jensen, Phantom Limb, in Wall and Melzack's Textbook of Pain., S.B. McMahon and M. Koltzenburg, Editors. 2006, Elsevier: Amsterdam. p. 961-71. [317].) (Artwork by Monica Javidnia.)

Pain after an amputation can be explained by plastic changes in the nervous system, induced by the enormous stimulation of pain circuits in the spinal cord and the brain that occurs during such operations. The patient is unaware of the pain because the neural activity that is generated by the surgical trauma is blocked by the surgical anesthesia, but that occurs high up in the pain pathways. Which neural structures are blocked by the anesthesia probably depends on the kind of anesthesia used. The abnormal nerve activity that is generated by the surgical trauma to nerves and other tissue acts on neural circuits in the spinal cord and perhaps in some structures in the brain that have not been blocked by the surgical anesthesia.

After the patient has recovered from the operation, deprivation of sensory input from the limb that is amputated due to severed peripheral nerves may activate neuroplasticity in the spinal cord and the brain, and this may cause the pain after the amputation. Some of these changes may cause bi-stable circuits that can remain in the abnormal condition, thus not reversing spontaneously over time to their normal function. This may explain the persistent pain and other phantom sensations that often occur after amputations. The sympathetic nervous system may be involved in creating the phantom pain and perhaps, in maintaining the pain [216].

Other forms of amputation pain are caused by a neuroma that occurs at the location where peripheral nerves are severed (stump pain). Such a neuroma consists of sprouts from the axons in the peripheral nerves that have been severed.

These sprouts are pain sensitive and mechanical and chemical stimulations may cause pain. A neuroma can also cause pain without any known stimulation. The likelihood of such sprouting can be reduced by a simple technique of splitting the nerve stump along the nerve and then putting the ends of the two parts together by anastomosis [22].

Also, the dorsal root ganglion (DRG) cells are affected by severing of a peripheral nerve making DRG cells generate spontaneous activity and making them sensitive to mechanical and chemical stimulation (such as noradrenalin).

Pain from the stump of a severed nerve is referred to the location of the amputation (the stump) while the pain that is a part of the phantom sensation may be referred to various locations on the amputated limb.

It has been suggested that after a nerve injury, specific cellular and molecular changes can affect the excitability of nerve cells and induce new gene expression, causing enhanced responses to future stimulation. Central inhibitory pathways may become deficient in the process and this can contribute to the mechanisms of central neuropathic pain [359].

# Deafferentation pain

Deafferentation pain is caused by lack of or reduction of normal sensory input that activate neuroplasticity that changes the function of specific parts of the central nervous system. Severance or damage to sensory nerves causing interruption of input to the CNS is known as deafferentation. Phantom limb pain is this a form of deafferentation pain. Deafferentation of the spinal cord or the brain can activate neuroplasticity and create plasticity disorders, such as chronic neuropathic pain (see Appendix A).

There is considerable evidence that injuries to peripheral nerves are especially powerful in initiating changes in the function of specific parts in the central nervous system (spinal cord and brain) through the expression of neuroplasticity.

An extremely severe form of deafferentation pain is anesthesia dolorosa, which is characterized by constant severe burning pain and reduced or absent sensation to innocuous stimulation. Anesthesia dolorosa occurs in connection with deafferentation through injury to nerves and it often affects the face [98, 254] but it can occur in other parts of the body [325, 425]. Anesthesia dolorosa from injury to the trigeminal nerve is a rare variant of face pain that may occur as a complication to partial section of the trigeminal nerve for treatment of trigeminal neuralgia (TGN) [254].

Anesthesia dolorosa occurs in connection with deafferentation pain through injury to nerves and it often affects the face [254], but it can occur in other parts of the body [325]. Anesthesia dolorosa from injury to the trigeminal nerve is a rare variant of face pain that may occur as a complication to a partial section of the trigeminal nerve for treatment of TGN [254]. It may occur from surgical sectioning of peripheral nerves or spinal nerve roots [325] although it has been claimed that anesthesia dolorosa is specific to the trigeminal system [425]. No known treatment is effective to treat that form of pain, although DBS recently has been found beneficial [395]. Electrical stimulation of premotor areas can relieve the pain from anesthesia dolorosa, which was assumed to be a form of deafferentation pain [98, 201, 275, 446].

Deafferentation pain is associated with hyperactivity of the somatosensory cortex. Rudolphus Llinas (1999) [237] presented a hypothesis to explain some of the symptoms of deafferentation pain. (The same hypothesis could also explain some forms of tinnitus [96]).

# Cortico-thalamic loop abnormalities in deafferentation pain

The reciprocal connections between sensory cortical areas and the sensory regions of the thalamus form loops where information can circulate. There is evidence that such circulating activity creates typical and specific patterns of the electrical activity of the brain (electroencephalographic, EEG) and magnetoencephalographic (MEG) activity that can be recorded from the brain in resting individuals. The pattern of the EEG has been shown to reflect various abnormalities and disorders. The MEG is a recent kind of measure that records the very small magnetic activity that is caused by neural activity of the brain.

Llinas (1999) showed that spontaneous magnetoencephalographic (MEG) activity in awake individuals suffering from neurogenic pain, tinnitus, Parkinson's disease, or depression was different from that recorded from individuals who did not have any of these symptoms [237]. Individuals with any one of these symptoms had increased low-frequency theta rhythmical activity in their magnetoencephalograms together with widespread and marked increase of coherence among high- and low-frequency oscillations.

These data were interpreted to indicate the presence of a thalamocortical dysrhythmia (Figure 8.6) and these investigators proposed that this dysrhythmia was responsible for the symptoms and signs of neurogenic pain, tinnitus, Parkinson's disease, and depression [237].

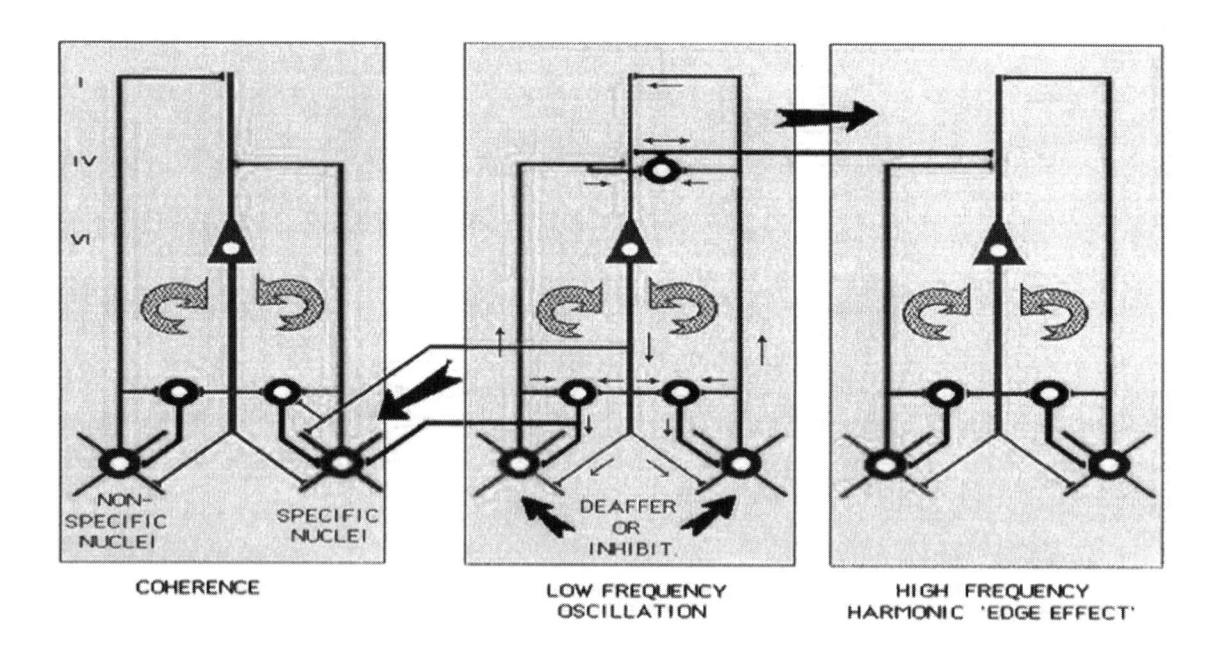

Figure 8.6 Diagram of the thalamocortical circuits that describes the hypothesis of thalamo-cortical dysrhythmia. Two thalamocortical systems are shown, the specific pathway to layer IV of the cortex that activates layer VI cortical neurons and feed-forward inhibition through inhibitory cortical interneurons. (From: Llinas, R.R., U. Ribary, D. Jeanmonod, E. Kronberg, et al., Thalamocortical dysrhythmia: A neurological and neuropsychiatric syndrome characterized by magnetoencephalography. Proc Natl Acad Sci., 1999. 96(26): p. 15222-7.) [237]

As illustrated in Figure 8.6, Dr. Llinas assumed that collaterals of the sensory projections to the cerebral cortex produce inhibition in the thalamus through the reticular nucleus of the thalamus. The return pathway (circular arrows on the right in Figure 8.6) re-enters the neural activity that is oscillatory in nature to specific- and reticularis-thalamic nuclei through layer VI pyramidal cells. The second loop involves nonspecific nuclei in the thalamus (part of the non-classical sensory pathways), projecting to the most superficial layer of the cortex (Layer I) and giving collaterals to the reticular nucleus of the thalamus. The conjunction of the specific and nonspecific loops is proposed to generate temporal coherence (center diagram in Figure 8.6).

Prolonged hyperpolarization of thalamic cells by altered synaptic input triggers low-frequency neuronal oscillation. Either disfacilitation, as occurs after deafferentation (as in neurogenic pain or tinnitus), or excess inhibition caused by over-activity in the pallidus of the basal ganglia (as occurs in Parkinson's disease) hyperpolarizes the cells sufficiently to deinactivate T-type calcium channels, resulting in thalamic oscillations in the theta range (4-7Hz).

Such oscillations can entrain corticothalamic loops (left graph in Figure 8.6), generating increased coherence as observed in the study [237]. At the cortical level, low-frequency activation of cortico–cortical inhibitory interneurons, by reducing the lateral inhibitory drive, can result in high-frequency, coherent activation of neighboring cortical modules, the "edge effect" (right graph in Figure 8.6).

# Perception of "self" and amputations

Sensory input from the body is normally the basis for our perception of the location of our body parts – this is an important component of what we call "self". The sensory input creates maps of the body in the brain, mostly apparent on the surface of the somatosensory cerebral cortex, but similar maps also exist in other parts of the brain and may be equally important.

This topographical representation of the body is normally updated constantly and the maps are adjusted by input from sensors in the skin, joints, tendons, and muscles. When a limb is removed by amputation, the maps still exist, but can no longer be updated.

The maps that were there before the operation are kept unchanged. That is what produces the feeling that the pain, itching, and other sensations come from specific locations of an amputated body part.

Awareness of a missing body part can, therefore, be explained because the mapping of the limb in the brain is not removed by the amputation. If the person had pain in the limb in question before it was amputated, the pain after the amputation can be explained by activation of an old map in the brain. If, for example, it is felt that an arm or leg is in an awkward position that may be painful, an amputee cannot move the perception of where an amputated limb is felt to be because the map of the amputated limb cannot be updated. Amputation of a body part means that regions of the brain that represent the body part in question no longer receive sensory input from the part that was amputated.

Studies have shown that regions of the brain that are deprived of their normal input and, thereby, become unused, may be invaded by sprouts of cells in adjacent areas [172]. For example, an amputation of a hand may cause sensations elicited by touching the face. The reason is that the face region of the somatosensory cortex is located anatomically close to that of the hand (see Figure 8.4).

The areas in the somatosensory cortex that are located near to the ones that represent the hand will take over (or "remap") the cortical region that no longer has input. Inspired by the results of Pons et al (1991) [333], Ramachandran [349] realized that phantom limb sensations could be due to "cross wiring" in the somatosensory cortex. Ramachandran and his colleagues demonstrated this remapping by showing that stroking different parts of the face led to perceptions of being touched on different parts of the missing limb [350]. Through magnetoencephalography (MEG), which permits visualization of activity in the human brain, these investigators verified the reorganization in the somatosensory cortex.

Ramachandran reasoned that if someone were to lose their right hand in an accident, they may then have the feelings of a phantom limb because the input that normally would go from their hand to the left somatosensory cortex would had been stopped. On the basis of this reasoning, Ramachandran designed the mirror treatment that now bears his name and which is in general use to relieve some of the symptoms of amputated body parts. It is described in Chapter 12.

As mentioned above, some individuals who have had a limb amputated feel that the amputated limb is locked in an odd position and the person is unable to move it. The reason that the perception of an amputated limb cannot be moved is that the body map cannot be updated [333]. The perception of the position of an amputated limb can be changed by the mirror treatment described by Dr. Ramachandran, thus, remedying the problem that the perception of the position of an amputated limb is locked in an odd position (see Chapter 12).

# Can pain influence body perception of "self"?

Pain has been shown to be associated with altered body perception (altered "self"). Dr. De Ridder described a patient who experienced severe deafferentation pain in the face (anesthesia dolorosa) and perceived that her right eye was displaced to a location below the real eye [97].

A patient (53 years, female) presented with a 10 year history of sharp, lancinating pain in the right upper (V1) distribution of the trigeminal nerves and a phantom sensation in the right middle distribution of the trigeminal nerve (V2) of the right eye being displaced down on the V2 distribution of the face (Figure 8.7). The patient had more than 30 surgical excisions of basal cell carcinoma on her right forehead. She experienced pain and the phantom sensation of her displaced eye after her first operation. The intensity of the pain had increased since then. Her pain was interpreted to be a form of anesthesia dolorosa. The displaced eye caused a misperception of surrounding objects and she often bumped into objects despite normal vision according to conventional tests.

She had hyperalgesia and loss of vibration and temperature senses in the right V1 area [97]. The location of the phantom eye could shift back to normal by applying the mirror test [348] (with the normal eye covered). All other clinical examinations, including ophthalmological examinations, were normal. The patient felt the sensation from tactile stimulation of the medial cornea and upper eyelashes as coming from the location of her phantom eye (in the right V2 dermatome).

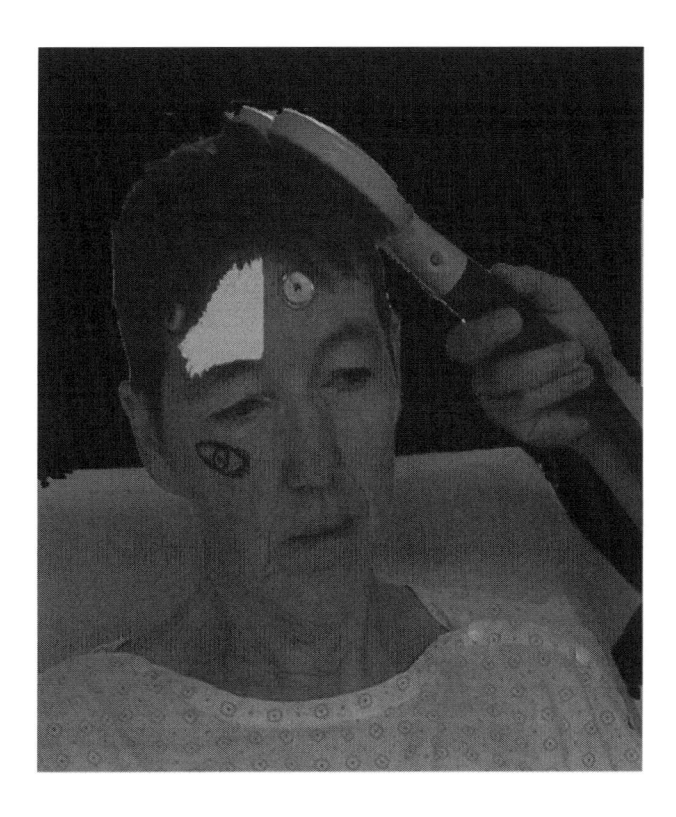

Figure 8.7 The patient who had a phantom eye located below and lateral to her right real eye undergoing transcranial magnetic stimulation (TMS). (Picture with permission of the patient.) (From De Ridder, D., G. De Mulder, T. Menovsky, S. Sunaert, et al., Electrical stimulation of auditory and somatosensory cortices for treatment of tinnitus and pain, in Progress in Brain Research, G.H. B. Langguth, T. Kleinjung, A. Cacace & A.R. Møller (Eds.) and V. Progress in Brain Research, Editors. 2007, Elsevier: Amsterdam p. 377-388 [97].

The pain was effectively relieved and the eye was no longer displaced following treatment with transcranial magnetic stimulation (TMS), which induced electrical current in her somatosensory cortex. The patient also no longer bumped into objects [97].

Stimulation of the cerebral cortex can be done non-invasively by applying impulses of a strong magnetic field to the surface of the skull (transcranial magnetic stimulation, TMS). The magnetic field is generated by passing strong electrical impulses through a coil (see Figure 11.4). When the coil is held close to the skull, the magnetic field induces an electrical current in the surface of the brain, thus making it possible to stimulate the cerebral cortex. The method is painless.

TMS caused a maximum reduction of 80 percent of the supraorbital pain and a complete disappearance of the phantom sensation. The suppression of the pain was obtained immediately after starting the TMS and had a residual effect whereas the phantom shifted back to its normal position only after a longer period of stimulation [97].

After it was found that stimulation of the cerebral cortex was an effective treatment, an electrode was implanted on the surface of the dura overlaying the somatosensory cortex. Stimulation through that electrode placement was effective in alleviating both pain and displacement of her eye for 6 years after which her problems returned. She again experienced neuropathic pain with allodynia and hyperpathia, which cannot be controlled by re-programming the electrical stimulation.

Two new electrodes were implanted on places determined by PET and fMRI scans on different locations from the first used electrode (one was placed anterior and the other posterior to the old electrode placement). The patient was free of pain only when both electrodes were stimulated. This means that electrical stimulation of brain structures is effective only for a limited time. This is also experienced in other use of electrical stimulation such as deep brain stimulation of nuclei in the basal ganglia for Parkinson's disease.

# Pain in connection with specific disorders

Many disorders have pathological pain as one of their symptoms. Examples include strokes, spinal injuries, multiple sclerosis, epilepsy, Alzheimer's disease, various forms of cancer, and Parkinson's disease. Muscle pain often occurs together with hyperactive motor disorders (see Chapter 9 Muscle Pain). Amputations of body parts, especially limbs (phantom limb pain), are associated with pain that may be long lasting as discussed above.

# Pain after strokes

Central pain following strokes (central post stroke pain, CPSP) [212] is a neuropathic pain syndrome characterized by both pain and sensory abnormalities in the body parts that correspond to the brain territory that has been injured. The sensory loss and hypersensitivity in the body regions of pain in people with CPSP indicate that the symptoms are caused by deafferentation, which has caused neuronal hyperexcitability. Lacunar strokes (strokes in deep parts of the brain), especially when it occurs in the thalamus causing the Dejerine-Roussy syndrome, are associated with severe pain and hypersensitivity (also known as thalamic pain syndrome). Ischemic strokes may create an immune reaction as discussed in Chapter 11. The immune reaction may contribute to the pain after strokes in addition to deficits and risk of death.

# Spinal cord injuries

Like spasticity, these forms of pain often develop some time after the occurrence of the injury. It has been reported that phantom sensations occur in as many as 90 percent of individuals with spinal cord injuries (SCI) [393].

Spasticity that often occurs after SCI may be perceived as muscle pain (see Chapter 9). About one third of the people with SCI rate their pain as being severe. SCI are often devastating for other reasons and pain is not usually the primary concern although it is a contributing factor for the reduced quality of life that most SCI victims experience. The pain is, in most instances, pathological pain caused by changes in the excitability of spinal neurons from the injury and from regeneration [392].

The pain seems to be independent of the level of the injury to the spinal cord. Neuropathic pain may be more common in connection with incomplete lesions of the spinal cord compared with complete transections. Typically, the pain stays relatively constant during many months. The pain is pathological pain caused by changes in the function of the spinal cord or the brain. Nociceptive (physiological) pain may develop because of urinary bladder and bowl insufficiency from paralysis causing urinary infections, bowl impaction, or kidney stones.

234 PAIN: Its Anatomy, Physiology and Treatment

The pain localized above the lesion, at the lesion, and below the lesion is typically different. Pain above the level of injury may be related to the sympathetic nervous system. Symptoms of CRPS may occur, but may not be directly associated with the spinal cord injury. CRPS in SCI victims may occur because of changes in the autonomic nervous system. Pain in SCI victims is typically localized at the spinal level of injury and typically within 2 dermatomes above and below the actual lesion (Figure 8.8A).

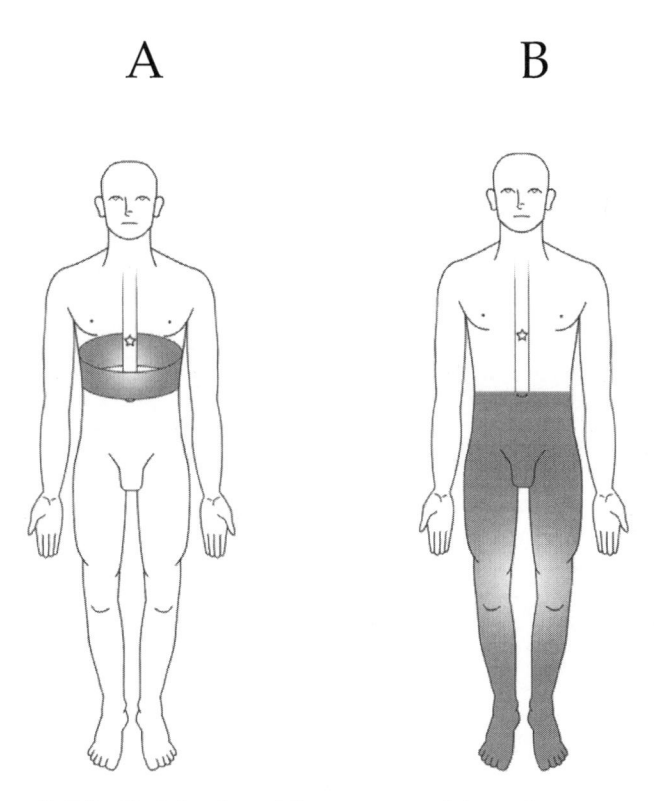

Figure 8.8 Individuals with neuropathic pain.
A: Typical pattern of neuropathic pain following spinal cord injuries (SCI) at T7. The shading represents the distribution of pain. (Artwork by Monica Javidnia.)
B: Typical pattern of below level distribution of pain following SCI at T7.
A & B are based on Siddall: Pain following spinal cord injury, in Wall and Melzack's Textbook of Pain, S.B. McMahon and M. Koltzenburg, Editors. 2006, Elsevier, Churchill, Livingstone: Amsterdam. p 1043-1055 [392]. (Artwork by Monica Javidnia.)

Pain below the level of injury typically is localized to large regions of the body below the lesion (Figure 8.8B); thus, a sign that activation of neuroplasticity plays an important role in the creation of this form of pain. The pain is similar to phantom pain or deafferentation pain and their different symptoms, such as allodynia, hyperpathia, hyperalgesia, and burning and shooting pain that may occur spontaneously or evoked by touching the skin [392].

# Parkinson's disease

Pain is an overlooked symptom of Parkinson's disease (PD). PD is regarded as a movement disorder and the focus has been on movement symptoms although it is known that many individuals with PD also have cognitive deficits. Pain has been reported to occur in approximately 40 percent of individuals with PD [124]. Pain may even be the first symptom of PD [155]. There is some evidence that inflammatory processes involving microglia reactions may also be involved in causing the central pain in PD [15, 147].

These forms of pain are pathological pain, but pain may also be caused by musculoskeletal problems related to poor posture, from neck or back arthritis, or from dystonia with sustained twisting or posturing of a muscle group or body part. These forms of pain may be physiological pain caused by stimulation of pain receptors. This means that pain in connection with PD may be a mixture of physiological pain and pathological pain.

# Alzheimer's disease

Alzheimer's disease is not normally associated with pain; at least, there do not seem to be any published papers regarding a higher incidence of pain in individuals with Alzheimer's disease than in individuals who do not have Alzheimer's disease. However, the cognitive deterioration that occurs in such individuals may mask pain conditions that are related to the disease as well as pain conditions that are unrelated.

It has been suggested that individuals with Alzheimer's disease have less sensitivity to painful stimuli because of the neurodegenerative disease. However, a recent study shows that this is not the case and individuals with Alzheimer's disease have been shown to have similar equal pain sensitivity as people who do not have Alzheimer's disease [80]. The study [80] pointed to inadequate treatment of pain in individuals with Alzheimer's disease.

Individuals with Alzheimer's disease can naturally have pain of the same causes as people who do not have Alzheimer's disease, but they are not receiving adequate treatment because of their (co-morbidity) Alzheimer's disease.

There is recent evidence that the immune system of the brain may be involved in creating the damage that causes the symptoms of Alzheimer's disease and these same related processes may cause central pain [15, 147].

# Pain and motor disorders

Muscle pain may also occur secondary to dystonia (a syndrome of abnormal muscle contractions that produce repetitive, involuntary twisting movements and abnormal posturing of the neck, trunk, face, and extremities according to Stedman's Electronic Medical Dictionary) (discussed in Chapter 9).

Pain in neck muscles is common in individuals with spasmodic torticollis and it also occurs in individuals with spasticity such as, for example, after spinal cord injuries.

# Neural structures especially involved in creating pathological pain

Many parts of the spinal cord and the brain are involved in creating pathological pain and recent research has shown that more parts of the central nervous system are implicated than earlier believed. The dorsal horn and the caudal trigeminal nucleus play important roles in creating central neuropathic pain. It is now known that the anterior cingulate, the amygdala, the insula lobe, the thalamo-cortical loop, and various parts of the cerebral cortex (premotor areas, PMA, and supplemental areas, SMA) are involved in different kinds of pain.

# The role of changes in the dorsal horn of the spinal cord

Central neuropathic pain is a phantom sensation that involves changes in the function of the spinal cord and the brain brought about by activation of neuroplasticity [488, 489]. These functional changes cause pain in addition to other symptoms such as abnormal cross modal interactions that may result in allodynia (sensation of pain from touching of the skin). Other changes that may be present together with pain are changes in neural processing causing hyperpathia (an abnormal reaction to minor pain stimulation involving prolongation and exaggeration of the pain sensation) and increased sensitivity to painful stimulations (hyperalgesia).

Like other central nervous system (spinal cord and brain) structures, the neural circuits in the dorsal horn that are involved in processing noxious stimuli are plastic, and reorganization of these circuits plays an important role in central neuropathic pain. Functional changes of these circuits are implicated in the maintenance of central neuropathic pain.

Changes in processing of noxious information in the dorsal horn of the spinal cord and the caudal portion of the trigeminal nucleus can explain many of the characteristic features of central neuropathic pain. The changes in the function and the organization of the dorsal horn neural circuits can be caused by both external and internal factors that activate neuroplasticity.

A correct balance between inhibition and excitation in the dorsal horn is important for normal functioning of the pain system [404, 495]. Sivilotti and Wolf (1994) [404] found that blocking of inhibition could lead to allodynia. Activation of most nerve cells involves both excitation and inhibition. The outcome (whether or not a cell becomes activated or not) depends on the balance between inhibition and excitation.

Changes in the mode (or state) of processing in the dorsal horn (and the caudal portion of the nucleus of the trigeminal nerve) that are associated with development of central pain are characterized by a change in sensitivity, a change in the way stimuli are processed, and a change in the anatomical location where information is processed. Distinct steps in these changes have been identified on the basis of studies in rats. (For a review of abnormal states, see Doubell (1999) and Sandkuhler (2009) [109, 371]).

According to Doubell and co-workers (1999), the processing of pain signals in the dorsal horn of the spinal cord (and the trigeminal nucleus) can operate in four main states [109] and operating in each one of these different states (or modes) results in characteristic symptoms.

State 1 is the normal state. The pain caused by activity in this state is physiological pain. Stimuli that activate low-threshold mechanoreceptors produce innocuous sensations such as that of touch, vibration, pressure, warmth, or cool. Activation of high threshold receptors produces localized pain sensations that are distinctly different from innocuous stimulations. The sensation of pain in this state is not accompanied by any noticeable emotional engagement.

State 2 represents a functional re-organization of the dorsal horn (and the trigeminal sensory nucleus) where suppression of the transmission of somatosensory information occurs, and the ability of high intensity stimuli to evoke a sensation of pain is reduced. The decrease in sensory transmission is caused by an inhibitory influence on neurons in the dorsal horn. The source of the inhibition can be peripheral, such as from activation of A$\beta$ fibers, or from the brain, such as a part of "fight and flight" reactions mediated by the noradrenalin (NA)-serotonin descending pathways (see Figure 3.23). It is believed that this is one of the many mechanisms through which the perception of painful stimuli can be suppressed. Stimulation of skin receptors, hypnosis, placebo effects, suggestions, distraction, and cognitive activity can activate these systems. Experiments in animals have shown that pharmacological agents, such as opioids, $\alpha$-adrenergic agents, and GABA$_A$ receptor antagonists (bicuculine), can promote the expression of state 2 in dorsal horn pain circuits.

State 3 represents a combination of increased excitatory synaptic transmission and decreased inhibition causing increased excitability of dorsal horn sensory cells, thereby facilitating or sensitizing their response to sensory stimuli. The result is that stimulation of sensory receptors elicits larger than normal neural (postsynaptic) activity in this mode. Low intensity stimulation that is normally innocuous causes pain (allodynia). Central sensitization occurs in this mode causing exaggerated pain experiences that outlast the duration of the noxious stimulation (hyperpathia) from moderate pain stimulation.

Mononeuropathies may promote the changes that occur in stage 3 and spinal cord stimulation can attenuate the hyperexcitability in the dorsal horn as found in studies in rats [494]. The existing nociceptive receptive fields of dorsal horn neurons may become extended through activation of ineffective (dormant) synapses [171].

State 4 represents permanent pathological pain. In this state, anatomical reorganization occurs with changes in morphology, including cell death, degeneration or atrophy of synapses, creation of new synapses, and modification of the contacts between cells and synapses. Aβ fibers that normally terminate in layers III-V of the horns of the spinal cord may invade the territories of C-fibers (lamina II) and make synaptic contact with cells that are innervated by C-fibers [109].

This may explain why normally innocuous stimulation can be perceived as being painful (allodynia).

In summary, Doubell's view on plastic changes in the spinal cord causing pain involved four states (or modes) in which the neural circuits in the dorsal horn can operate. State 1 is the normal state of the function of the dorsal horn of the spinal cord (and the trigeminal nucleus). State 2 represents a decreased gain regarding noxious stimulation. State 3 represents transient and functional increased gain. Finally, state 4 is a (anatomically) permanent state of increased pain and redirection of information. Changes from state 1 to states 2 or 3 involve mainly changes in synaptic efficacy. Changes to state 4 are different because they involve structural (morphological) changes. Therefore, the changes in state 4 are more difficult to reverse than of the changes that occur in states 2 and 3.

# Wide dynamic range (WDR) neurons

Wide dynamic range (WDR) neurons are involved in creating central neuropathic pain through plastic changes. WDR neurons receive input from several different types of sensory nerve fibers, polymodal C-fibers, Aδ fibers that mediate pain information (heat), and high threshold mechanoreceptors. These nerve fibers are collaterals of those that terminate on cells in lamina I and II of the dorsal horn of the spinal cord. The WDR neurons also receive input through Aβ fibers that are collaterals to those that innervate low threshold mechanoreceptors and which travel on the same side of the spinal cord to reach the dorsal column nuclei. The input from Aβ fibers provides both inhibitory and excitatory input to the WDR cells (A in Figure 8.9). Other collaterals to those nerve fibers terminate on inhibitory interneurons, the axons of which terminate on cells in lamina II of the dorsal horn.

240 PAIN: Its Anatomy, Physiology and Treatment

The excitability of WDR cells increases when C-fiber input is increased such as occurs when pain receptors are stimulated (C in Figure 8.9). When the input from the Aβ fibers decreases, excitation of these cells increases because the normal inhibitory influence decreases (B in Figure 8.9). This happens when nerves have been severed (deafferentation).

Prolonged pain may lead to an increased response of WDR neurons from the C-fiber input they receive [39, 266, 434, 491]. Stimulation of pain receptors, for example by inflammation or peripheral nerve injuries, may cause or promote such sensitization through the expression of neuroplasticity. The properties of these cells change and their firing rate increases when the excitation increases. The WDR neurons normally have a maximal firing rate of 350-400 impulses per second, but when affected by plastic changes, their firing rate can reach 700 impulses per second.

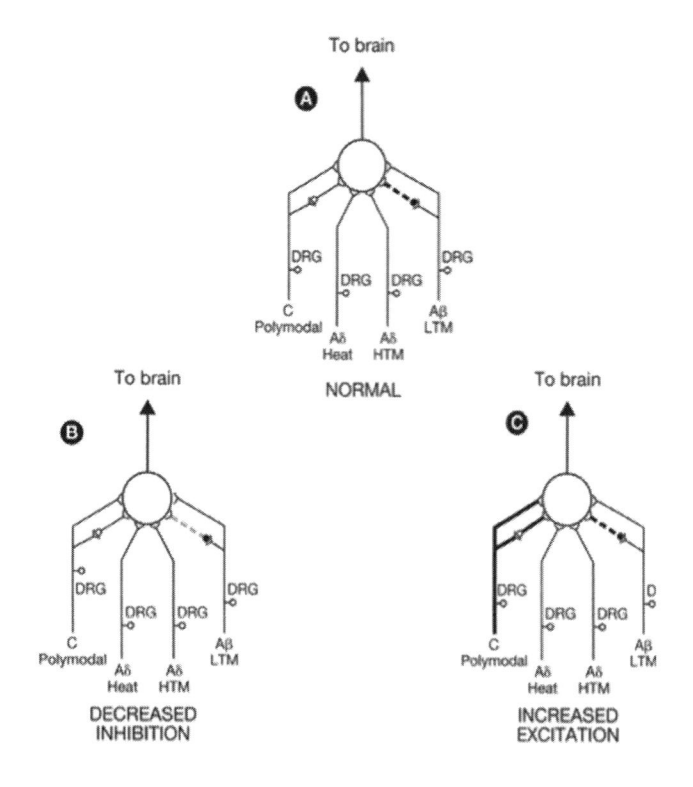

Figure 8.9 Wide dynamic range neurons that are subjected to plastic changes that can cause central neuropathic pain. A: Normal situation; B: Decreased inhibitory input from low threshold mechanoreceptors (LTM) through Aβ fibers causing reduced inhibition; C: Increased excitatory input from polymodal receptors through C-fibers. HTM: High threshold mechanoreceptors. (Modified from Price, D.D., S. Long, and C. Huitt, Sensory testing of pathophysiological mechanisms of pain in patients with reflex sympathetic dystrophy. Pain, 1992. 49: p. 163-173.) [335]

# Role of other parts of the brain

New research shows an increasing number of sites in the brain outside the normally recognized pain circuits that are involved in pain. These sites include structures such as the insula lobe, the premotor and supplemental motor cortices, [19] and the thalamo-cortical loop [237]. Affective symptoms, such as depression, often accompany severe pain, and this may be explained by the establishment of new connections in pain pathways and by enhancing (amplifying) transmission in existing pathways. In these respects, central neuropathic pain has many similarities with other hyperactive sensory disorders such as tinnitus [62, 285, 299], which also involves many parts of the brain and which are often accompanied by symptoms and signs of mood disorders such as depression [224].

# Motor cortical areas

Other evidence of involvement of the structures outside the traditional pain pathways comes from treatment of patients with pain using electrical stimulation of the cerebral cortex. Thus, it has been shown that electrical stimulation of premotor areas (PMA) and supplementary motor areas (SMA) [275, 446] can reduce pain, suggesting involvement of motor areas in pain perception. Even electrical stimulation of primary motor areas (MI) has been reported to provide beneficial effect on some forms of pain [12].

Some investigators [131] have hypothesized that motor cortex stimulation is effective because it increases regional cerebral blood flow in the ipsilateral ventrolateral thalamus in which corticothalamic connections from the motor and premotor areas predominate. The extent of pain alleviation also correlates with the increase of blood flow in the cingulate gyrus [52]. Whether the observed changes (in blood flow) are caused by the stimulation or by the changes in the function of some brain structures because of the stimulation is not clear.

It may seem strange that motor areas of the brain are involved in pain and that activating such areas by electrical stimulation can control pain. Arle and Shils [12] have suggested that motor cortex stimulation activates superficial (layer I) neurons in the motor cortex and that they connect to somatosensory cortices (SI) and that could be the route through which the motor cortex can suppress pain sensation.

# Limbic structures

Pain often has two different effects on a person, namely a phantom perception of pain and a negative effect that can be described as suffering [188]. Pain is often associated with affective symptoms such as depression and various kinds of fear as are other hyperactive disorders such as tinnitus.

The medial portion of the thalamus is involved in physiological pain and it is also likely to be involved in pathological pain, providing subcortical (direct) connections to limbic structures such as the lateral nucleus of the amygdala [227], the supplementary motor areas (SMA), and the prefrontal cortex (see Figure 3.14).

# The insula lobe

The insula lobe is a little known structure that is located deep in the brain, under the temporal lobe and adjacent to the frontal lobe [417]. It has recently been associated with many different sensations such as feeling ill and strange feelings from visceral structures.

The insula cortex has also been associated with negative emotional experiences. The right anterior insula is involved in awareness of visceral matters, thus, providing a neural substrate for different subjective qualities of pain feelings [88, 389].

Evidence has been presented regarding the judgment of the degree of pain indicating that the insular cortex may be the anatomical location of the awareness of some qualities of pain [19]. Using fMRI, it was found that encoding of nociceptive stimuli activated different regions of the insular lobe than encoding of innocuous stimuli such as vision [19, 416].

New ways of studying the function of structures deep in the brain, such as the insula, have evolved through the development of neurosurgical methods in the treatment of severe epilepsy. These methods involve implantation of many electrodes in specific structures of the brain and then recording from these structures. Electrical stimulation is also used to identify the anatomical location of epileptic foci. In one study, extensive recordings and stimulations from as many as 123 electrode sites in the same patient have yielded a wealth of basic information about the function of such structures as the insular lobe [416, 417].

# The role of the sympathetic nervous system on pain

The sympathetic nervous system can modulate pain (decrease or increase pain) and it can cause pain. In the periphery, activity of the sympathetic nervous system can increase the sensitivity of receptors as discussed in Chapter 3.

Centrally, increased sympathetic activation can influence the excitability of dorsal horn neurons that receive pain signals from the body as well as neurons in the caudal trigeminal nucleus that receive pain information from the head. Sympathetic activation can reduce pain sensation as it does for instance in the "fight and flight" reaction.

The "fight and flight" reaction typically occurs after severe traumatic events such as severe accidents or in connection with gunshot wounds where a person does not experience any pain before arriving at the hospital.

Pain conditions that are directly related to sympathetic neural activity are known as sympathetic maintained pain (SMP) [39, 184]. Partial nerve injury can cause injured and uninjured nerves to express α-adenoceptors causing such axons to discharge in response to circulating epinephrine and norepinephrine. Sympathetic afferent fibers enter the dorsal horn of the spinal cord and their activity can modulate neural transmission in pain circuits of the dorsal horn. Sprouting sympathetic nerve fibers that project to the dorsal root ganglia (DRG) may also be involved in causing SMP.

The role of the autonomic nervous system is normally perceived as beneficial, such as by serving to maintain homeostasis, etc. Activation of the sympathetic nervous system can, however, be harmful which occurs when it is involved in the creation of several kinds of pain. An example is sympathetically maintained pain that is a complex condition that involves many parts of the central nervous system.

# The sympathetic nervous system may provide positive feedback in pain circuits

An example of positive feedback in a biological control system is when the sympathetic nervous system becomes activated by pain and sympathetic-fibers release norepinephrine near mechanoreceptors, increasing their sensitivity as discussed in Chapter 3.

This increases pain, which increases sympathetic activation. This creates a positive feedback loop that can lead to sympathetically maintained pain (SMP). In general, positive feedback easily causes instability. Specifically, positive feedback aggravates the symptoms of disorders such as those that are associated with the activation of the sympathetic nervous system.

While positive feedback is rare in biological systems, negative feedback is common in biological control systems as well as in man-made systems. The Renshaw inhibition that consists of feedback from motor axons to the $\alpha$-motoneuron as inhibition is a typical example of negative feedback in a biological system. An example of positive feedback was shown in Chapter 6 (see Figure 6.8).

# Complex regional pain syndrome, CRPS I and II

The autonomic nervous system cannot only modulate pain, but it can cause symptoms of diseases such as by causing sympathetically maintained pain (SMP). The sympathetic nervous system is involved in specific disorders such as complex regional pain syndromes, CRPS I and II. (CRPS I was earlier known as reflex sympathetic dystrophy (RSD) and CRPS II was known as causalgia.)

The terms reflex sympathetic dystrophy (RSD) and causalgia have been used as a general description of pain where the sympathetic nervous system is involved. More recently more a different terminology has been adapted. RSD has been replaced by the term complex regional pain syndrome (CRPS Type I). The symptoms of CPRS Type I follow noxious events and include spontaneous pain and possibly allodynia and hyperpathia. Skin edema and abnormal sudomotor (sweat glands activated by sympathetic nerves) activity in larger anatomical regions of the body [375] is a frequent component of CRPS I.

The term "causalgia" has been used earlier to describe pain where the sympathetic nervous system was involved. The term causalgia has been replaced by the term CRPS Type II, which relates to syndromes that are more anatomically localized than those of CRPS Type I, which are often observed following peripheral nerve injury. CRPS II may include allodynia and hyperpathia and skin edema but in more localized body regions than that of CRPS Type I [272, 375].

Specifically, the symptoms of these two diseases are "burning" pain, abnormal sweating, increased skin sensitivity, and changes in skin temperature, which can go in both directions, either warmer or cooler than the opposite extremity. The skin is typically blotchy, purple, pale, or red; thus, several symptoms that can be related to abnormal activation of the sympathetic nervous system.

Skin edema and abnormal sudomotor (sweating) activity typically are present in all forms of increased sympathetic activation. Changes in skin texture, including the skin appearing shiny and thin, are also typical. Abnormal regulation of blood flow, edema of skin and subcutaneous tissue, active and passive movement disorders, allodynia, and hyperpathia are typical symptoms.

Sweating is also a typical sign and it is sometimes excessive. Changes in nail and hair growth patterns along with swelling and stiffness in affected joints are typical symptoms. The symptoms normally affect only one limb, but it may spread to other parts of the body over time.

The most important cause of the symptoms from the involvement of the autonomic nervous system is distortion of the information processing in the spinal cord [179]. There are many factors that can make that occur. The effects of such abnormal processing in the spinal cord are many (Figure 8.10). Pain of some form is the general outcome, but also abnormal motor functions can result. Activation of the sympathetic nervous system is perhaps the most visible of these different effects of the abnormal processing that occurs in the spinal cord.

246 PAIN: Its Anatomy, Physiology and Treatment

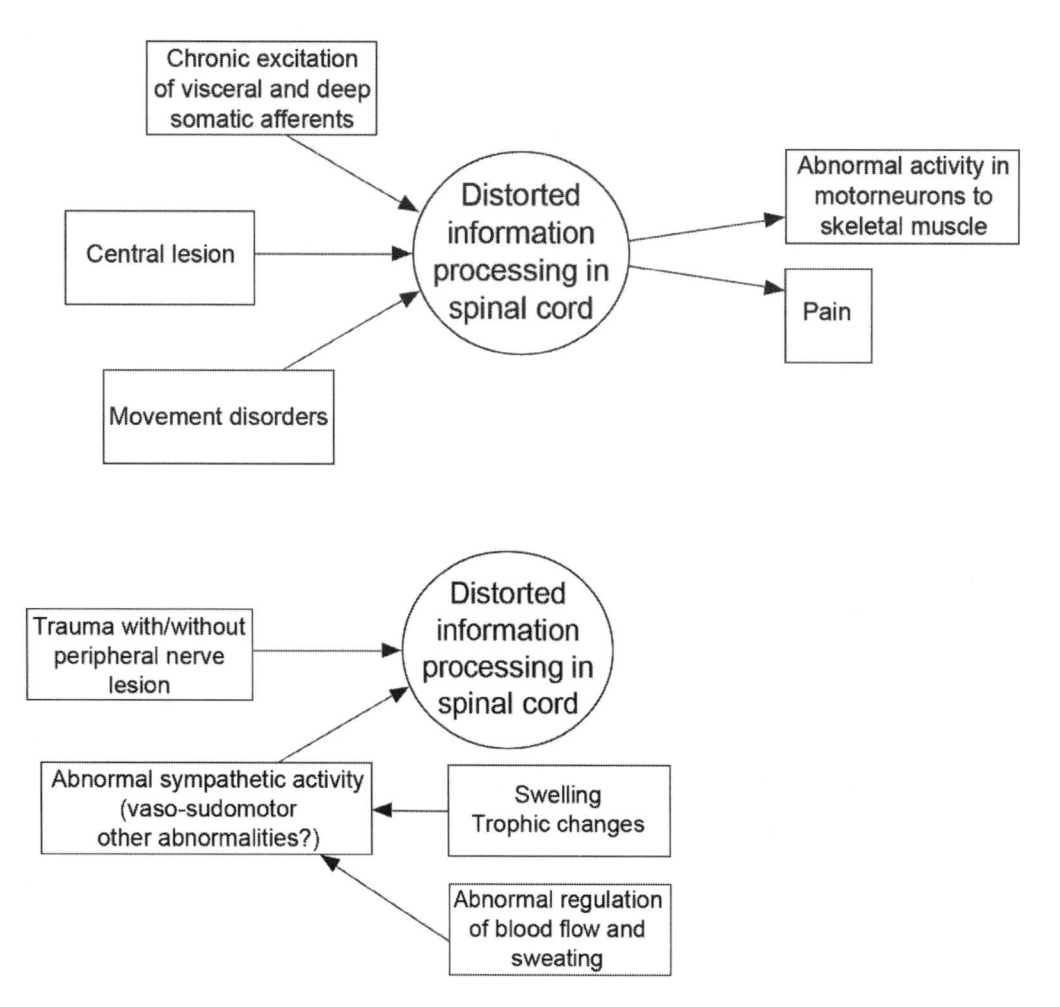

Figure 8.10 Contemporary hypotheses of neural mechanisms involved in generating CRPS I and II following trauma. Adapted from Jänig, W., The puzzle of "reflex sympathetic dystrophy": mechanisms, hypotheses, open questions, in Reflex sympathetic dystrophy: a reappraisal, W. Jänig and M. Stanton-Hicks, Editors. 1996, IASP Press: Seattle. p. 1-24 [179]. (Artwork by Monica Javidnia.)

Complex regional pain syndromes (CRPS) I and II are examples of how a dysfunctional nervous system can cause symptoms and signs of disease. Complex regional pain syndromes, CRPS I and II, are specific disorders where the sympathetic nervous system plays an important role. In general, both CRPS I and II are chronic pain conditions with continuous, intense pain, which gets worse over time.

Traumas of various kinds are the most common causes, but movement disorders may also cause processing of information in the spinal cord to become abnormal (Figure 8.10). Circulating adrenergic substances (mostly adrenaline) can increase the sensitivity of central pain neurons and promote plastic changes in wide dynamic range (WDR) neurons. Pain sensations can be increased by secreting noradrenaline from sympathetic nerve fibers close to cells in the dorsal horn neurons.

Sympathetic afferent fibers enter the dorsal horn of the spinal cord and their activity can modulate neural transmission in pain circuits of the dorsal horn. Sprouting sympathetic nerve fibers that project to the dorsal root ganglia may also be involved in causing sympathetically maintained pain.

Activation of the sympathetic nervous system can increase pain that is caused by the stimulation of pain fibers (physiological pain). The sympathetic nervous system is involved in modulating the sensitivity of the central (spinal cord and brain) parts of the pain systems. Here the sympathetic nervous system may modify existing pain conditions.

The symptoms of CRPS I typically occur after harmful events (such as trauma) and include spontaneous pain and possibly allodynia and hyperpathia. Over time, these symptoms typically aggravate and the pain spreads to include the entire arm or leg, even though the initiating injury might have been only to a finger or toe.

Pain can sometimes travel to the opposite extremity and may be heightened by emotional stress. CRPS type II is generally more localized than CRPS type I. CRPS type II was earlier referred to as causalgia. It is typical for both CRPS I and II that the diagnosis of either one is discarded if some other cause of the symptoms can be found.

It is not known exactly what causes CRPS. While the symptoms are usually started by trauma of some kind, similar kinds of trauma occur frequently without causing CRPS. This means that something else – one or more additional factors – must be present in order for CRPS to develop. It is a common observation that the manifestation of a disease does not depend on a single factor, implying that more than one factor is often necessary to cause symptoms and signs.

Regarding CRPS, it is not known what this or these "additional factors" may be, but it has been suggested that anomalies of pain receptors may make them especially sensitive to the norepinephrine that is released from C-fibers when the sympathetic nervous system is activated. Other hypotheses involve the immune system. As is discussed in other parts of the book, there are now more and more indications that the immune system of the central nervous system (activation of microglia and astrocytes) is involved in many symptoms and signs from the nervous system [183, 259, 478] .

Recent studies have shown that CPRS is associated with morphological changes in the brain. Geha and collaborators showed that gray matter morphometry and white matter anisotropy in people with CRPS are different from matched controls[138]. Atrophy was present in the right insula, right ventromedial prefrontal cortex (VMPFC), and right nucleus accumbens and there were changes in the left cingulum-callosal bundle. White matter connectivity in these regions showed signs of re-organization consisting of changes in branching patterns and there was signs of increased connections from VMPFC to the insula and decreased VMPFC connections to the basal ganglia. The observed regional atrophy related to pain intensity and duration but the strength of connectivity between specific atrophied regions related to anxiety.

The sympathetic nervous system gives some forms of central neuropathic pain their characteristics. Using low back pain as a model, Apkarian and his co-workers have found an anatomical marker in the brain for chronic pain [246]. Recent concepts regarding the pathology of many forms of chronic pain involve learning and memory circuits in the brain.

# Other complex pain conditions

Many kinds of pain are complex; some forms of pain occur together with other symptoms such as fibromyalgia and myofascial pain, which will be discussed in Chapter 10. Often, pain is a combination of physiological and pathophysiological pain. Low back pain is an example of a common form of pain that is complex and carpal tunnel syndrome is another example.

Some of these have often been referred to as nerve entrapment disorders, but mostly erroneously. This was discussed briefly in Chapter 5. A more detailed discussion follows below.

## Low back pain

There are many forms of back pain [238]. Low back pain can have the form of sharp, shooting pain such as with sciatica, but more often, the pain has the form of an aching pain that is aggravated in some body positions, from sitting in a certain way, etc. Sciatica is a symptom rather than a specific diagnosis [451]. Sciatica is probably best described as a form of low back pain that is characterized by shooting pain in a leg.

We discussed lower back pain and carpal tunnel syndrome in chapter 5 because injuries to a single nerve (mononeuropathies) are involved but the pathology of these common disorders is more complex than just pathology of a nerve or nerve root.

The cause of many forms of low back pain is likely to be a mixture of several different pathologies. It is now agreed that both nociceptive (physiological pain) and central neuropathic mechanisms (pathological pain) are often involved [126]. The causes of the different forms of back pain are also most likely different. Thus, sciatica causing distinct strong pain and chronic back pain that are characterized by aching and burning pain seem to have different causes.

Back pain may occur after a specific event, but often, no cause can be identified. The pain may start as acute pain that is most likely physiological pain, but after some time, a central pain component is likely to develop (pathological pain) having the form of aching pain, thus, pathological pain caused by activation of neuroplasticity.

Nerve root compression (nerve entrapment) is a common hypothesis for the cause of low back pain as was discussed in Chapter 5. Imaging studies (MRI) show signs of nerve root compression that often occur with increasing age when the foramina (opening in the bone) from spinal stenosis become smaller and compress the nerves that pass through the foramina. This would mean that low back pain would be what is called a nerve entrapment disorder.

However, there are several reasons why it is unlikely that the common forms of back pain are caused by compression of a (normal) mixed nerve (or nerve root). Compression of mixed nerves (or nerve roots) mostly affects the function of large myelinated fibers (Aα and Aβ) that communicate somatic sensation and motor commands while the smaller myelinated fibers (Aδ) and unmyelinated (C) fibers that communicate pain are only slightly affected (see Chapter 3). (The opposite is the case for administration of local anesthetics that mainly affect small unmyelinated fibers, C-fibers).

As we discussed in Chapter 5, acute mechanical insult to a mixed nerve would cause numbness, tingling, or perhaps stingy pain and motor weakness because it mainly affects large myelinated nerve fibers. Constant compression would cause decreased sensation and perhaps numbness and muscle weakness due to compression of large myelinated nerve fibers [220].

Interference with the axoplasmatic flow may also occur [220]. Small diameter myelinated fibers and especially unmyelinated (C) fibers are not noticeably affected by mechanical compression. This may explain why sensation can be lost from compression of a nerve (causing numbness) while maintaining pain sensation. We also discussed in Chapter 3 and 5 that compression of a nerve only affect the small diameter nerve fibers that are involved in causing pain when another factor is present; that second factor being inflammation, injury or vitamin B deficiency.

Muscle spasm is often associated with low back pain and often some of the pain may be caused by muscle contractions that turn painful. Constantly contracted striate muscles cause pain (tonic contractions) and are not easily observed.

The clinical experience that back pain often can be treated successfully by benzodiazepines supports the hypothesis that muscle contraction is a component of low back pain.

# Sciatica

The term sciatica commonly refers to a radiculopathy (disease of a nerve root), involving one of the lower extremities and related to disc herniation (DH). However, nerve roots from $L_1$ to $L_4$ may be involved. The prevalence of sciatica is poorly known.

Suggestions are made on how to improve accuracy of capturing sciatica in epidemiological studies. In a recent review of 23 published studies [219], only two used clinical assessments for assessing sciatic symptoms. The definitions of sciatica used in these 23 studies varied widely. Sciatica prevalence from different studies ranged from 1.2 percent to 43 percent.

The term sciatica is often used (incorrectly) to describe any pain arising from the lower back and radiating down to the leg. Often, what is known as low back pain (or sometimes sciatica) is referred pain from the lower back, unrelated to DH or nerve-root compression. The sciatica type of back pain is most likely caused by trauma to $A\delta$ fibers of a nerve root or by stimulating $A\delta$ fibers in a nerve and perhaps $A\beta$ and $A\alpha$ as well.

This is supported by studies in working populations with physically demanding jobs, which consistently report higher rates of sciatica compared with studies in the general population.

Recently, the interest has been directed to the DRG rather than the nerve root. Bulging vertebral discs may compress DRG [10]. Studies in animals (rats) have shown that chronic compression of cell bodies (CCD) in the dorsal root ganglion, DRG, makes the DRG become hyperexcitable, and some exhibit ectopic, spontaneous activity (SA) [241]. Inflammatory mediators have a potential role in modulating the excitability of DRG neurons and, therefore, may contribute to the neuronal hyperexcitability after CCD. Chronic compression of the DRG has a different effect than compression of a nerve root. It can increase the effect of substances that are associated with inflammation such as bradykinin, serotonin, prostaglandin $E_2$, and histamine (an "inflammatory soup", IS) [241].

Experimental studies have shown that administration of such substances becomes more effective in inducing electrophysiological changes in DRG neurons after compressing the DRG. This means that compression of DRG increases the sensitivity to inflammatory processes. Compression of the cell bodies of DRG together with mediators of inflammation, such as the IS, may be the cause of some forms of pain that have been attributed to nerve compression. Other studies have shown the importance of another known pain mediator, the tumor necrosis factor alpha (TNF-$\alpha$). Root compression that occurs in people who do not have pain could be explained by the absence of inflammatory mediators.

Several recent studies have shown that both inflammation and compression of DRG are important for the development of the symptoms of sciatica. Inflammatory reactions to fluid that may be leaking from ruptured vertebral discs could be a factor in the creation of symptoms (pain) in sciatica [92]. Animal models have shown indications that the TNF-$\alpha$ is involved, but its contributions to sciatica symptoms in humans is not clear [200, 451].

Estimates of the prevalence of sciatica vary considerably between studies. This may be due to differences in definitions, methods of data collection, and perhaps populations studied. The involvement of inflammatory processes is also supported by the experience of back pain treatment that shows that administration of anti-inflammatory medications, such as NSAID and steroids, is beneficial in the treatment of back pain. Thus, it is yet another situation where it has recently become evident that inflammatory (and immune) reactions are important for the manifestation of many disorders.

## Periformis sciatica

A rare form of sciatica is caused by the sciatic nerve being compressed by a small muscle, the periformis muscle giving numbness and weakness in in a leg and perhaps some pain. This problem is caused because the sciatic nerve travels very near this muscle and in some individuals it actually passes through the muscle. This form of sciatica (periformis sciatica) is easily treated by very simple physical exercise that anybody can do at home but the danger is that an MRI most often shows compression of spinal nerves (also) and that can result in surgical operations that have no benefit because as mentioned above, many people have compression of spinal nerves without any pain.

# Causes of low back pain

It has been pointed out above that there is considerable evidence that common low back pain is not caused by mechanical compression of spinal nerve roots. Despite considerable evidence to the contrary, mechanical compression of nerve roots (root pain) is the common explanation for the cause of low back pain.

While nerve compression indeed may play a role in sciatica especially for causing the numbness and weakness in a leg, it probably plays a much lesser role than what is commonly interpreted from imaging studies in chronic and common forms of back pain.

Imaging studies in individuals with low back pain often show impressive changes, including compressions of nerve roots, and these observed changes are often taken as the cause of the pain although similar abnormalities are present in individuals who do not have pain [168]. This means that coincidences (of abnormalities) have been mistaken for causes of the pain (coincidence mistaken for causality).

There are large differences between the acute effect of nerve compression and the chronic effect, and the effect naturally depends on the degree of compression. For example, acute strong compression of the sciatic nerve, such as may occur when sitting with crossed legs or when resting the upper parts of the legs on a hard surface, causes weakness, numbness, and tingling, but not pain, is in good agreement with the fact that compression of a mixed nerve mainly affects large myelinated axons and may interfere with the axoplasmatic flow, causing ischemia [220].

This means that compression of mixed nerves, including spinal nerve roots, would be more likely to cause deficits, such as numbness and motor deficits (paresis or paralysis), than burning or throbbing pain that is common in various forms of low back pain including spinal stenosis. When a nerve root is compressed in individuals with low back pain, it is more likely to be coincidental than being the cause.

These signs do indeed occur in connection with back and neck problems causing motor deficits (weakness) and some surgeons only operate on persons with these signs, not on people who present with pain only. This decision is supported by neuroscience as well as the experience of poor results of decompression operations.

The physiological pain component of common low back pain may be caused by axon sprouts within a degenerated disc, by an otherwise damaged vertebral disc[49], or by the action of inflammatory mediators (inflammatory neuropathic root pain) originating from a degenerative disc that may cause pain even without any mechanical compression.

Outgrowth of unmyelinated axons in damaged vertebral discs may be a cause of some forms of back pain [49], but this is more likely to be the cause of the pain than many people experience after one of more surgical operations for back pain. There is evidence that low pH favor such outgrowth of unmyelinated fibers in intervertebrate disks[236]. [236]Such operations naturally cause damage to both bone and soft tissue with outgrowths of unmyelinated nerve fibers that are pain sensitive [49]. The same is likely to occur as a result of trauma to axons that innervate tissue that are traumatized during surgical operations. This may explain (at least partly) why many individuals have pain for long periods of time after surgical operations, including those for low back pain.

This means that the earlier prevailing assumption that common low back pain, including sciatica, and carpal tunnel syndrome are caused by mechanical compression of spinal nerve roots, which is obvious from commonly used imaging studies, is too simplistic and partly erroneous. These misinterpretations of the cause of some forms of pain, such as in low back pain, as well as that of other kinds of "nerve entrapment" pain has lead to treatments that are ineffective (see Chapter 12) resulting in many people have been suffering unnecessarily.

It is yet another example of "sure" facts that often causes trouble. Mark Twain's old saying:

*"It ain't what you don't know that gets you into trouble. It's what you know for sure that just ain't so"*

This is applicable to many forms of the management of pain.

What is regarded as established knowledge about low back pain, namely that it is caused by compression of nerve roots is, in fact, incorrect. Instead, the truth is that low back pain and carpal tunnel syndrome are far more complex disorders than just symptoms that are caused by a simple compression of a nerve root.

The occurrence of compression of spinal nerves roots may not the cause of the symptoms. A combination of (at least) two factors is necessary to cause symptoms; compression of neural tissue, such as the cells of the DRG, is one such factor and inflammatory mediators are other factors that must be present in order for pain to manifest.

## Other forms of back pain

Low back pain also occurs in individuals with spondylitis (inflammation of one or more vertebrae) [238, 471] and together with spinal stenosis (narrowing of the openings in the bone through which the spinal nerves enter the spinal canal). These abnormalities are detected using imaging techniques such as MRI. However, the abnormalities that are revealed from MRI scans are not necessarily the cause of the pain that the patients actually experience [239] and that can explain the poor outcome of treatment using surgical techniques to enlarge the holes to relieve the compression of nerve roots.

## Carpal tunnel syndrome

Pain and other symptoms are believed to be caused by entrapment of the median nerve or pressure on the nerve [255, 407]. Carpal tunnel syndrome is, therefore, commonly regarded as a nerve entrapment disorder, but is subjected to similar misunderstandings as for low back pain regarding the role of physical compression of a peripheral nerve or nerve root. However, carpal tunnel syndrome may occur without any detectable morphological signs of nerve entrapment or any other detectable morphological abnormalities. The disease is the second most common industrial injury disease in the U.S.A. [407].

Many different treatments in addition to surgically decompressing the nerve, such as splinting, cortisone injections, massage, and immersion of the hand in water, are in common use. There are strong indications that the cause is more complex than just a mechanical compression of a peripheral nerve, probably involving changes in the function of the central nervous system. Carpal tunnel syndrome is worsened by psychosocial factors such as boredom, stress, job dissatisfaction, monotonous routines, and insecurity. Again, this is an indication of the involvement of the central nervous system.

The hypothesis that carpal tunnel syndrome may involve the central nervous system is supported by studies of temporal integration. An individual who developed carpal tunnel syndrome during a study of temporal integration of painful stimuli [300] developed changes in temporal integration that occurred during the 9-month period where the symptoms of the carpal tunnel syndrome (pain and tingling) developed (Figure 8.11). At the end of this period, the threshold of pain sensation from electrical stimulation of the skin on the arm resembled that of individuals with central pain symptoms from upper limbs (Figure 8.11). During this period, the threshold for pain also decreased markedly while the threshold for tingling stayed nearly unchanged.

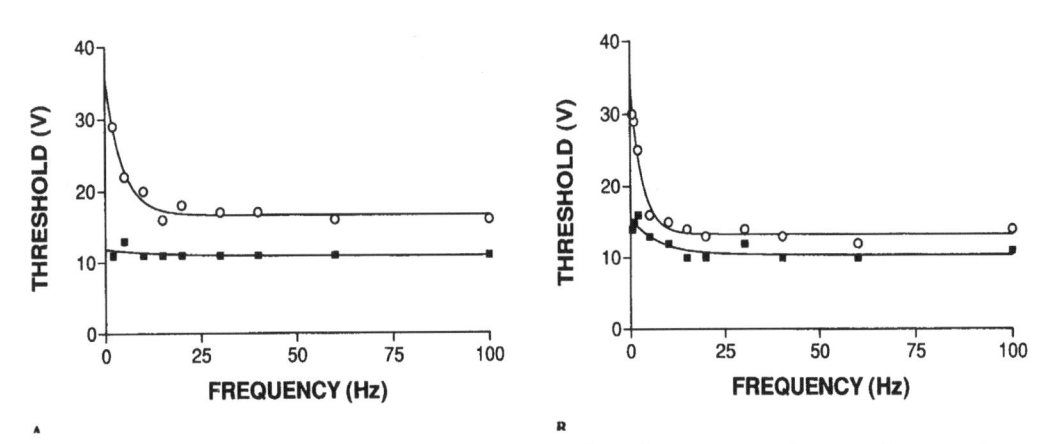

Figure 8.11 Temporal integration during development of carpal tunnel syndrome. Temporal integration of sensation and of pain in response to electrical stimulation applied to the skin of the forearm (as in Figure 8.3) in an individual who developed pain from carpal tunnel syndrome. Left graph: Results obtained before the person noticed any pain. Right graph: Similar results obtained 9 months later when the person had pain in the wrist and was diagnosed with carpal tunnel syndrome. (From Møller, A. R. and T. Pinkerton (1997). "Temporal integration of pain from electrical stimulation of the skin." Neurol. Res., 19: 481-488. [300].)

# Entrapment of other nerves

Entrapment of other nerves is also suspected to cause pain and other symptoms. Ulnar entrapment is associated with symptoms in the distribution on the hand of the ulnar nerve (the fifth digit and the lateral aspect of the fourth) and is the second most common entrapment neuropathy [255, 407]. Similar symptoms are found in the distribution areas of other peripheral nerves such as the sciatic and common peroneal nerves (for an overview of mononeuropathies, see [255]).

## In summary:

Thus, it is likely that many of the symptoms from what is known as entrapment of peripheral nerves or nerve roots only occurs when the nerve in question has been damaged or inflamed and that later stages of such pain are, in fact, caused by changes in the function of the spinal cord or the brain through activation of neuroplasticity, possibly induced by abnormal activity in the peripheral nerve in question.

This abnormal activity (including lack of activity) affects the function of the nerve's sensory nucleus, and it can make it hyperactive through activation of neuroplasticity. However, as discussed above, the pathophysiology of common back pain is more complex than just being caused by mechanical compression of spinal nerve roots and there is generally a poor correlation between MRI (structural) findings and symptoms [168, 221].

# Microvascular decompression disorders

Trigeminal neuralgia (TGN) and hemifacial spasm (HFS) [132-135] are typical microvascular compression disorders where the symptoms are relieved by moving a blood vessel off the root of the respective nerve (trigeminal and facial nerves) [23, 25]. TGN and two other similar pain disorders, glossopharyngeal neuralgia (GPN) and intermedius neuralgia, were discussed in Chapters 3 and 5.

These disorders are characterized by the fact that the symptoms can be relieved with a high degree of success (approximately 85%) by moving a blood vessel (artery or vein) off the nerve root in an operation known as a microvascular decompression (MVD) operation [23, 25, 284, 286].

More than 50 percent of individuals have similar close contact between a blood vessel and a cranial nerve root, but no symptoms [424]. This means that objective tests, such as imaging of various kinds, may not identify the individuals who could benefit from MVD operations.

In these diseases, there is evidence that the close contact between a blood vessel and a nerve root is just one of two or more factors that need to be present to get signs of a disease (symptoms) [284, 297]. Removing one of these several factors that must be there together to cause symptoms can cure the disease as demonstrated in the treatment of hemifacial spasm. The same reasoning applies to other microvascular compression disorders (as well as to many other disorders). Studies [284, 297] have shown evidence that the symptoms of a MVD disorder (hemifacial spasm, HFS) are caused by plastic changes in the respective nuclei.

For a long time, the cause of the pain was thought to be the direct effect of the close contact with a blood vessel [132, 315], but studies of hemifacial spasm (HFS) during MVD operations have indicated that the cause of the symptoms of this kind of disease is not the vascular contact with a cranial nerve as such, but changes of function of structures in the central nervous system [284, 297]. The impressive anatomical abnormalities (close contact with blood vessels) have masked information about the role of other factors; the most noticeable are plastic changes in the function of the respective nuclei.

That the microvascular compression diseases can be cured by moving a blood vessel off the respective nerve root means that the contact with a blood vessel is important although it is not the direct cause of the symptoms. It is believed that the hyperactivity of central structures (first the respective nucleus) is caused by activation of a form of neuroplasticity or kindling, but exactly how that occurs is not known.

It is possible to create symptoms in animals (rats) that are similar to hemifacial spasm by stimulating the facial nerve electrically daily for several weeks [385]. Bringing a blood vessel in contact with the facial nerve alone did not cause symptoms of HFS, but when a blood vessel was brought in contact with the facial nerve that was slightly injured, the animal showed similar signs as individuals with HFS [223], indicating that the "second factor" to vascular contact might be slight injury of the respective nerve.

It was believed earlier that it was the mechanical "pounding" of an artery onto the root of a cranial nerve that caused the problem, but it was later found that even small veins (that do not pulsate) could cause the symptoms [186]. The pathology was far more complex involving activation of neuroplasticity causing hyperactivity of the respective nucleus [284, 297] .

Studies of hemifacial spasm using intracranial recordings and stimulations in patients undergoing microvascular decompression operations showed evidence that the symptoms came from the facial motonucleus [297], which was shown in these intraoperative studies to be hyperactive [298]. The results of these studies indicated that vascular contact with the nerve root was necessary for causing symptoms, but not sufficient. In order to cause symptoms, a "second factor" was necessary [284]. That vascular contact was necessary explained why the symptoms (spasm) disappeared after moving the vessel off of the nerve root.

That vascular contact was not sufficient to cause symptoms explained why not every individual who had vascular compression had spasm. In fact, many individuals had similar vascular contact with cranial nerve roots without having any symptoms [424]. Because both factors seem to be necessary for symptoms to manifest, it was sufficient to release the vascular compression to cure the disease. This is why microvascular decompression (MVD) operations are so efficient in treating trigeminal neuralgia and hemifacial spasm [24, 25].

# Transformations from acute pain into chronic pain

Acute pain often turns into chronic pain and physiological pain can turn into pathological pain. It is believed this is the common way that central neuropathic pain is started. How acute pain can turn into pain that lasts a long time has recently been studied, both in humans and in animals. Thus, Apkarian and coworkers [10] have used data from studies in humans and animals to develop a unified working model of the mechanism by which acute pain turns into a chronic state (Figure 8.12).

The model depicted in Figure 8.12 takes into account knowledge about the parts of the brain that are involved in these two different kinds of pain and their reorganization.

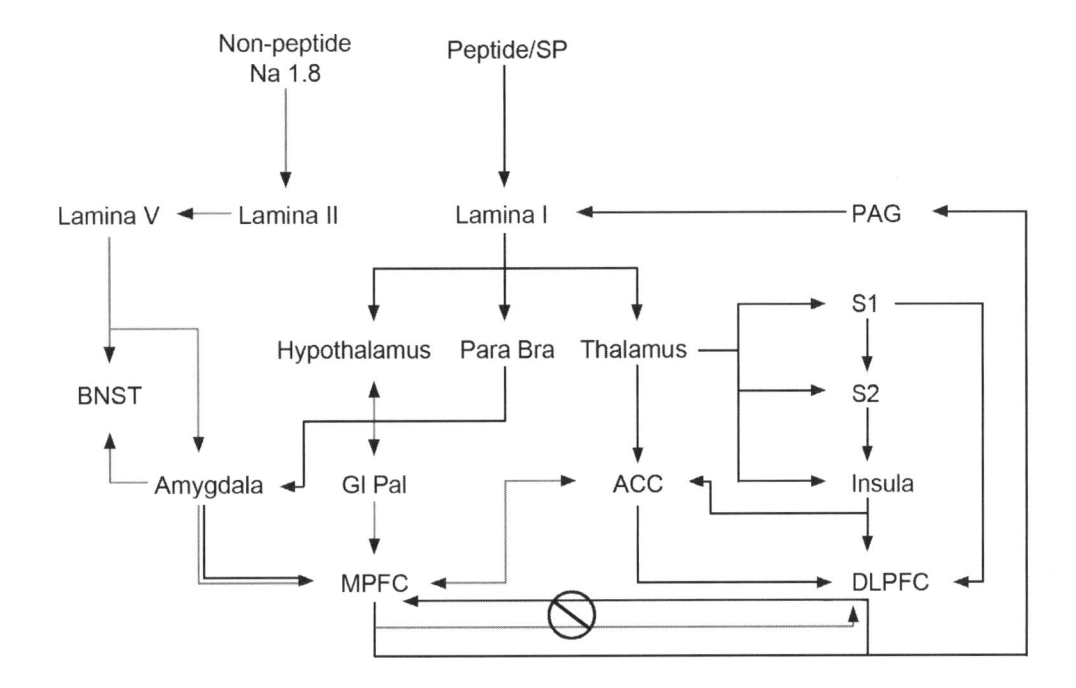

Figure 8.12 A simplified working diagram of a hypothesis of a theory of chronic (pathological) pain. Amyg: Amygdala; ACC: Anterior cingulate cortex; S1: Primary somatosensory cortex; S2: Secondary somatosensory cortex; BNST: Brainstem; HYP: Hypothalamus; mPFC: Medial prefrontal cortex; DLPFC: Dorsolateral prefrontal cortex; PAG: Periaqueductal gray (Adapted from: Apkarian, A. V., M. N. Baliki, et al. (2009). "Towards a theory of chronic pain." Prog Neurobiol. 87(2): 81-97. [10].) (Artwork by Monica Javidnia.)

The model depictured in Figure 8.12 includes matters such as pain persistence and injury types [10]. The model is based on the work of many investigators and it includes the main aspects of central pain (pathological pain). Information about the segregation of afferent input in the spinal cord, brainstem, and thalamus is from Braz et al., 2005 [45]; cortical connectivity is derived from Price, 2000 [334] and Apkarian et al., 2005 [11]. The model is based on data from functional MRI (fMRI) studies of a clinical pain patient population and basically an expansion of a diagram originally proposed by Melzack and Casey 1968 [263].

Figure 8.12 illustrates a hypothesis about interactions between structures in the basal ganglia (Gl Pal), amygdala (Amyg), and medial prefrontal cortex (mPFC) that constitute the emotional, motivational, and hedonic (pleasure) components that these authors [10] hypothesize influence the quality of perceived pain and also modulate nociceptive processing at the spinal cord level through descending pathways.

The authors hypothesize [10] that the pathways in the lower part of the diagram (faint lines) are strengthened in chronic neuropathic pain and that the pathways in the upper part of the diagram (black lines) are more involved in acute pain. The descending pathway indicates that the periaqueductal gray (PAG), in fact, comprises a multiplicity of descending projections (from Apkarian et al 2009 [10]).

# Cancer pain

Cancer is often associated with chronic pain. Some investigators have regarded cancer pain as a special form of pain. Earlier, different treatment regiments were used for cancer pain from that used for similar pain in patients who did not have cancer, but similar pain. Now this is no longer the case and cancer pain is mostly treated in a similar way as other forms of pain (see Chapter 12).

However, it is possible that at least some forms of cancer pain may be different from non-cancer pain, such as regarding the immune reaction it evokes. Immune cells secrete many substances that can activate and sensitize primary afferent pain nerve fibers and this may play a role in some forms of cancer pain. Pursuant to these peripheral changes, secondary pain neurons in the spinal cord have been shown to have increased spontaneous activity and enhanced responsiveness to heat, cold, and noxious mechanical stimuli in many individuals with cancer pain [384].

# CHAPTER 9
# Muscle Pain

# Abstract

1. Muscle pain (myalgia) caused by muscle contractions has two forms, one that is caused by contractions elicited by activity in motor nerves and one form that is not.

2. Muscle pain may be caused by excessive contractions, by muscle spasm, and by exhaustion.

3. Lack of blood supply to muscles is a common cause of muscle pain often affecting leg muscles when walking (claudication).

4. Pain receptors in muscles are free nerve endings mainly found near muscle end plates. They respond to various chemicals and are innervated by Aδ fibers.

5. Muscle spindles that are sensitive to shortening (contractions) of the muscles can also mediate pain from muscles.

6. Activation of receptors in tendons, joints, ligaments, and muscle fascia can also cause pain.

7. Pain from persistent muscle contractions often add to other forms of pain in disorders such as low back pain, tension headaches, etc.

8. Constant contractions, muscle tone, and increased mechanical stiffness may be caused by viscoelastic changes and it may occur without activity in motor nerves and without the normal electrical activity of muscles.

9. Fibromyalgia is associated with muscle pain, but the muscles are normal and the pain is generated in the central nervous system. Chronic widespread pain is an entity that includes fibromyalgia.

10. Myofascial pain is a chronic pain condition that has similarities with fibromyalgia, but it is different in that it has trigger points.

11. Chronic fatigue syndrome is characterized by extreme fatigue and may be interpreted as muscle pain. This is also a disorder of the nervous system, but the muscles have normal function.

12. Abdominal pain is often caused by contractions of smooth muscles.

# Introduction

There are two main types of muscles, striated and smooth muscles. Skeletal muscles are striated muscles and so are muscles of the head. Muscles in visceral organs, such as the intestines, are smooth muscles as are muscles in blood vessels of the body. Heart muscles are somewhat in between striated and smooth muscles. Striated muscles can contract only for a certain time whereas smooth muscles can contract indefinitely. This chapter will discuss pain that is associated with striate muscles.

# Pain from striate muscles

There are two main forms of muscle pain (myalgia): one where the pain is associated with muscle contractions and the other where pain occurs independently of muscle contractions. Muscle contractions can be caused by neural activity in the motoneuron or contractions can be elicited without activation of the motonuclei. Contractions that are too small to be observed by visual examination can sometimes cause pain.

There are free nerve endings acting as pain receptors throughout muscles and they may mediate pain under different circumstances [215, 313]. These pain receptors are mainly found near muscle endplates (endplate zones). They are innervated by Aδ fibers like the nociceptors found in the skin and they may play a role in causing pain from excessive muscle contractions [148]. Several kinds of noxious stimuli, such as chemicals and mechanical stimulation, can activate the same nociceptors [148, 505] which are also sensitive to endogenous substances, such as those released during inflammatory processes and injuries. Serotonin, together with bradykinin [268], can cause increased sensitivity to mechanical stimuli (pressure) as shown in animal experiments [148]. Inflammation of muscles (myositis) can also cause pain.

# Muscle tone

Some muscles may, at some point, be constantly contracted, known as muscle tone. Muscle tone is a continuous and passive partial contraction of muscles. Muscle tone also appears as the muscle's resistance to passive stretch while the muscle is not contracted voluntarily. Muscle tone is important for maintaining posture. The normal muscle tone of skeletal muscles is initiated by unconscious activation of muscles by neural activity in motor nerves or by the muscle itself without neural activation (see Figure 9.1).

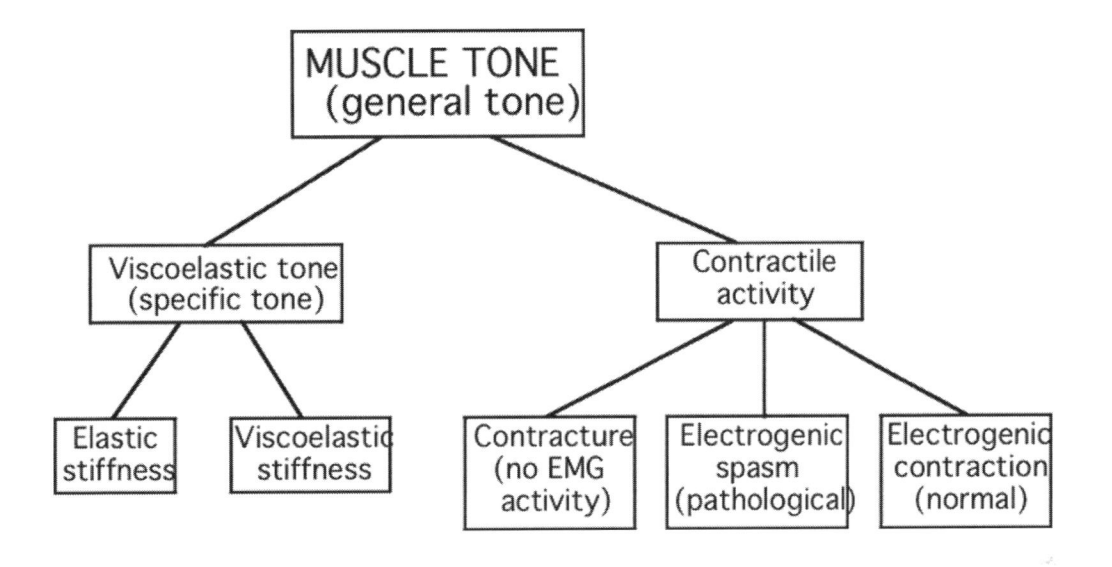

Figure 9.1 Different causes of muscle tone (Modified from: Møller, A. R. (2006). Neuroplasticity and disorders of the nervous system. Cambridge, Cambridge University Press [288]; based on Simons, D. G. and S. Mense (1998). "Understanding and measurement of muscle tone as related to clinical muscle pain." Pain. 75(1): 1-17 [396]. (Artwork by Monica Javidnia.)

The resting state of a muscle depends both on the activation of the contractile apparatus from the motor nerve and on the basic viscoelastic properties of the muscle tissue. The other form of contraction that causes increased mechanical stiffness of the muscles is not induced by activity in the motor nerve that innervates the muscle in question. Such increased mechanical stiffness does not cause electrical activity in the muscle (electromyographic, EMG, activity) and it can only be determined by physical examination. It can be measured quantitatively as a resistance against a slowly applied force.

Resting muscle tone has been assumed to be caused by a low rate of firing of motor nerves, thus, caused by activity of α motoneurons. However, this assumption seems to rest on a misconception according to Simons and Mense [396] who credited Walsh (1992) [464] for clarifying the misconception that muscle tone was normally caused by electrical activation of the contractile apparatus of muscles.

The terms muscle tone and muscle tension, are sometimes used synonymously, but some authors [396] regard muscle tone to mean only viscoelastic changes in a muscle when it occurs in the absence of neural activity from the motor nerve.

# Nature of muscle pain

Muscle pain is different from somatic pain. Muscle pain has different characteristics and causes than visceral pain and somatic pain, which is caused by stimulation of pain receptors in the skin, joints, and tendons. There are essentially two main kinds of muscle pain (Figure 9.1), namely pain associated with viscoelastic tone of a muscle and pain associated with contractions of muscle elements.

# Anatomical and physiological basis for muscle pain

Little is known about the physiological and anatomical basis for pain from muscles. It is known that there are several types of nerve fibers and receptors involved, such as free nerve endings that may play a role in causing pain from muscles. Muscle spindles have receptors that are innervated by large diameter myelinated axons (12-20 micron) that are primarily involved in the feedback of the state of a muscle (its length and rate of change in length). There are also sensors in tendons (Golgi organs) that sense the tension in the tendons, which are innervated by large diameter nerve fibers as well. It has been suggested that the sensors of the muscle spindles also play a role in communicating pain.

Nerve endings of large fibers (6-12 micron axons) that are not involved in muscle spindles are believed to mediate deep touch, thus innocuous stimuli. Finally, there are two kinds of free nerve endings (2-6 micron and 0.5-2 micron axon diameter) that are believed to mediate pain from chemical stimuli and temperature. The larger axons are believed to be important for the normal response to temperature and exercise. The smaller fibers are believed to mediate pain in general.

# Cause of muscle pain

The term myalgia is used to describe muscle pain of many causes, including some complex forms of pain involving the central nervous system such as fibromyalgia, myofascial pain, and chronic fatigue syndrome. Spasticity and tension headaches are also caused by functional changes in the central nervous system.

Muscle pain may occur from exhaustion due to excessive use of muscles for a long period (i.e. intensive physical exercise). Muscle pain often occurs from muscle spasm. Pain from muscles is often the primary complaint in disorders of muscle spasm such as spasmodic torticollis. Muscle spasm and spasticity (increased tonus of muscles and increased resistance to passive stretch) often occurs some time after spinal cord injuries. Tension headaches are other examples of muscle pain. These kinds of headaches often include trigger points on various muscles of the head and neck from where touching can start the headaches (Figure 9.2). The muscle pain in these disorders is not caused by diseases of the muscles, but the symptoms are caused by contractions induced by motor nerve activity. An often-overlooked cause of pain is the steady contraction of muscles that often occurs in stress related forms of pain such as tension headaches. Some of the pain in low back pain often comes from muscle contractions and the pain induces stress, which causes more pain, thus creating a viscous circle.

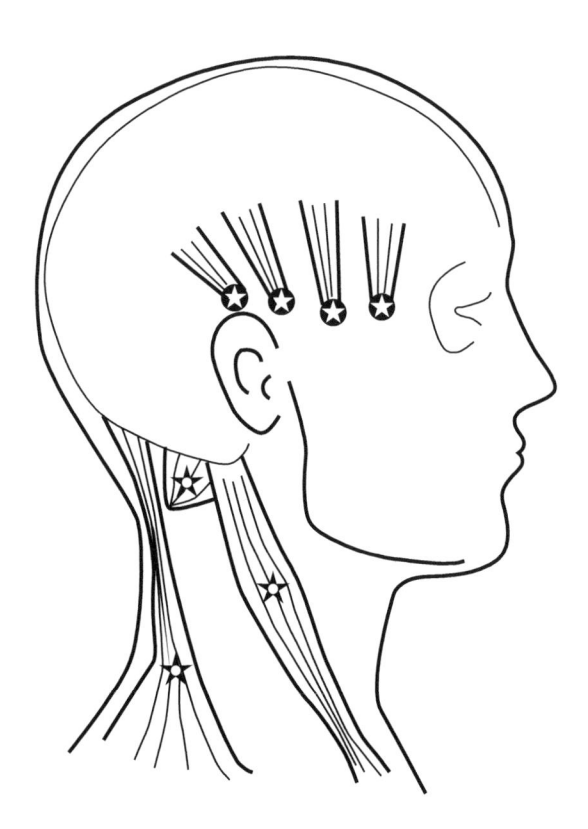

Figure 9.2 Tension type headaches often involve trigger zones in the temporalis, suboccipital, sternocleidomastoid, and upper trapezoid muscles. (Modified from Simons, D. G. and S. Mense (1998). "Understanding and measurement of muscle tone as related to clinical muscle pain." Pain. 75(1): 1-17. [396])

Diseases of muscles can cause muscle pain, but many forms of muscle pain are not related to muscle contractions, and many forms of muscle pain are not caused by any detectable muscle disorders. The diagnosis of muscle pain is complicated because of the different causes and different expressions of muscle pain. Patients' descriptions of muscle pain vary greatly, which complicate the diagnosis further [313].

Proprioceptors in tendon organs and receptors in joints, ligaments, and muscle spindles may cause pain in excessive muscle contractions by activating specific neural circuits, some of which are not normally active. This may be a form of cross-modal interaction that occurs in neuropathic pain causing allodynia. Local processes in the spinal cord can cause steady contractions of muscles (muscle tone) and that can also affect the sensation of pain from muscles. Many of the common forms of pain from muscles lack comprehensive coverage in textbooks and muscle pain is, therefore, often overlooked as a cause of common forms of pain such as low back pain.

# Muscle spasm

Involuntary contractions of muscles such as muscle spasms (or cramps) and spasticity are often associated with pain. Twitching of muscles, constant contractions (tetanic contractions), and tonic contractions can cause pain. Involuntary muscle contractions that cause pain are often loosely described as cramps, contractures, spasms, or tetanus without making precise reference to the accurate definitions of these terms [171, 313].

Painful muscle contractions may be associated with electromyographic (EMG) activity, which is a sign that the contractions are caused by $\alpha$ motoneuron activity. However, muscle contractions may also result from chemical causes such as changes in the extracellular fluid or electrolytic imbalance [226]. Muscle spasms may be caused by disorders of muscles, but most forms of painful muscle contractions are caused by abnormal activity in the nervous system causing increased activation of $\alpha$ motoneurons.

# How muscle contractions can cause pain

Normal use of muscles is not associated with pain – pain only occurs in abnormal use of muscles. Abnormally increased muscle activity contributes to many forms of pain such as low back pain and tension headaches. The forms of muscle spasms that cause pain are usually tonic contractions.

Muscle spasms occur in disorders such as spasmodic torticollis, Trismus, stiff-man syndrome, and nocturnal leg cramps, but even tension headaches belong to this group of disorders.

Overuse is perhaps the most common cause of muscle pain, but there are many other causes of muscle pain. Strain injuries or sprains are also common causes of muscle pain. Cramps of various kinds cause muscle pain. Claudication (actually meaning "limping") is an example of a disorder that has pain from muscles and in particular, the use of muscles as one of its symptoms.

The pain is caused by too little blood flow that manifests during exercise. It is often poor circulation in the legs that causes the pain, but claudication can also occur in the arms.

Inflammatory disorders, such as dermatomyositis, cause muscle weakness and pain. Infections with the staphylococcus bacteria can affect muscles and cause muscle pain. Viral infections, such as the most typical influenza, have muscle aches as one of the classical symptoms. Tendinitis (inflammation of tendons) can also give pain that may be referred to muscles. Inflammation of muscles (myocitis) causes muscle pain.

A rare, but serious, disorder of muscles that has muscle pain as one of its symptoms is rhabdomyolysis. This is a condition where muscle fibers break down and different components of the debris enter the bloodstream, creating a potentially life threatening condition. It is a known side effect from the use of statin drugs for lowering cholesterol. In these situations, pain is an important warning signal. Muscle spasm (or cramps) can be caused by muscle fatigue, electrolyte disturbances such as hypokalemia, hypocalcaemia, and by low blood glucose.

Various forms of muscle cramps, such as restless legs syndrome, cause pain. Nocturnal leg cramps [245] are involuntary painful contractions usually occurring in a calf muscle at night when in bed. The cause (pathophysiology) of leg cramps is poorly understood. A common hypothesis claims that the metabolic syndrome is involved.

A study [245] comparing the occurrence of leg cramps in people with a metabolic syndrome and in individuals who did not have a metabolic syndrome showed only a small difference (60 percent vs. 50 percent had frequent leg cramps). Leg cramps are more frequent in females than males and seem to be more frequent during pregnancy. These cramps have been associated with many conditions of a metabolic nature, but some of these could very well be coincidence rather than causal relationship. It is different from the restless leg syndrome, but may have similarities.

It has been suggested that the cause of leg cramps is psychosomatic, vascular, muscle related, and neural related. These theories have been applied to clinicians' assessment of patients with these complaints [187]. However, there is considerable evidence from neurophysiologic research that muscle cramps are caused by excitation of spinal motor neurons controlled by the input they receive. As is not uncommon, obsolete theories about pathophysiology and treatments often live their own life for long periods in clinical practice.

The "stiff-man" syndrome is a rare condition that is characterized by slowly progressive stiffness of axial and proximal leg muscles and occasional painful muscle spasms. It is a disorder of a spinal or brainstem origin [226] and is characterized by antibodies to glutamic acid decarboxylase (GAD) in a majority of individuals with these symptoms.

Trismus is involuntary closing of the jaw due to tonic spasms of the muscles of mastication. Spasmodic torticollis [332] is a chronic neurologic disorder that involves neck muscles that contract involuntarily, causing the head to turn to the left, right, upwards, and/or downwards. There are two kinds, one where the head turns only to one side and another type where the head turns to both sides [307].

Pain is a common symptom in hyperactive motor disorders such as spasmodic torticollis, spasticity from spinal cord injuries, and other disorders where spastic muscle contractions occur. Spasmodic torticollis is also known as "cervical dystonia". Both agonist and antagonist muscles may contract simultaneously during dystonic movements. It is a source of pain because of the persistent muscle contractions. Since the muscle contractions are so obvious in these disorders, these symptoms often take the attention away from the pain that is associated with the muscle contractions, but pain is often patients' main complaint in such disorders. People with other forms of hyperactive movement disorders, such as Tourette's syndrome, also often complain about muscle pain.

One likely pathway for maintaining pain from muscle contractions consists of neurons in the dorsal horn (or trigeminal nucleus) that receive input from nociceptors in muscles and which activate sensory cortical neurons through a thalamic pathway. As in so many other pain conditions, the sympathetic nervous system is involved in many forms of muscle pain. Input from the sympathetic nervous system increases $\alpha$ motoneuron excitability and, since pain increases sympathetic activity, a vicious circle may be created which can increase or maintain pain after the original cause of the pain has been eliminated.

# Muscle pain that occurs together with other disorders

Many disorders have muscle pain as one of several symptoms. The most characteristic disorders where pain is referred to muscles are fibromyalgia, chronic fatigue syndrome, and myofascial pain. Fibromyalgia and myofascial pain are perhaps the two best-known disorders that present with muscle pain without any disorder of the muscles that can be found. The term fibromyalgia is defined as a chronic and widespread muscle pain for at least three months, tenderness that is deep, but soft tissue is normal. Myofascial pain is referred to both the involvement of muscles and the fascia. Myofascial pain is associated with trigger points. It causes limited range of motion of the affected muscle and regional body pain and stiffness. It is also referral of pain from a trigger point.

The names of many of these disorders are misleading because their names were created before it was known that the disorders were not disorders of muscles, but complex disorders of the central nervous system. Ambiguous definitions of disorders are common. The American College of Rheumatology had published attempts to arrive at a standard definition for fibromyalgia and they have coined the term chronic widespread pain (CWP), which includes fibromyalgia. However, fibromyalgia is currently defined as the presence of both chronic widespread pain (CWP) and tender points which must be present at an examination of 11 of 18 tested body points and only approximately 20 percent of individuals with CWP have a sufficient number of tender points to be regarded as having fibromyalgia. The other 80 percent of individuals with less tender points have no clear clinical diagnosis, but their pain is most certainly not due to inflammation or damage of structures, nor is it likely to be peripheral in nature. This means that it is referred to as central neuropathic pain.

Common for these disorders is that pain is only one of many different symptoms. Due to the many often diffuse and varying symptoms, these disorders have either been neglected, given ineffective treatments, or the patients have been remitted to psychiatrists.

# Fibromyalgia

Fibromyalgia is a common, often debilitating and intractable, chronic, generalized pain condition. The symptoms of fibromyalgia [31, 413, 414] are more or less diffuse, being chronic and widespread muscle pain. Symptoms of fibromyalgia may appear after a physical trauma, surgery, infection, or significant psychological stress or they may occur without any known cause and gradually become worse over time.

Women are much more likely to develop fibromyalgia than are men. Fibromyalgia is characterized by chronic widespread musculoskeletal pain and related symptoms along with multiple painful tender points. Effective treatment is hindered by a lack of understanding of the cause of the disease.

The pathogenesis of fibromyalgia is poorly understood, although the current concept views the syndrome as the result of central nervous system malfunction resulting in amplification of pain transmission and interpretation.

Recent evidence suggests that genetic and environmental factors may play a role in the cause of fibromyalgia as it does in other related syndromes. It has been suggested that also the vagus nerve may play an important role in the cause of the disease [234].

Fibromyalgia has been regarded as a muscle disorder (and therefore, the name), but no signs of muscle disorders have been found [413, 414]. Symptoms of depression and other affective disorders are an important component of fibromyalgia as is fatigue [31]. Paresthesia (odd sensations such as tingling, pins and needles, etc.) typically occurs distally and bowels are generally irritable. Headaches will originate in the occipital region, and sleep disturbances and fatigue are significantly present. Unlike myofascial pain, there are few physiological and biochemical abnormalities. However, it has been shown recently that people with myofascial pain often have deficits in vitamin $B_{12}$, folic acid and trace elements such as zinc[322]. This means that it would be beneficial for people with myofascial pain to take supplements of B12, folic acid and perhaps trace elements such as often found in the common multivitamin tablets.

Symptoms such as those of fibromyalgia are common in individuals who have an autoimmune disease [77, 89, 366, 484]. Fibromyalgia itself has been regarded as an autoimmune disease [61]. This may be yet another reminder that the immune system is heavily involved with many poorly understood conditions including some pain disorders.

People with fibromyalgia are much more likely to have other symptoms such as tension headaches, temporo-mandibular joint (TMJ) disorders, irritable bowel syndrome, anxiety, and depression. It is not known if these symptoms are a part of fibromyalgia, contributing factors to the disease, or whether they are totally independent, thus occurring as a coincidence.

Most clinicians and investigators will now agree that the disorder known as fibromyalgia is not a single entity, but a complex group of diseases that have some symptoms in common. However, the symptoms of what is diagnosed as fibromyalgia may differ from person to person and it may change from time to time. Recent studies indicate that the disorder is better characterized as a complex pain syndrome [31].

The pathophysiology of fibromyalgia has been debated [143] and the view of the mechanisms behind the symptoms has changed. It is now generally accepted that the anatomical location of the abnormalities that cause the symptoms of fibromyalgia is the central nervous system. There is considerable evidence that neuroplasticity is involved in creating the complex symptoms of fibromyalgia [31]. This means that fibromyalgia, and probably disorders such as myofascial pain and chronic fatigue syndrome, may be regarded to be plasticity disorders [288]. Plastic changes in the central nervous system (spinal cord and brain) could explain the altered pain processing such as central sensitization of pain processing that is now believed to be the main cause of the symptoms and signs of fibromyalgia [31, 39]. This, together with abnormal functioning of peripheral pain mechanisms, may explain the many, sometimes confusing, symptoms of fibromyalgia.

# Chronic widespread pain

Chronic widespread pain (CWP) is an entity that includes fibromyalgia [77]. Some of the best estimates of the prevalence of chronic widespread pain are shown in Table 9.1. It is seen that the prevalence of chronic widespread pain in population studies varies between 7.3 percent and 13.5 percent. The most of the almost one-to-two variation between the studies is probably caused by different definitions of pain included in the studies.

Studies of prevalence are based on questionnaires and the formulations of the questions vary, causing some of the variations in the results. It is seen that the prevalence is approximately 12 percent of adult populations. When epidemiology is concerned, the definition of the disease in question is important. The pain in all of these studies was defined according to one standard, the one by the American College of Rheumatology, and that is one of the reasons for the lower variations in the results in this study compared with other studies.

## TABLE 9.1

| STUDY | SAMPLE | CHRONIC WIDESPREAD PAIN |
|---|---|---|
| Schochat & Raspe (2003) | 2253, 35-74 years, Germany | 13.5 percent |
| Bergman et al (2001) | 2425, 20-74 years, Sweden | 11.4 percent |
| Hunt et al (1999) | 1953, 18-65 years, UK | 12.9 percent |
| White et al (1999) | 3395, 18-75+ years, Canada | 7.3 percent |
| Wolfe et al (1995) | 3006, 18-80+ years, USA | 10.6 percent |
| Croft et al (1993) | 1340, 18-85 years, UK | 11.2 percent |

Table 9.1: Prevalence of chronic widespread pain (CWP) in population studies. In all studies, the definition of chronic widespread pain was that of the American College of Rheumatology. (Data from Macfarlane, G.J., G.T. Jones, and J. McBeth, Epidemiology of pain, in Wall and Melzack's Textbook of Pain, S.B. McMahon and M. Koltzenburg, Editors. 2006, Elsevier: Amsterdam [242].)

The prevalence of pain is poorly described by single numbers because it depends on a person's age and it is different for men and women [242].

It is interesting that the prevalence of widespread pain is largest in the age interval of 60-69 years and that it is almost twice as frequent in females compared with males [77] (see Figure 2.6). Studies of the prevalence of these kinds of symptoms are complicated by the many neurobiological, psychological, and behavioral factors that can cause chronic central pain.

CWP is a group of disorders that includes different kinds of pain. The prevalence is different for different kinds of pain, and the prevalence's dependence on age is different for different kinds of pain.

# Myofascial pain

Myofascial pain is a poorly defined syndrome that has few objective signs, and the diagnosis must be made based on the patient's history and the presence of trigger zones. Both muscles and fascia are assumed to be involved. Reduced range of motion, local pain, and muscle tenderness are common symptoms that occur together with pain. Myofascial pain has local/regional pain patterns with singular muscle spasms. Myofascial pain generally results in referred pain and regional paresthesia, and generally will not cause fatigue. The cause of the pain is uncertain, but may be inflammatory; however, some investigators believe that it is psychosomatic.

Myofascial pain is muscle pain with tenderness. Like trigeminal neuralgia, myofascial pain syndrome typically has trigger points from which pain attacks can be elicited [41, 170, 171, 174, 444]. Myofascial trigger points are described as being sensitive spots on a muscle where a palpable "taut" band of muscle fibers (or painful lumps) can be identified [170, 171]. Trigger points can be located not only at the place to which the pain is referred, but also to locations that are distant to that of the perceived pain.

There is also evidence that the trigger points are regions of a muscle with a "local twitch response" (LTR) associated with loci of high sensitivity that have developed as a result of minor injuries. People with myofascial pain have both active and latent "trigger points", both locally and regionally. It has been shown that such "latent trigger points" [445] occur in 50 percent of asymptomatic individuals [174, 408]. These loci can be converted into active trigger points by some external event, which causes them to aggregate and sensitize their pain receptors.

Leakage of calcium and other substances may activate nearby muscle fibers resulting in the formation of a taut band. The EMG activity that can be recorded from these "taut bands" is very localized and is not caused by endplate potentials [174]. It has, therefore, been hypothesized that the EMG activity at the trigger points is caused by contractions of intrafusal muscles caused by sympathetic activity [174] (Figure 9.3). This means that the LTR may be a polysynaptic reflex [174].

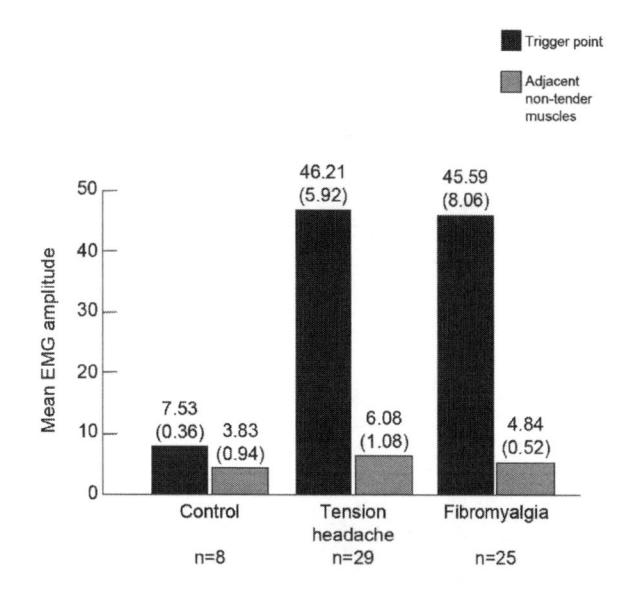

Figure 9.3 Recordings from a muscle at a trigger point and at an adjacent non-tender muscle. (Data from Hubbard, D. R. and G. M. Berkoff (1993). "Myofascial trigger points show spontaneous needle EMG activity." Spine. 18(13): 1803-1807 [174].) (Artwork by Monica Javidnia.)

Studies have shown that various kinds of treatment directed to such trigger points can alleviate the pain [170]. Treatment of myofascial pain utilizes anesthesia of the trigger point (see Chapter 12).

# Differences and similarities between fibromyalgia and myofascial pain

Although both fibromyalgia and myofascial pain are muscle pain disorders involving complex pathophysiology of the central nervous system, they have differing clinical distinctions. The pattern of pain is more generally localized in fibromyalgia (usually with a minimum of 11 tender points) than it is in myofascial pain where the pattern is more local or regional and it can even be isolated to a single muscle. Myofascial pain has trigger points from where pain can be elicited [171].

Trigger points are absent in fibromyalgia. Tender points are widespread in fibromyalgia, but not a feature of myofascial pain. Fatigue is a common feature in fibromyalgia, but not in myofascial pain. Paresthesia (tingling and other sensations that are not caused by physical stimulations) is present regionally in myofascial pain, but distal in fibromyalgia. Headaches are forms of referred head pain in myofascial pain whereas headaches are located to the occipital region in fibromyalgia. Irritable bowel syndrome occurs frequently together with fibromyalgia, but not with myofascial pain (Table 9.2).

TABLE 9.2

| Clinical Features | Myofascial Pain | Fibromyalgia |
|---|---|---|
| Pain Pattern | Local or regional | Generalized |
| Least Distribution | A signal muscle | 11 tender points |
| Trigger Points | Local, regional (& stiffness) | Not a feature |
| Tender Points | Not a feature | Common, widespread |
| Paresthesia | Regional | Distal |
| Headaches | Referred head pain | Occipital origin |
| Irritable Bowel | Not a feature | +++ |
| Muscle Spasm | +++ | ++ |
| Twitch Response | ++ | - |
| Referred Pain | +++ | - |
| Swelling Sensation | + | ++ |
| Fatigue | + | ++++ |
| Sleep Disturbance | +++ | ++++ |

Table 9.2: Summary of clinical distinctions between myofascial pain syndrome and fibromyalgia syndrome. (Data from: Russell, I. J. and C. S. Bieber (2006). Myofacial pain and fibromyalgia syndrome. Wall and Melzack's Textbook of Pain. S. B. McMahon and M. Koltzenburg. Amsterdam, Elsevier, Churchill, Livingstone: 669-681 [366].)

# Chronic fatigue syndrome

Chronic fatigue syndrome is a complicated disorder that is characterized by extreme fatigue of unknown cause. Chronic fatigue syndrome also includes pain. Theories range from viral infections to psychological stress. It is a group of disorders rather than a single entity that involves many unknown factors together with stress, boredom, unsatisfying work or home conditions, etc. Chronic fatigue syndrome is a poorly defined term that is often used to describe disorders with unknown causes and which does not fit into other descriptions.

# Other diseases that have pain as one of their symptoms

Pain is common in Parkinson's disease and it may be perceived as muscle pain. Hanagasi and coworkers [155] have shown that pain occurs as the first symptom in individuals who later develop Parkinson's disease, and that as many as 65 percent of individuals with Parkinson's disease report pain. The reported prevalence of pain in individuals with Parkinson's disease varies and some authors report much smaller numbers. There are several reasons that prevalence data must be interpreted with caution. One reason is that many people who do not have Parkinson's disease also have pain. This means that for some of the individuals with Parkinson's disease who report pain, the pain may be independent of their Parkinson's disease. The pain may occur not as a cause, but as a coincident symptom (it is not uncommon in clinical medicine to fail in distinguishing coincidence from cause). Another reason is the definition of pain varies as it also does in studies of the prevalence of pain.

# CHAPTER 10

# Inflammatory Pain and the Immune System

# Abstract

1. Most kinds of inflammation are accompanied by pain.

2. The pain can be caused by the inflammation itself or from the immune reaction.

3. Inflammatory pain can last a short time or it can last a long time (chronic pain).

4. Pain from inflammatory processes in the body has been categorized to be between physiological and pathological pain, having properties of both these large groups of pain.

5. Rheumatoid arthritis is an example of a common cause of chronic pain from inflammatory processes.

6. Inflammatory pain is caused by activation of pain receptors by substances generated in the inflammatory process. The most important substances that are involved are two ions ($K^+$, $H^+$), bradykinin, histamine, prostaglandins $E_2$ (PGE2), 5HT (serotonin), ATP, and nitric oxide.

7. IL-10 (an anti-inflammatory cytokine) can reduce allodynia and hyperalgesia by suppressing the production and activity of TNF-$\alpha$, IL-1$\beta$, and IL-6.

8. The discovery that the spinal cord and the brain have their own immune system changed the view of the role of inflammation on pain.

9. The discovery of the immune system of the central nervous system involving microglia and astrocytes has wide consequences for understanding many forms of pain as well as for other disorders such as strokes.

10. Early development of an (innate) immune system reveals characteristics that are common for the developed (adaptive) immune system, as we know it, such as neural control of the immune system and the fact that there is an optimal strength of the immune system.

11. The finding that a common drug, minocycline, can reduce the effect of the immune reaction such as those from dying cells is of great importance. Also, anti-inflammatory drugs such as NSAID are effective in reducing activation of microglia and thereby, reducing the damage caused by inflammatory processes.

# Introduction

Pain from inflammatory processes has often been categorized as being somewhere between physiological and pathological pain – not belonging to either one, or belonging to both of these main groups of pain (see Figure III.1). Most kinds of inflammation are accompanied by pain. Inflammation plays several important roles in pain. Inflammation affecting the body can cause pain. Recently, it became known that the central nervous system has its own immune system. The immune system of the central nervous system involving microglia seems to be involved in pathological pain.

Inflammation that affects the body has many forms. The word inflammation is Latin and means "set on fire". It gets its name from the vascular reaction that often causes redness of the skin. The reactions are caused by "pathogens" (from Greek, pathos, meaning "suffering, passion"). Chemicals of various kinds can also cause similar reactions.

Inflammation of the skin, joints, and tendons are common causes of pain. Rheumatoid arthritis (RA) is an example of chronic inflammation of joints causing pain. It is associated with symptoms of pain, fatigue, and sleep disturbances that can overlap with or mimic symptoms of depression. Inflammation of peripheral and cranial nerves are common causes of pain. It includes many different kinds of inflammation. Pain from nerves (neuritis) is regarded to be physiological pain and is covered in a separate chapter (Chapter 5). There is now evidence that one of the factors that can initiate pathological pain is injury to peripheral nerves.

Inflammation that affects internal organs (visceral inflammation) is different from that which affects joints, muscles, skin, tendons, and nerves. Rheumatoid arthritis (RA) is also an example of what most people agree is chronic pain. Other pain disorders that usually last a long time are related to malfunctions of the central nervous system such as fibromyalgia and myofascial pain. Inflammatory pathways may hold the key to a link between depression and RA, and cytokines have been a major target of research in this area. Reviews on some of the most recent research and commentary on this complex relationship can be found in [53].

It has been known for a long time that bacteria and viruses can infect the spinal cord and the brain by causing inflammation of the linings of the brain and the spinal cord (meningitis) as well as spinal cord and brain tissue (encephalitis). Only recently did it become evident that the central nervous system has an immune system and it can, therefore, cause a reaction to inflammatory processes [204].

Inflammation can also be caused by a reaction to chemical and biological substances in the environment such as pollen (known as allergies). An overreaction of the immune system to body tissue of various kinds, known as an autoimmune reaction, can also occur. Such autoimmune reactions are reactions against the body itself. Thus, it has been recognized that the involvement of inflammatory processes in causing pain is much more complex and more extensive than earlier thought. Also, the reaction to inflammatory processes by the immune system is more complex than earlier thought. While the redness, swelling, etc. from peripheral inflammation is well-known, the reaction of the central nervous system's immune system is complex and so far, poorly understood.

Immune reactions can cause pain. Independent of the cause, immune reactions are associated with the liberation of specific chemicals, such as prostaglandins, causing common tissue reactions, such as swelling and redness. The same substances may also activate nervous tissue and contribute to the pain. The immune reactions may be caused by chemicals that are liberated from injured or dead cells resulting from injuries.

Pain from inflammation of body structures is caused by liberated substances and activated specific pain receptors. Immune reactions may be involved in cancer pain because immune cells that react to cancer cells produce and secrete mediators that activate and sensitize pain receptors (nociceptors).

The effect of inflammation that causes pain can last a short time, resolve on its own as a result of the immune system, or be helped by administration of antibiotics. The manifestations of inflammation, swelling, change in blood circulation, etc. can be alleviated by administration of anti-inflammatory drugs such as corticosteroids or non-steroidal anti-inflammatory drugs (NSAID) (see Chapter 12).

Inflammation makes tissue become more sensitive to painful stimulation (hyperalgesia) and innocuous stimulations may produce a sensation of pain (allodynia). Inflamed tissue may also generate pain without external stimulation.

Earlier, the role of inflammatory processes in pain was regarded to be limited to inflammation of body structures such as acute and chronic inflammation. Now, it is known that the central nervous system has its own immune system. Microglia cells and astrocytes mediate the immune reactions in the central nervous system. This means that glia cells are involved in pain of the central nervous system.

Presently, there are more and more indications that the immune system is involved in many symptoms of disease [183, 259, 478]. Only recently has it become evident that the activity of the immune system of the central nervous system may be an important factor in the creation of central neuropathic pain [176]. The discovery that the spinal cord and the brain have immune reactions has revealed a complex involvement of the immune system of the central nervous system in many forms of pain. For example, evidence has been presented that inflammatory processes, in connection with ischemic strokes, can destroy brain tissue during a period after the acute effect of a stroke.

In this chapter, we will first discuss the effect of inflammatory processes in body tissue and viscera, including peripheral nerves, as causes of pain. We will then discuss inflammatory processes in the central nervous system and then, in a third part of this chapter, we will discuss the immune system and its role in causing and modulating pain.

# Mechanisms of inflammatory pain

While inflammatory pain is caused by the activation of pain receptors, the tissue is not normal and, therefore, the pain is regarded as being pathophysiological [38]. Tissue injuries release molecules from damaged cells that activate chemical pathways and various substances released in the resulting chain of events can activate receptors of pain or affect the sensitivity of the pain receptors (peripheral sensitization).

The main players in these events are ions (K⁺, H⁺), bradykinin, histamine, prostaglandins E$_2$ (PGE2), 5HT (serotonin), adenosine triphosphate (ATP), and nitric oxide (NO). Inflammation of the skin, joints, and muscles are common causes of pain. Inflammation around the teeth is especially prone to produce pain and this pain is often poorly defined and perceived as aching. Muscles and joint pain, such as in RA, are common causes of chronic pain.

Pain associated with nerves is common and the causes can be trauma, inflammation, or diseases such as diabetes. Trauma (including surgically induced trauma) and inflammation can affect a single nerve, as do some forms of viral induced inflammation. Many nerves can be affected such as in diabetes and alcohol related neuropathies. Compression of nerves or nerve roots is common and has often been regarded as a cause of pain.

However, compression of nerves or nerve roots mainly affects large myelinated nerve fibers causing tingling when affecting sensory nerves and motor weakness when affecting motor nerves, not pain, which is mediated by small diameter axons.

Low back pain also occurs in individuals with spondylitis (inflammation of one or more vertebrae) [238, 471] and together with spinal stenosis (narrowing of the openings in the bone through which the spinal nerves enter the spinal canal). However, as discussed in other places in this book, similar nerve compression occurs in individuals who do not have pain.

Chemoreceptors are sensitive to substances from inflammation or ischemia and are regarded as being pain receptors. Substances that are released during inflammatory processes and injuries can activate or sensitize pain receptors. Serotonin can cause hyperalgesia to mechanical stimuli when combined with bradykinin [148, 268].

Inflammation and the subsequent immune reactions may cause pain. Pain may be accompanied by allodynia (innocuous stimuli to produce pain). Depending on the condition of the nervous system, inflammatory processes in the body may also cause hypersensitivity to pain (hyperalgesia), or an abnormal reaction to mild painful stimuli (hyperpathia).

Unmyelinated axons can grow into scar tissue, such as from trauma to bone of the spinal cord, and cause central pain [49]. This occurs after traumatic injuries including surgical operations on the spine, often causing long-lasting pain.

Chemical irritation of internal organs (viscera) can result in pain as can inflammation. It is debated whether there are specific pain receptors in the viscera. There is evidence that visceral pain is caused by the activation of non-specific wide dynamic range receptors (often bare axons) rather than specific pain receptors [70, 351] (see Chapter 7).

# Peripheral nerves

Pain from the stumps of nerves that have been surgically severed, for example, in amputations, or nerves that have been damaged in accidents are common for causing long term severe pain. Means to prevent that from happening has been described [321].

Administration of tumor necrosis factor $\alpha$ (TNF-$\alpha$) applied to a peripheral nerve also caused pain in animal studies [458]. The pain reaction is increased when such an inflammatory substance is combined with mechanical (physical) injury.

That the reaction in the form of pain is mediated by the immune system is supported by the finding that corticosteroids and the immunosuppressant cyclosporine decrease the induced hyperalgesia.

It has been shown in animal experiments that chemicals released from chromic gut sutures can cause injury to peripheral nerves [257] with a subsequent inflammatory reaction, creating increased sensitivity to pain (hyperalgesia).

# The role of the immune system in pain

It has recently become evident that the immune system in general plays a role in pain. The immune system can cause pain, modulate pain, and affect the action of such chemicals as opioids. There is, therefore, a reason in a book on pain to consider some basic properties of the immune system. Recently, interest in the innate (early or inborn) immune system has resulted in some unexpected discoveries, some of which are applicable to our (adaptive) immune system.

It has been known for a long time that physiological pain can be caused by inflammation of many structures of the body. As was mentioned in Chapter 1, inflammatory pain is often regarded as a separate form of pain that can be classified as both physiological and pathological pain (see Figure III.1). Rheumatoid arthritis (RA) is an example of chronic pain caused by inflammation.

For a long time, it was assumed the inflammatory processes and subsequent immune reactions only affected structures of the body, but there is now increasing evidence of the role of the central nervous system immune system in chronic pathological pain [183, 208, 249, 259]. The central nervous system has an immune system that is often involved in pathological pain. Involvement of the immune system explains some of the effects of corticosteroids and NSAID as relievers of central pain. The findings that the immune system plays an important role in many forms of pain will undoubtedly lead to the developments of new treatments for pain.

There are strong requirements on the immune system. If it is not sufficiently effective (strong), then it will not be able to identify and eliminate all virus, bacteria, and fungi to which the organisms may be exposed. If it is too strong, in will attack the organism's own tissue, causing autoimmune diseases. The innate (inborn or natural) immune system was developed very early in evolution and studies of the immune system in a 1 mm long nematode revealed the need for such a balanced approach to fighting intruders.

The innate immune system is programmed to defend the host from infection by other organisms, it acts promptly, and it cannot change the way it does that. To do that, the cells of the innate system must be able to recognize and respond to disease factors. This is slightly different from the adaptive immune system, which exists in vertebrates. This much more developed immune system can "learn" to recognize new disease factors and learn and remember how to respond. The innate system does not confer long-lasting or protective immunity to the host, but it provides immediate defense against infection. It is found in all classes of plants and animal life. The innate immune system is an evolutionarily older defense strategy than the adaptive immune system that is present in vertebrates.

The normal physiology of immune defense involves the unfolded protein response (UPR), which occurs when unfolded or misfolded proteins accumulate in the endoplasmic reticulum. The UPR has also been implicated in several human diseases such as diabetes, cancer, neurodegenerative diseases, and inflammatory diseases. The nervous system controls the activity of a non-canonical UPR pathway required for innate immunity in Caenorhabditis elegans. The results of recent studies [423] suggest a molecular mechanism by which the nervous system may sense inflammatory responses and respond by controlling stress-response pathways at the organismal level.

# Evolution of the immune system

The earliest type of immunity ("innate immune system") seems to exist in all living multicellular species that have been studied. It is the nervous system that regulates immunity even in early evolution of species. It was recently shown that a 1mm long worm nematode, the C. elegans [423, 443], has an immune system that is controlled by its nervous system (Figure 10.1).

When exposed to infectious agents, the nematode's innate immune system activates responses and coordinates the defense against the insult. The same system enhances the repair of tissue injury.

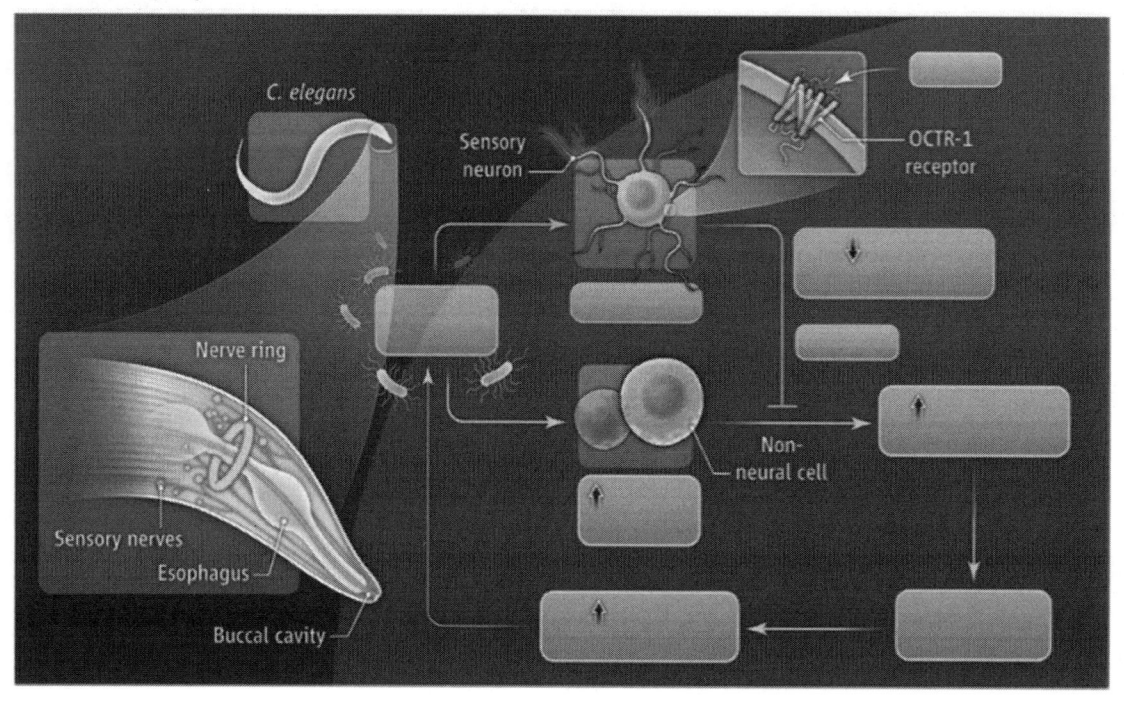

Figure 10.1 Illustration of how an infection of a nematode, C. elegans, is fended off by the innate immune system. (From Tracey, K. J. (2011.) "Ancient Neurons Regulate Immunity." Science. 332: 673-674. Reprinted with permission from AAAS [443].)

Thus, even phylogenetic, very early organisms such as a 1 mm long nematode, C. elegans, have a developed immune system [423]. It seems obvious that a strong immune system is advantageous when it comes to protecting an organism from bacteria and virus invasions. It is also obvious that too strong an immune system has disadvantages in that it can cause autoimmune diseases such as arthritis, diabetes type 1, etc.

This is evident from many different multicellular organisms and it has been shown that the immune system in a primitive organism is balanced, not too strong and not too weak. Thus, it seems to have been recognized already that early in the evolution of organisms, immune systems should be strong, but not too strong.

The main purpose of the innate immune system is to recognize "self" from "non-self" ("non self" meaning "microbial non-self," recognition of "missing self," and recognition of "induced or altered self"). The immune system also has the ability to destroy and eliminate what the system finds to be "non-self" or intruders of the organism. In order to do so, vertebrate animals use the strategies of immune recognition that can be described in terms of recognition of microbial "non-self".

The innate immune system recruits immune cells to sites of infection, through the production of chemical factors, including specialized chemical mediators called cytokines (chemicals secreted by glia cells and which communicate between cells). The innate immune system activates the so-called complement cascade to identify bacteria, activate cells, and promote clearance of dead cells. The innate system also identifies and removes foreign substances that may be present in organs, tissues, the blood, and lymph by specialized white blood cells.

Sun et al (2011) [423] showed that the old (innate) immune system was controlled by the nervous system. In mammalians, the (adaptive) immune response is also controlled by the nervous system, mainly the vagus nerve innervating the spleen and by other organs releasing acetylcholine. Acetylcholine is an old molecule that blocks cytokine production in innate immune cells [466]. Vagus stimulation suppresses innate immunity as shown in experiments where lesions in this pathway were shown to enhance innate immune responses to pathogens and injuries [442].

The hypothesis that immune reactions in the central nervous system play a role in pathological pain and in the way analgesics work [154] has been met with skepticism, as is common for new and novel "out of the box" hypotheses and new approaches to old problems. This hypothesis may bring up memories of what happened when it was first suggested that some forms of stomach ulcers (peptic ulcers) were caused by bacterial infections (Helicobacter pylori) [251]. This discovery was met with tremendous skepticism, but it finally won acceptance and a PubMed search now (2011) shows more than 8,000 articles with that as a topic. It resulted in Barry Marshall and Robin Warren being awarded the 2005 Nobel Prize.

The nematode mentioned above has only 320 nerve cells and neural control of the immune system. Since acetylcholine is the transmitter, we can learn more regarding the neuroscience and the treatment of pain. Infection of *C. elegans* with a communicable agent stimulates the innate immune response and activates the synthesis of new proteins.

To restore protein homeostasis, other proteins are activated. Sensory neurons regulate (decrease) the innate immune response to infection by blocking specific protein responses in non-neuronal cells. A specific receptor, the OCTR-1 receptor, in the sensory neurons is required for this effect. The adaptive immune system, on the other hand, is activated through a process known as antigen presentation.

It was evident from studies of the nematode discussed above that too strong an immune system can damage normal tissue and organs, potentially killing the organism it is designed to protect. That the immune system involves a critical balance between being effective in fending off intruders and in not being so strong that it damages the organism is evident throughout the ascent of species, including humans. This was evident very early in evolution from the innate immune system in the nematode described above. Our own immune system is not strong enough to protect against all kinds of infections, but it is so strong that it can attack our own organs such as causing diabetes type 1 and RA, for example.

It is interesting that this problem was manifest so early in evolution as shown by the above-mentioned example and that it still is at a similar state. Now, as obviously then, life is a balance between the two threats of insufficient innate immune responses—which would allow pathogens to prevail—and overabundant innate immune responses—which would kill or impair the own organism.

Another interesting revelation is that neurons in this ancient small nematode worm can regulate innate immunity. We know that the nervous system in many ways controls the immune system in vertebrates, but the above-mentioned study in a nematode showed that the nervous system regulated the immune response mechanism very early in evolution.

# The role of the immune system in strokes and other insults

Ischemic strokes are often associated with pain. Immune reactions occur after strokes where the products generated in the ischemic tissue by dead cells elicit an immune reaction in the tissue surrounding the ischemic region (penumbra). An ischemic stroke is a major insult to a specific part of the central nervous system that is often accompanied by pain. The effect is not limited to the region that was initially destroyed by ischemia, but the destructive effect spreads gradually to neighboring areas. The tissue that surrounds the core of the infarction (the penumbra) becomes affected by the toxic substances from dead cells leading to an inflammatory reaction causing subsequent cell death. Such inflammatory processes that occur in connection with ischemic strokes can destroy brain tissue in the penumbra, thus, extending the damage beyond the region that was initially affected by the ischemia.

It has been suggested that administration of an antibiotic, minocycline [207, 498], or a selective COX-2 enzyme inhibitor, such as Celebrex, could prevent some of the damage that occurs in the period after the primary damage from ischemic strokes. Studies have supported these hypotheses and shown less damage to brain tissue after strokes when minocycline has been administered shortly after. Again, it is a question of accepting treatments that are results of thinking "outside the box".

Immune reactions of the brain may also be involved in creating the damage that causes the symptoms of Alzheimer's disease as indicated by the finding that there is an increased accumulation of microglia in the brain of individuals who have Alzheimer's disease [68]. These same related processes may cause central pain [15, 147] . It is interesting that individuals who have such common diseases as diabetes type 2 also have a much higher risk of neurological diseases such as various forms of dementia and Alzheimer's disease.

# The role of glial activation in pathological pain

In general, it seems possible to improve the treatment of pathological pain by using drugs that decrease inflammation [498]. Glia cells play an important role in the maintenance of neuronal homeostasis in the central nervous system. A kind of glia cells, the microglia, is part of the immune system of the spinal cord and the brain.

Astrocytes and microglia are activated by neuronal activity and by substance P, glutamate, and fractalkine [478]. Activation of these glia cells can lead to activation of other glia cells and neurons. Microglia and astrocytes have been found to be active in inflammatory processes of different kinds such as injuries to the spinal cord and brain and invasions of microorganisms (bacteria or virus). Microglia are activated by nerve damage of different kinds. The activation of microglia causes activation of astrocytes. The activation of microglia is transient and that of astrocytes is much longer. These glia cells enlarge (hypertrophies) when activated and begin to produce many different chemicals such as inflammatory cytokines, chemokines.

It is now accepted that glia cells, especially microglia, are involved in the immune system of the spinal cord and the brain. While altered functioning of nerve cells is an important factor in creating pathological pain, there is recent evidence that activation of astrocytes and microglia plays a role in creating the pain through their participation in immune reactions of the spinal cord and the brain.

Knowledge on microglia biology and microglia functions in disease has increased during the past 20 years, exceeding the expectations formulated when the microglia "immune network" was introduced. More than 10,000 articles regarding microglia have been published during this time [147].

While microglia and astrocytes play an important role in the immune system of the central nervous system, they also play important roles in the development of pain hypersensitivity (hyperalgesia) through central sensitization following nerve injuries. Activation of microglia alters activity of the opioid systems and the resistance (tolerance) to morphine. This means that microglia is involved in pain.

Targeting glial activation is a clinically promising method for treatment of neuropathic pain [278]. The results of many studies support the hypothesis that modulation of glial and neuroimmune activation enhance morphine analgesia [176, 278].

This means that anti-inflammatory medication, may offer a possibility for controlling neuropathic pain. Substances, such as propentofylline, pentoxifylline, and fluorocitrate, decrease microglial activation and inhibit proinflammatory cytokines, thereby suppressing the development of neuropathic pain. The experimental drug, MK801, and antibiotics, such as minocycline, a cousin to the well-known antibiotic, tetracycline, have been found to counteract the activation of glia cells [501]. Some glial inhibitors, which are safe and clinically well tolerated, are potentially useful agents for the treatment of neuropathic pain and for the prevention of tolerance to morphine analgesia.

Control of microglial activity is, therefore, a hot topic now and much effort is being devoted to searches of substances that can activate anti-inflammatory cytokines like interleukin – 10 (IL-10). IL-10 has been shown to reduce allodynia and hyperalgesia by suppressing the production and activity of the tumor necrosis factor alpha (TNF-$\alpha$), IL-1$\beta$, and IL-6.

Glia cells produce immune factors that are believed to play an important role in the transmission of pain signals in the spinal cord and the brain. Microglia and astrocytes release a family of proteins called "proinflammatory cytokines" and these substances are important mediators of exaggerated pain. Microglia can express molecules, such as cell surface receptors, intracellular signaling molecules, and diffusible factors involved in nerve injury-induced pain behaviors and hyperexcitability of dorsal horn neurons [147, 176]. Uncontrolled activation of microglia cells under neuropathic pain conditions seems to induce the release of substances that facilitate pain transmission such as proinflammatory cytokines (interleukin - IL-1$\beta$, IL-6, tumor necrosis factor alpha (TNF-$\alpha$), complement components (C1q, C3, C4, C5, C5a), etc. [278]).

Understanding how spinal microglia control pain may provide us with exciting insights into pain mechanisms, which may be important for developing better treatments of neuropathic pain [176]. (This is discussed in Chapter 12.) These new findings regarding the role of glia cells may have a wider importance than that regarding pain and it has been suggested that glia cells may play roles in other behavioral phenomena [478]. While traditional therapies for pathological pain have focused on neuronal targets, the newly acquired understanding of glia cells as a mediator of exaggerated pain as new therapeutic targets may result in the development of new treatments (see Chapter 12).

# Pain that occurs in autoimmune diseases

There are perhaps a hundred autoimmune disorders that affect humans, most of which are rare. Some of the most common ones are associated with some forms of pain. Of the common autoimmune disorders, perhaps the best known is rheumatoid arthritis (RA), but many other diseases are suspected to be autoimmune disorders. Other common ones are inflammatory bowel diseases and scleroderma, but also diabetes type I is an autoimmune disorder. Of those that are specifically associated with pain is RA. It is also RA that now is treated with immunosuppressive drugs with some success; thus, supporting the hypothesis that at least some of the symptoms are caused by an overactive immune system.

Autoimmune disorders are mainly caused by a "misdirected immune response" in which the immune system of a person attacks the person's own cells and tissues, such as those in joints and connective tissues.

# The role of the immune system in opioid tolerance

Song and Zhao (2001) [412], in experiments in rats, showed that glia cells are actively involved in opioid tolerance. Specifically, these investigators found hypertrophy (enlargement) of astroglial cells (astrocytes), but no proliferation or migration.

There is evidence that the immune system, microglia, and astrocytes are involved in creating opioid tolerance (decreased efficiency of opioids as pain relievers after long term use). Proinflammatory cytokines seem to interact with opioid receptors making them less sensitive. Glia cells have opioid receptors and opioids can, therefore, activate glia cells. This makes up for some complex functioning regarding the effect of opioids on pathological pain.

When morphine was administered in combination with fluorocitrate, which is a specific and reversible inhibitor of glial cells, spinal tolerance to morphine analgesia was partly attenuated. This was believed to be the first evidence for the role of glial cells in the development of morphine tolerance in an animal [412]. Later, it was shown in other experiments that tolerance to opioids could be reduced by administrating drugs, such as minocycline (an antibiotic of the family of tetracycline) [279], which also could reduce opioid induced apoptosis (cell death) [159].

The immune reactions can also affect general systems, such as the sympathetic nervous system, that may become activated. This, in turn, suppresses the immune system of the body and may thereby cause diseases, such as pneumonia, secondary to strokes that may be fatal [270].

# CHAPTER 11

# Modulation of Pathological Pain

# Abstract

1. Central sensitization (increased gain) can cause increased sensitivity to painful stimulation (hyperalgesia), allodynia (pain from normally innocuous stimulation such as light touch), secondary punctuate or pressure hyperalgesia, after sensations, and hyperpathia (exaggerated and prolonged response to mild pain stimulation).

2. Peripheral nerve activity can modulate pathological pain. Electrical stimulation of peripheral nerves (transdermal electrical nerve stimulation, TENS) is used in management of many forms of pain including chronic neuropathic pain.

3. Activity in the sympathetic nervous system can both increase and decrease the intensity of pathological pain.

4. Adrenergic substances circulating in the blood can affect the sensitivity of pain circuits in the brain and the spinal cord.

5. The vagus nerve can influence pathological pain, in a natural way as mediated from visceral receptors, and artificially by electrical stimulation of the vagus nerve (vagus nerve stimulation, VNS) used for controlling many forms of pain.

6. Attention and other mental activity can affect processing in the neural circuits that are involved in pathological pain.

7. Prostanoids (various types of prostaglandins and thromboxanes that are arachidonate metabolites) are important for normal and pathological functions of the pain nervous system and they can both increase and decrease the activity in many different neural circuits.

8. The immune system of the spinal cord and the brain can modulate pain. Immune reactions in the central nervous system are mediated by microglia and astrocytes.

9. Microglia and astrocytes when activated, secrete substances that act on nerve cells including those in the parts that are involved in pain.

10. Anti-inflammatory substances, such as NSAID and especially an antibiotic, minocycline, can decrease the immune reaction.

11. Activated glial cells cause a decrease in the effect of opioids in relieving pain, which can be reversed by administration of minocycline.

12. Prostaglandins and other members of its family of prostanoids can influence pain processing in the central nervous system and thereby, modulate physiological as well as pathological pain.

13. The reward system of the brain involving pathways from the tectum to the middle part of the insula and nucleus accumbens can influence central pain. Also, the anterior cingulated gyrus is involved.

# Introduction

As discussed in Chapter 6, there are extensive neural circuits that serve to modulate physiological pain. Pathological pain may also be modulated through the same neural circuits as those that modulate physiological pain. In addition, pathological pain may be modulated by other structures of the brain and by substances in the blood.

Modulation of pathological pain includes many aspects of neural coding, including increasing as well as decreasing activity in neural circuits involved in processing of pain signals in the spinal cord and the brain. It includes changes in temporal integration and redirection of information through activation of neuroplasticity.

This chapter will discuss internal mechanisms that control pathological pain. External control, which also may be called modulation, is what is normally known as treatment and that is discussed in Chapter 12.

# Peripheral control of central pain

The fact that stimulation of peripheral nerves through acupuncture or transdermal electric nerve stimulation (TENS) can relieve central pain (see Chapter 12) is a sign that peripheral structures can modulate central pain [405]. While the mechanisms for peripheral modulation of physiological pain are understood, the effect on pathological pain is poorly understood. There are extensive descending pathways that are involved in control of pain. The anatomy of these pathways was described in Chapter 3 in connection with physiological pain. Some of these pathways are also important for modulation of pathological pain.

Intense C-fiber stimulation, such as occurs from tissue inflammation and peripheral nerve injury, can sensitize spinal dorsal horn neurons leading to the enhancement of pain. Input from the periphery caused by trauma can cause changes in processing in the spinal cord and the brain manifested by secondary hyperalgesia. This and other effects of modulation of pain signals in the spinal cord and the brain were first described and explained by Woolf in 1983 [486]. These matters have since been discussed and the topic extended by many investigators, summarized in a recent article by Woolf [487].

# Central sensitization

Various forms of central sensitization are involved in creating abnormal conditions that cause a sensation of pain without stimulation of pain receptors [39, 243]. Central sensitization is a form of modulation of pain. It manifests as pain hypersensitivity, allodynia, secondary punctuate or pressure hyperalgesia, after sensations, and hyperpathia. The change in temporal summation that occurs in pathological pain may also be related to central sensitization.

It is not known if some individuals have a higher inherited risk for developing central sensitization than others, and if so, whether such individuals would also have an increased risk in developing pain hypersensitivity and other symptoms associated with pathological pain. Clinically, it would be an advantage to be able to identify patients with higher risks of central sensitizing in order to select the best treatment for pain management.

296 PAIN: Its Anatomy, Physiology and Treatment

Different kinds of afferent activity from peripheral sources can trigger changes in function that manifest as long-lasting increases in the excitability of spinal cord neurons, profoundly changing the gain of the somatosensory system [487]. Central sensitization causes many changes in the function of pain circuits in the spinal cord and the brain such as a reduction in pain threshold, an increase in responsiveness, prolonged aftereffects of painful stimuli (hyperpathia), and an expansion of the receptive fields for pain on the skin. These changes are the basis for secondary hyperalgesia where the responses of stimulation of non-injured areas of skin that are adjacent to injured skin produce pain. Central sensitization also includes effects such as altered temporal summation.

Central sensitization can account for secondary hyperalgesia to mechanical and heat stimuli from burn injuries to the skin. Unlike peripheral sensitization, central sensitization involves the central nervous system, specifically the dorsal horn. Central sensitization is the only phenomenon that is involved in punctuate hyperalgesia that depends on the activation of Aδ fibers. Central sensitization also gives rise to exaggeration of the wind-up phenomenon, which is a form of temporal summation assumed to develop when C-fibers discharge in response to sustained stimuli at a high frequency.

Central sensitization of pain circuits may occur in the dorsal horn of the spinal cord (and in the cranial nerve V (CNV) nucleus) and from above the spinal cord (brain) [489, 491]. The molecular aspects on sensitization are shown in Figure 11.1. The cells in the dorsal horn of the spinal cord that receive afferents from pain receptors are influenced by many different transmitters. Of these, the NMDA receptor, is the most important.

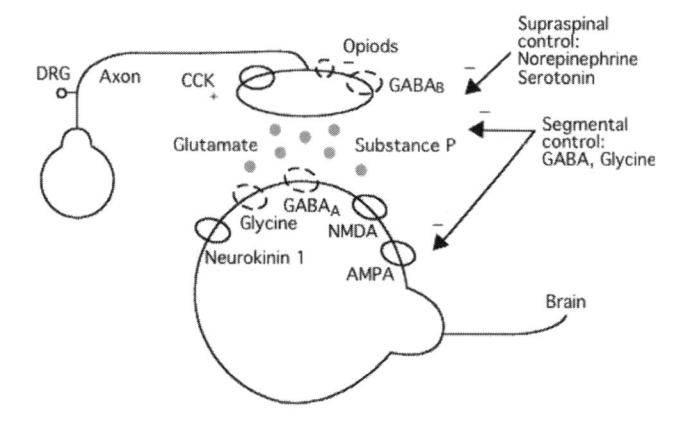

Figure 11.1 Central sensitization. Modified from Møller, A.R., Neuroplasticity and disorders of the nervous system. 2006, Cambridge: Cambridge University Press [288] Based on Bolay, H. and M.A. Moskowitz, Mechanisms of pain modulation in chronic syndromes. Neurology, 2002. 59(5 Suppl. 2): p. S2-7 [39]. (Artwork by Monica Javidnia.)

# Central action of the sympathetic nervous system

Central sensitization refers to the increased "gain" in central pain circuits. This can occur in the dorsal horn of the spinal cord and is mediated by prostaglandin $E_2$ (PGE2). Repeated stimulation of C-fibers can lead to increased efficacy of excitatory synapses and decreased efficacy of inhibitory synapses.

Figure 11.2 shows how activation of the sympathetic nervous system can sensitize pain circuits. Circulating catecholamine can increase the sensitivity of central pain neurons promoting plastic changes in pain circuits in several parts of the brain involving neurons with various functions such as the wide dynamic range (WDR) neurons.

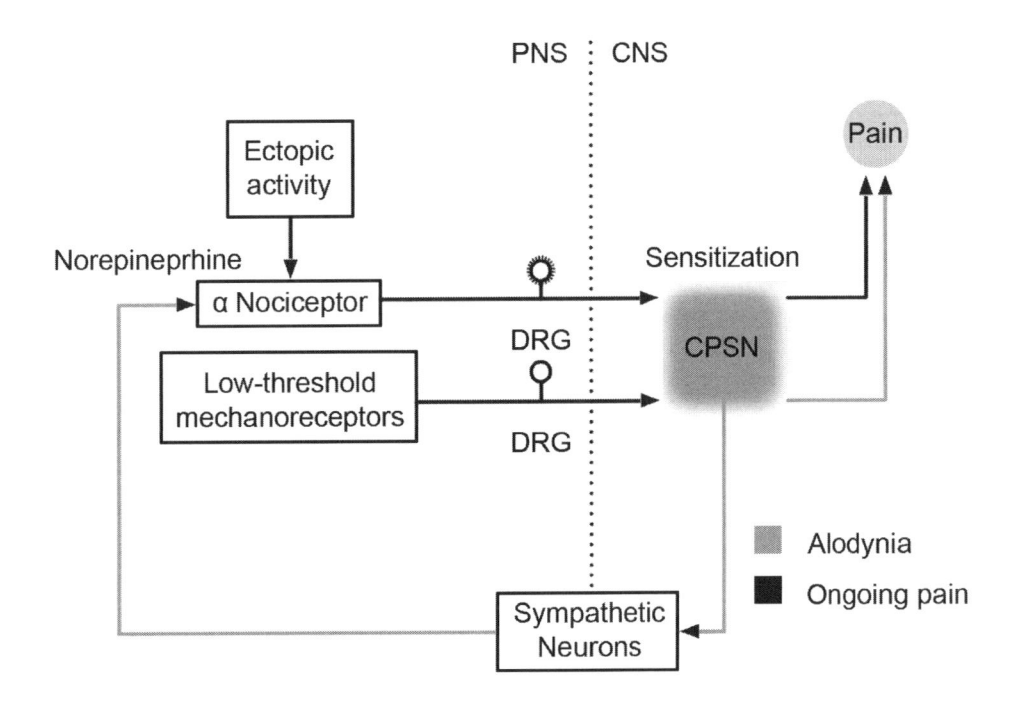

Figure 11.2 Model of the development of hyperalgesia in sympathetically maintained pain. CPSN: Central pain signaling neuron; PNS: Peripheral nervous system; CNS: Central nervous system. (Adapted from Meyer, R.A., M. Ringkamp, J.N. Campbell, and S.N. Raja, Peripheral mechanisms of cutaneous nociception, in Wall and Melzack's Textbook of Pain, S.B. McMahon and M. Koltzenburg, (Eds.), Editors. 2006, Elsevier: Amsterdam. p. 3-34[274].) (Artwork by Monica Javidnia.)

Neuroimaging techniques have been used in many studies to visualize the main brain areas involved in pain modulation. One study, using neuroimaging to determine the modulating effect of the autonomic nervous system (ANS), has provided much valuable information about the extensive and close interactions that occur between many different systems of the brain. One example is the interaction between pain circuits in the brain and the ANS [231]. Activity in the ANS plays a major role for achieving the best adaptive response to pain experiences.

Circulating adrenergic substances in the blood can increase the sensitivity of central pain neurons. Stress of various kinds and exposure to threatening situations can also modulate pain signals. Pain is often suppressed after traumatic accidents and even after a severe injury; the person may not feel any pain for a period immediately after the injury. The ability of cells in specific regions of the brain to control common functions is enormous and often underestimated.

# Hyperactivity via the adrenal medulla

Vagal afferents from the small intestine have inhibitory influence on central input to the pre-ganglionic neurons that innervate the adrenal medulla. Thereby, the vagus nerve controls the production of adrenalin in the adrenal gland. Circulating adrenalin increases the sensitivity of pain receptors [181].

# Central control of pain

Even pure mental activities (thoughts or attention) can affect the perception of pain. Positron emission tomography (PET) scan studies have shown that attention to pain can increase its perceived intensity and distraction decreases its perceived intensity. Belief that a treatment is beneficial decreases the perceived pain intensity (placebo effect). This means that expectancy plays a key role in the processing of pain.

The power of attention to pain on brain activity from painful stimulations was demonstrated in an experiment using PET-scans described in Chapter 2 (illustrated in Figure 2.5). In this experiment, a painful (heat) stimulus was presented together with a tone while the participant was asked to pay attention to either the pain stimulus or the tone.

When the participant paid attention to the painful stimulation, the PET scan showed activity over the somatosensory cortex while this sign of activity disappeared when the person was asked to pay attention to the tone and instead, activity showed up over the auditory cortex. This was taken as an indication that a person's attention could switch activity from one location in the brain to another. This has been incorporated in the modified gate hypothesis model [459] (Figure 11.3).

**Immediate Gate Control**

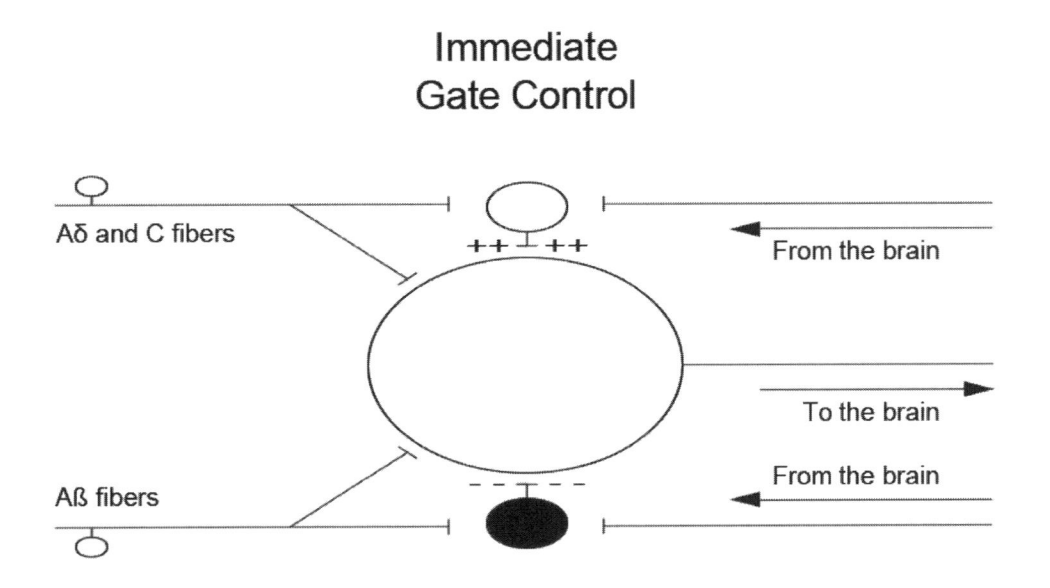

Aδ and C fibers
Aß fibers
From the brain
To the brain
From the brain

Figure 11.3. A modified version of Melzack's and Wall gate hypothesis showing three stages of control of pain impulses. Modified from: Wall, P., Pain: The Science of suffering. Maps of the Mind, ed. S. Rose. 2000, New York: Columbia University Press. [459]. (Artwork by Monica Javidnia.)

The modified gate control hypothesis shown in Figure 11.3 includes influence from the central nervous system on the activity that is transmitted in the main ascending pathways for acute pain (the spinothalamic tract, STT) to the brain. The modified gate hypothesis has three stages. In the first stage (A in Figure 11.3), pain impulses from Aδ and C-fibers arrive at cells in lamina I or II of the horn of the spinal cord. Aδ fibers terminate in cells in lamina I of the dorsal horn of the spinal cord; C-fibers terminate on cells in lamina II, the axons of which terminate on cells in lamina I. Cells in lamina I send impulses to cells in lamina V. From there, the impulses travel to the brain through the STT. In this stage, signals from the brain can modify the firing of the cells in lamina V that send axons to the brain in the STT.

Stimulation of pain receptors can affect neural activity in the STT by exaggerating the firing of excitatory cells in the dorsal horn that send axons to the STT (on the top of the diagram in A) or it can slow the firing when an inhibitory cell is activated by large myelinated fibers (Aβ). This is similar to what was described in the original gate hypothesis [264].

The cells which receive input from the brain and which can influence the firing of the main cells also receive input from C-fibers. This becomes of importance when there is a long, strong input from C-fibers such as occurs with persistent, severe pain from injuries or burns (B in Figure 11.3). The C-fibers then secrete chemicals that increase the firing of the main cells, increasing the activation of the STT fibers.

In the third stage of gate control (C in Figure 11.3), the chemicals that are transported to the spinal cord by the C-fibers increase the excitation of the main cells as the impulses in C-fibers did in the situation illustrated in B in Figure 11.3. In addition, there is now an increased influence from the small excitatory cells that may now fire by themselves and further increase the firing of the main cells. This situation describes some of the events that occur when nerves have been severed such as in amputations (discussed in Chapter 12). In this situation, the inhibitory cells that receive input from Aβ fibers are turned off.

Thus, this modified gate hypothesis explains how descending pathways from the brain can sensitize pain receptors (peripheral sensitization) or block pain impulses from reaching the brain in the spinal cord, such as often occurs after trauma. This reaction is a part of the "fight and flight" reaction that explains the freedom of pain that a person may experience in the short period immediately following a serious trauma.

# Central sensitization from prostaglandins and other prostanoids

Tissue damage is followed by liberation of many kinds of molecules. Earlier, the focus was on small molecules such as Prostaglandin $E_2$ ($PGE_2$), which still is assumed to be important for sensitization of peripheral as well as central parts of the pain pathways. Prostaglandins are blocked by aspirin, indomethacin, and common NSAID (COX inhibitors). Elimination of the sensitizing from prostaglandins is (only) one of the pain relieving effects of aspirin and other NSAID.

It is not only prostaglandins that can modulate neural activity in pain circuits in the spinal cord and the brain, but also other members of the prostanoid family have similar effects [310]. Prostanoids include various types of prostaglandins and thromboxanes that are arachidonate metabolites.

Prostaglandins and other prostanoids exert strong effects on cells in the entire pathways of pain, thus affecting transmission of pain at many levels of the pain pathways. Prostanoids are released in response to many kinds of physiological and pathological stimuli and in general, these substances are important for the normal function of the many basic systems of the body where they help keep homeostasis [310]. The prostanoids are important in that they can both sensitize and de-sensitize cells in pain pathways.

The normal biosynthesis of prostanoids starts with the enzyme cyclooxygenase. This enzyme is inhibited by aspirin-like common medications (NSAID) used to treat everyday pain (aspirin and other NSAID). NSAID reduce fevers (antipyretic effect) and they reduce inflammation and pain. Prostanoids act on a family of G-protein-coupled receptors, designated prostaglandin D (PGD) receptors, prostaglandin eicosanoid (PGE) receptor subtypes EP1-EP4, PGF receptors, PGI receptors, and TX receptors to elicit their actions.

Recently, the effects of prostanoids have been studied using mice that do not have these receptors ("knock-out mice") [310]. Studies by Narumiya, 2009, [310] have also shown that prostanoids can have the opposite effect of what is normally associated with prostaglandins and other prostanoids, which is sensitization of cells in pain circuits.

It was earlier believed that prostanoids had little effect on immune reactions. This was based on the observation that aspirin and other NSAID that inhibit the synthesis of the prostanoids had little effect on immune reactions. Studies using the "knock-out" mice, however, showed that the prostanoids indeed have effects on the immune system [370]. Immune reactions associated with specific defense cells, such as T helper (Th) cells, Th1, Th2, and Th17, contribute to defense against bacteria and viruses that invade the body, but they also cause diseases (immune diseases). The various functions of different kinds of T cell subsets are mainly regulated by specific cytokines. However, recent studies have revealed that prostanoids, including various types of prostaglandins (PGs) and thromboxane (TX), are also involved in regulating the function of T cells. Prostanoids exert their actions by binding to their specific receptors [370]. It was earlier believed that prostanoids (especially prostaglandin PGE2) suppressed the immune system, but studies using "knock-out" mice have revealed a far more complex action by these prostanoids.

Prostanoids seem to collaborate with cytokines to regulate proliferation of T cells, their differentiation, and their functions. Thus, PGE$_2$ has been found to facilitate Th1 cell differentiation and Th17 cell expansion in collaboration with IL-12 and IL-23, respectively.

Studies using "knock-out" mice also showed that prostanoids could do the opposite of what there were earlier believed to do. Thus, prostanoids seem to have both pro-inflammatory and anti-inflammatory effects. This dual action of prostanoids can explain some common immune and allergic reactions.

Other studies [432] pointed to the effect of inhibition of COX enzymes exerted by aspirin and other NSAID in inhibiting the COX enzyme with its effect on pain sensitivity. The study showed that COX inhibition also affects the metabolism of endocannabinoids that have modulatory effects on many basic functions such as appetite, mood, and memory, in addition to affecting pain sensation.

These investigators [432] concluded that inhibition of endocannabinoid breakdown and reversal of inflammation evoked spinal hyperexcitability by COX-2 inhibitors is more related to the effect on endocannabinoid mechanisms than to the inhibition of spinal prostaglandin synthesis. Because endocannabinoids can relieve pain, inhibition of the COX enzymes in the spinal cord may have pain-relieving effects through mechanisms other than by inhibition of the synthesis of prostaglandins such as by inhibiting the breakdown of endocannabinoids.

This has become evident after it was found that the central nervous system has its own immune system where microglia and astrocytes play similar roles as T-cells play for the immune system of the body.

# The role of activation of microglia in central sensitization

Many studies have shown that activated glia cells, particularly astrocytes and microglia, play an important role in central sensitization of pain and that administration of minocycline prevents the activation of microglia cells. Glia cells have also been shown to be strongly implicated in the states of pathological pain [147, 176, 259, 278].

Glial cells are abundant in the central nervous system (spinal cord and brain), but only relative recently has it been known that specific glial cells, such as microglia and astrocytes, are involved in pain. Activation of central immune cells plays a key role in causing pain hypersensitivity, but the exact nature of the afferent input that triggers the activation of microglia and other glial cells within the central nervous system remains unclear.

It has also recently become evident that larger molecules released from immune cells and glial cells seem to play a role as mediators of persistent pain while acting at various locations of the nervous system. Pro-inflammatory cytokines and neurotrophic factors seem to be able to change the response properties of both peripheral and central pain neurons [259]. Microglia especially seem to play an important role in pathological pain [176]. The receptors and secreted substances of glial cells are now known to have major influences on neural function [15, 147, 176, 278, 501] including those involved in pathological pain.

Minocycline, a semisynthetic second-generation tetracycline that exerts neuroprotection, has been shown to be an effective inhibitor of the activation of glial cells as in an immune reaction. Administration of minocycline has been shown to prevent sciatic inflammatory neuropathy and intrathecal HIV-1gp120 associated pain behaviors [500].

It prevents microglial activation and disease progression in experimental allergic encephalomyelitis, an animal model of multiple sclerosis, and other neurodegenerative diseases, such as amyotrophic lateral sclerosis (ALS) and Parkinson's disease. Activation of glial cells can also be inhibited by the administration of drugs such as naloxone, naltrexone, minocycline, pentoxifylline, propentofylline, AV411 (ibudilast), and interleukin 10 (could be useful in treatment of post-herpetic neuralgia, PHN).

High doses of topical vitamin D appear to offer particular promise because vitamin D has the ability to both reduce glial inflammation and reduce nitric oxide production. However, studies have not been conclusive to some extent because of design problems [28].

Other studies [360] have concerned the modulating effects that glial cells have and evidence has been presented that the substances secreted by glial cells may cause central sensitization and pain.

In yet another study [500], it was shown that administration of minocycline could decrease pain that occurs after a herpes infection. Neuralgia that occurs after a herpes infection (post-herpetic neuralgia, PHN) is a chronic pain syndrome and one of the most common complications of herpes zoster.

It has been hypothesized that lesions of the peripheral afferent pain pathways and damage to afferent ganglia in the spinal cord induced by the inflammation are factors involved in PHN, but that does not seem to be the entire explanation for the symptoms. Increased understanding of the role of microglia and astrocytes in pain has suggested that activation of glia may play a role in the central sensitization that occurs in PHN [500].

There is evidence that minocycline might attenuate post-herpetic neuralgia by specifically inhibiting the activation and metabolism of glial cells [500]. It is interesting that minocycline seems to be selectively active as a modulator of pathological pain; it has been shown that it does not affect acute pain [161].

## The action of minocycline is complex

A recent study [324] showed that minocycline had no effect on the early events of peritoneal inflammation (vascular permeability, inflammatory cell infiltration, and release of pro-inflammatory cytokines) in acetic acid or zymosan-injected mice. These results were interpreted to show that glia is not involved in acute pain, such as peritonitis, nor in the development and maintenance of hypersensitivity following chronic constriction injuries of the sciatic nerve in rats. Chronic administration of minocycline (10 or 30 mg/kg, i.p.) for 7 days prior to nerve injuries significantly prevented the development of neuropathic pain. Interestingly, it further delayed the development of hypersensitivity. In contrast, single injections of minocycline failed to reverse hypersensitivity when administered during the development of neuropathic pain. No significant effects were observed on hypersensitivity when treatment was started once neuropathic pain was established. Pre-treatment, but not post-treatment, with minocycline markedly attenuated increased pro-inflammatory cytokine release and oxidative and nitrosative stress in rats with mononeuropathy.

Chronic administration of minocycline, when started early before a peripheral nerve injury, could attenuate and further delay the development of neuropathic pain. That minocycline has no effect on acute peritoneal inflammation or nociception is a sign that glia are not involved because this is the known way that minocycline affects pain.

## Activation of glial cells influences opioid pain relieving effects

Opioids activate glial cells and activation of glial cells causes a decrease in the effect of opioids in relieving pain [175]. Animal studies (rats) have shown that the putative microglial inhibitor, minocycline, reduces many of the side effects of morphine when used as pain relievers, such as induced respiratory depression and activation of the brain's reward system.

When minocycline was administered systemically together with morphine, morphine-induced respiratory suppression was reduced and the pain reliving effect of morphine was increased. The authors concluded that these results supported that morphine can directly activate microglia in a minocycline-suppressible manner and suggest that minocycline modulates many of the normal effects of morphine such as depressing respiration, reward, and increasing its pain reliving effect. This is just one of the complex influences that the immune system of the central nervous system has on the modulation of pain.

# Role of descending pathways

It was discussed in several places in this book that descending facilitation from the rostro-ventromedial medulla (RVM) can modulate the ascending impulse traffic that is elicited by painful stimulation. The RVM circuits are also important for pathological pain where it plays an important role in the maintenance of chronic pain states [360], although it is unclear how exactly that occurs. A recent study in Sprague-Dawley rats [360] showed that glial activation in the RVM might promote descending facilitation from the RVM in connection with inflammatory pain. It was also shown that microinjections of minocycline could inhibit glia activation. Also, fluorocitrate, or the p38 mitogen-activated protein kinase (MAPK) inhibitor SB 203580, produced signs of reduced behavioral hypersensitivity that was caused by the experimentally induced inflammation; thus, supporting the hypothesis that some forms of pain are associated with activation of glia cells in the RVM system.

# Influence on LTP and LTD from glia activation

Activation of pain receptors can trigger a prolonged, but reversible, increase in synaptic efficacy in central pain pathways, namely the phenomenon of central sensitization [487, 490] and that has importance for central sensitization of pain circuits.

It was shown in a recent study [161] that C-fiber evoked sensitization was accompanied by significant microglial activation (increased Iba-1 immunoreactivity throughout the dorsal horn at 24 and 48 hours and significant up-regulation of markers of microglial activation: IL-6 and Mcp-1 at 3 hours and Mmp3, CSF-1 and CD163 at 24 and 48 hours). This study [161] also showed that pre-treatment with minocycline (40 mg/kg, i.p.) prevented the C-fiber evoked sensitization and microglial activation.

Animal studies [504] have shown that pretreatment with the microglia inhibitor, minocycline, reversed the effect of high frequency nerve stimulation which normally induces long-term potentiation (LTP). After administration of minocycline, the same stimulation induced long-term depression (LTD). This study also showed that the inhibitory effects of minocycline on spinal LTP were reversed by spinal applications of rat recombinant tumor necrosis factor-alpha (TNF-$\alpha$).

The high frequency stimulation failed to induce LTP of C-fiber evoked field potentials in TNF receptor-1 knockout mice and in rats pretreated with TNF-$\alpha$ neutralization antibody. These authors [504] suggested that in spinal dorsal horn activation, microglia might control the direction of plastic changes at C-fiber synapses and TNF-$\alpha$ might be involved in the process.

# Mental activity can modulate pathological pain

It was discussed in connection with modulation of physiological pain that the brain can influence the processing of pain signals in the spinal cord. It was shown in Chapter 2 that mental activity could affect the activation of several different brain areas when a painful stimulation was presented to a person together with a tone.

Just focusing attention on the tone switched the activation from the somatosensory cortex to the auditory cortex as evidenced from a PET scan (Figure 2.3) [59]. Also, pathological pain is subject to similar modulation from brain regions that are concerned with high mental functions. Studies have shown that attention and a person's emotional state may affect the perception of pain differently [454] and that the mechanisms underlying these two forms of pain modulation are at least partially different. Attention and emotions have also been shown to alter the perception of pain and its affective component differently and it has been concluded that two different brain circuits are involved [454]. Recall that the two different qualities of pain, escapable and inescapable pain, engage two anatomically different parts of the periaqueductal gray (PAG).

That hypnosis can modulate pain is another sign that high brain centers can exert modulatory influence on pain. Since hypnosis is used in treatment of pain conditions, we will discuss the effect hypnosis has on pain in Chapter 12.

## Bidirectional neural systems control nociception

The findings described above led to the contemporary concept about pain, namely that of a bidirectional central control of nociception that cannot only decrease or alleviate pain, but that can also facilitate pain and facilitate pathological states of hyperalgesia following peripheral tissue damage.

Facilitation of pain may be purposeful and beneficial to a person, for example, by making an individual pay increased attention to an injury, encouraging protection of the region of trauma. However, these facilitatory functions may be activated beyond the time of healing and might cause pain that is neither purposeful nor beneficial to an individual person.

## Other effects of mental activities

Similar abilities of mental activities to modulate body functions have been shown to occur in sensory systems and in motor systems. One of the clearest demonstrations of how just thinking can affect motor functions is illustrated in Figure 11.4. This demonstration of conscious control of motor functions that were elicited by electrical stimulation of the motor cortex in a conscious individual is perhaps one of the clearest demonstrations of the power of high central functions (a person's free will) for controlling a basic body function.

Electromyographic (EMG) responses from muscles in the hand were recorded to demonstrate the strength of the contraction. The participant was first asked to not think about the hand (the result of the cortical stimulation is seen in the top tracing of Figure 11.4).

Then, the participant was asked to concentrate on the hand in question (the response is seen in the next tracing, which is much larger than the first one). This means that just thinking of the hand where muscles were brought to contract by cortical stimulation is sufficient to change the strength of the contraction of hand muscles. The lowest two tracings in Figure 11.4 demonstrate that the effect is reproducible.

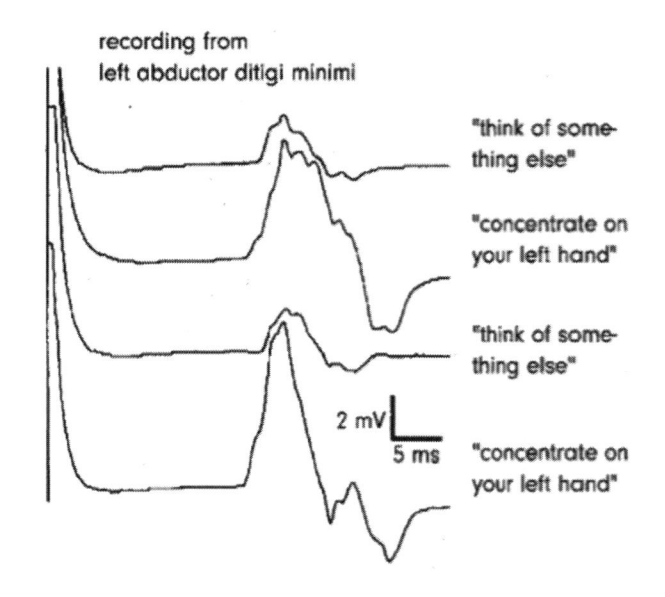

Figure 11.4. Illustration of facilitatory and inhibitory influence from high CNS levels on the response of a muscle in the hand of an awake human subject in response to transcranial magnetic stimulation of the motor cortex (From Rösler, K.M., Transcranial magnetic brain stimulation: a tool to investigate central motor pathways. News Physiol. Sci., 2001. 16: p. 297-302. [363]).

The willful control of the motor response was demonstrated by eliciting a contraction of muscles on the hand by electrical activation of the motor cortex (induced by applying an impulse of a magnetic field, such as that seen in Figure 11.5).

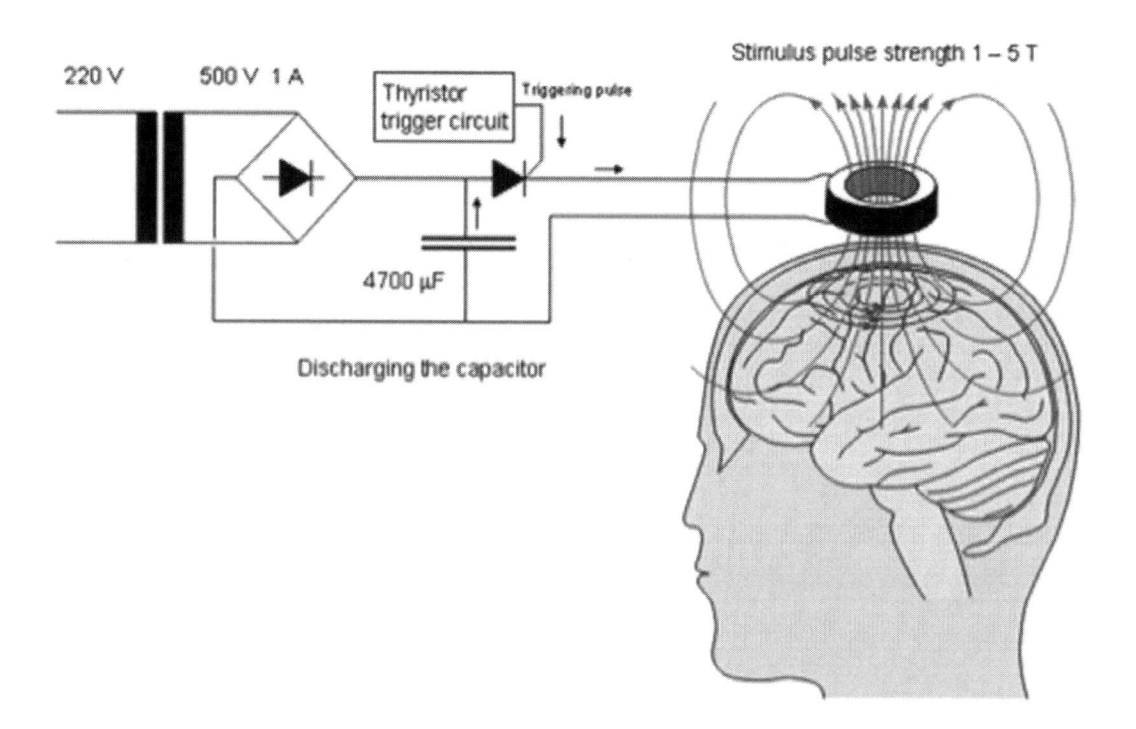

Figure 11.5. Illustration of how impulses of strong magnetic fields are generated by discharging a capacitor through a wire coil. The magnetic field induces an impulse of electrical current in the surface of the brain such as the cerebral cortex. (Modified from: Kleinjung, T., B. Langguth, and E. Khedr, Transcranial magnetic stimulation, in Textbook of Tinnitus, A.R. Møller, et al., Editors. 2010, Springer: New York. p. 697-710 [211].)

# The reward system of the brain and pain

It is well known that pain is associated with neural activity in many different parts of the brain. It may be a surprise to find that these areas of the brain that are involved in pain include the areas that are associated with rewards. These parts include the mid-limbic structures, with pathways from the ventral tegmental area though the medial forebrain structure to the nucleus accumbens. The primary transmitter is dopamine. Also, parts of the insula are involved. The limbic system includes the amygdala and the anterior cingulate gyrus, all of which are associated with emotional matters, including fear.

That these structures have more than one function (polymorphism) may impact on many aspects of pain such as, for example, pain tolerance and sensitivity, and indeed, the way pain impacts a person. This means that what is called the reward system of the brain, in fact, also involves unpleasant experiences.

It is hypothesized that these parts of the brain are predisposed for both intolerance and tolerance to pain. It has also hypothesized that the genetics of polymorphism provide a unique therapeutic target to assist in the treatment of pain. Thus, Chen et al, 2009, [74] have proposed that pharmacogenetic testing of certain candidate genes (i.e., μ receptors, PENK, etc.) will result in pharmacogenomics solutions personalized to the individual patient with potential improvements in clinical outcomes.

Cholinergic neurons and nicotinic acetylcholine receptors (nAChRs) are involved in the engagement of the reward system of the brain in matters such as pain and other matters regarding neuroprotection [281]. Nicotinic systems also have well-known roles in drug abuse (for a review, see Miwa et al 2011, [281]). These authors discuss how these contemporary advances open up possibilities for the development of treatments for many different diseases such as Parkinson's disease, diseases that are characterized by cognitive decline, epilepsy, and schizophrenia.

# CHAPTER 12
# Treatment of Pathological Pain

# Abstract

1. Treatment of pathological pain is in many ways different from treatment of physiological pain.

2. Many drugs that are effective in the treatment of physiological pain are not very effective in the treatment of pathological pain.

3. Other kinds of drugs are used for management of pathological pain such as drugs that are also used for treatment of depression, gabapentin (Neurontin), pregabalin (Lyrica).

4. Studies have shown that natural substances such as Omega-3, B vitamins and vitamin D3 has shown to be beneficial in the treatment of pathological pain of various kinds.

5. Cannabis or substances derived from cannabis are effective in treatment of many forms of chronic pain. Risk of addiction that has created legal problems that hampers use of cannabis.

6. The way medications are administrated is important for their effect, but this part of medical treatment is normally delegated to the patients with minimal instructions from health care professionals. Incorrect administration of pain medication is often the cause of poor effect of the medication.

7. Carpal tunnel syndrome has similarities with low back pain in that it is believed that the cause is mechanical compression (entrapment) of a peripheral nerve (in this case, the nerves at the wrist). However, the pain can be equally well treated by means other than surgical decompression.

8. Treatments, other than drugs, are increasing in use. Examples include various forms of neuromodulation induced by electrical stimulation of skin receptors such as transdermal electric nerve stimulation (TENS) or specific structures in the spinal cord and the brain such as the dorsal column of the spinal cord, premotor areas, and somatosensory cortical areas.

9. More recently, electrical stimulation of the vagus nerve has been described for controlling pain. The vagus nerve has many functions, one of which relates to the cholinergic system of the brain that promotes plastic changes similar to that of the nucleus of Meynert.

10. Deafferentation pain and pain in connection with amputations (phantom limb syndrome) are difficult to treat successfully.

11. Acupuncture and hypnosis are effective in relieving some forms of pain in some individuals.

12. Hypnosis has been reported to be effective in relieving some forms of pain in some individuals with chronic pathological pain. It is in limited used mainly because of the necessary guidance from a professional with experience in this technique.

13. Trigeminal neuralgia can be treated with a high degree of success by microvascular decompression of the trigeminal nerve root, partial sectioning of the trigeminal nerve, injection of glycerol around the trigeminal ganglion, and by medications such as carbamazepine, phenytoin, baclofen, gabapentin (Neurontin), or pregabalin (Lyrica).

14. Changes in lifestyle, including physical exercise, are also effective in relieving some forms of pain.

15. Modification of the perception of "self" has been shown to be effective in treating the symptoms of phantom limb syndrome. The treatment provides a means to update the map in the brain of an amputated body part such as a limb.

16. The risk of acquiring specific forms of pain, such as low back pain and hip and knee pain, is affected by a person's bodyweight and lifestyle in general.

17. Physical and general fitness may reduce the risk of acquiring some forms of pain such as low back pain, carpal tunnel syndrome, painful diabetes neuropathy, alcohol neuropathy, etc.

# Introduction

Treatment of central neuropathic pain is in many ways one of the most perplexing tasks regarding pain treatment. Management of pathological pain is challenging for the primary care physician and even for specialists in pain management. Pathological pain has long been recognized as one of the more difficult types of pain to treat. The first obstacle is, in many cases, to establish that a patient's pain is pathological pain and not physiological pain. Pathological pain is often referred to specific body parts and it may, thereby, resemble physiological pain.

A multidisciplinary assessment and approach to management and better understanding of the malfunction that causes the pain are essential for restoring the quality of life in individuals with severe pathological pain. While medical (drug) therapy is important, the presently available treatments cannot provide adequate pain relief for many individuals without causing severe adverse effects. Some natural substances such as cannabis are effective in treating many forms of pain but little used because of legal problems and because the believe that man-made substances are safer and more effective than natural substances. Some of the methods described in Chapter 7 for treating physiological pain may also be useful to treat pathological pain.

Like with treatment of many other disorders, a person's lifestyle, including physical exercise and adequate nutrition including vitamins, Omega-3, etc., is important for successful management of pathological pain.

The cause of many forms of pathological pain includes peripheral sensitization, activation of the sympathetic nervous system, central sensitization of different kinds, and activation of neuroplasticity. Many forms of pain, such as some kinds of low back pain and carpal tunnel syndrome (some of the single most costly disorders in many industrialized nations), are often combinations of physiological and pathological pain.

Many of the treatments used for pathological pain are not pain relievers (analgesics). Drugs that are effective in the treatment of pathological pain include antidepressants, such as nortriptylin, and its successors. It has even been suggested that Omega-3 can replace NSAID in causing pain relief [250].

Administration of medications of the NSAID family that inhibit the synthesis of prostaglandins may reduce immune responses in the spinal cord and the brain and thus, these drugs may reduce pathological pain by suppressing synthesis of prostaglandins. Progress in understanding the role of the immune system of the brain has also inspired the use of many other anti-inflammatory drugs in the treatment of pathological pain.

Drugs with complex and poorly known actions, such as gabapentin and pregabalin (Lyrica), are commonly used to treat pathological pain. Also, GABA$_B$ agonists, such as baclofen, are used for the treatment of some kinds of pathological pain.

Vitamin D may be important because of its effect on the immune system. While all of the drugs used for the treatment of pathological pain have more or less severe side effects, vitamins, except vitamin A, have no known side effects even when administered in large dosages.

Many forms of pain have no known cause. The aim of the treatment of such pain, known as idiopathic pain, should be the pain itself. Pain caused by functional changes such as central neuropathic pain may be called idiopathic pain although it is suspected, but not proven by any objective test, that the pain is caused by activation of neuroplasticity. Such pain can be treated by means that affect neuroplasticity as discussed later in this chapter.

An approach that incorporates pharmacological and interventional strategies and some non-pharmacological management strategies includes patient education, physical rehabilitation, psychological techniques, and complementary medicine [75]. Pharmacological strategies include the use of first-line agents that have been supported by randomized controlled trials. The approach should be tailored to the family physician and it should include suggestions regarding referral to pain specialists for additional assessment, interventional techniques, and rehabilitation.

# Diagnosis

The diagnosis of pain and determination of its cause are hampered by the absence of objective signs and the fact that there are no objective tests that can measure the severity with which it affects a person. In fact, there are no tests that can confirm that a person has pain at all. This is especially a problem regarding pathological pain. Diagnosis of what causes a person's pain must, therefore, often be made on the basis of the person's description of the pain. In the present state of medical care, physicians and surgeons seem to rely more on objective findings, such as imaging studies, than what a patient is describing about his/her problems. As we have seen from Dr. Melzack's experience, people's descriptions of their pain vary.

When imaging tests, such as MRIs, are evaluated for a diagnosis of, for example, back pain, it is often ignored that what is regarded as abnormalities in fact occur in many individuals without giving any symptoms. Conventional diagnostic methods applied to pathological pain may, therefore, provide misleading information. For example, the structural changes that are observed to compress spinal nerve roots may, in fact, often occur concomitant to the patients' complaints of pain, but not as a cause of the problems. This is a typical example of not distinguishing between coincidence and cause, and this error is especially common regarding the diagnosis of disorders that do not have distinct objective signs such as central neuropathic pain and some forms of tinnitus ("correlation does imply causation").

It should be kept in mind that MRI and other imaging tests describe structures and not functions. This means that imaging studies can only detect changes in structure and not the cause of symptoms. Blind trust in imaging studies has led to many treatments that have not been beneficial to the patient or it has led to no treatment when the disease had no detectable structural abnormalities that appeared on imaging tests.

# Incorrect diagnosis

An abnormality that is detected by imaging techniques may not be the cause of a patient's complaint. Signs of abnormalities in objective tests, such as MRI, CT scan, and various other forms of imaging tests, may occur coincidentally and not be the cause of the pain. An example of this is common low back pain.

If the same abnormality occurs in many individuals who do not have the symptoms, there are reasons to believe that the detected abnormality is not the cause of the patient's symptoms, or it can be an abnormality that only gives symptoms when it occurs together with another abnormality.

Microvascular compression of cranial nerves is an example of a condition that is associated with specific diseases, the diagnosis of which has caused much confusion. Microvascular compression of the root of cranial nerve V is associated with trigeminal neuralgia, hemifacial spasm when the root of cranial nerve VII is affected, cranial nerve IX for glossopharyngeal neuralgia, and when it occurs with nervous intermedius for geniculate neuralgia, deep ear pain may result [284].

As was discussed in Chapter 8, vascular compression (or rather vascular contact) alone does not cause the symptoms, but another factor is necessary (the "second factor") to cause symptoms. This factor (or factors) must be present together with the close contact between a blood vessel and a nerve root in order to cause symptoms [284, 297]. There is evidence that suggests that this second factor may be inflammation of one kind or another and/or the subsequent immune reaction.

This, and the involvement of neuroplasticity, can explain why several different treatments are successful in alleviating the pain associated with microvascular compression disorders. Disorders, such as complex regional pain syndrome type 1 and 2 (CRPS 1 and 2), involve many systems including the somatosensory system, autonomic systems, and motor systems, and the symptoms are of a broad range and often many.

Diagnosis is usually made by excluding other causes that may have similar symptoms that people with suspected CRPS present with. The following tests have been suggested: quantitative sensory testing (QST), autonomic testing that includes quantitative sudomotor axon reflex test (QSART) for sweating abnormalities, the cold presser test in conjunction with thermographic imaging to observe the vasoconstrictor response, and laser Doppler flowmetry to monitor background vasomotor control [415]. What such tests could tell about the cause of a patient's symptoms is often difficult to understand.

This all means that not only correct interpretation of tests such as imaging studies is necessary for obtaining a correct diagnosis, it is also necessary to know something about the pathophysiology of the disease.

# Which body part has the abnormal function that can cause pain?

In addition to concerns about which kind of pain a person has, it is also important to know which part of the body is affected. It would be very helpful in the treatment of pathological pain to know which parts of the brain were involved and to know if there is a "pain center" in the brain. There is increasing evidence that pain, like many other functions, is distributed over many different parts of the brain. Thus, pathological pain is likely to engage many different structures in the body. It would also be important to know at which structure to aim treatment.

For treatments of pain, it is often important to know which structures in the spinal cord and the brain are malfunctioning, causing the pain. A malfunctioning structure may cause pathological signs in other structures, which may be interpreted as being pathologic. Treatment of these structures will, therefore, not produce any relief of the pain. Finally, the output of normally functioning parts of the central nervous system may be abnormal because of abnormal input. Treatment should not be aimed at such parts.

The symptoms of pain, therefore, may not always come from the structures that are malfunctioning. If the pain is felt in an arm, but the structures that are malfunctioning are in the brain or the spinal cord, it does not help to treat the arm. Referred pain is an example of pain that is felt as coming from parts of the body that are perfectly normal.

There is no benefit from treatment that is aimed at structures that seem to behave abnormally due to abnormal input. In this way, causes of some forms of pain have similarities with those of other diseases such as, for example, diabetes type 2. Diabetes type 2, which often causes pain in the form of diabetes neuropathy, is an example of a disease that engages a sequence of structures and functions such as illustrated in Figure 12.1.

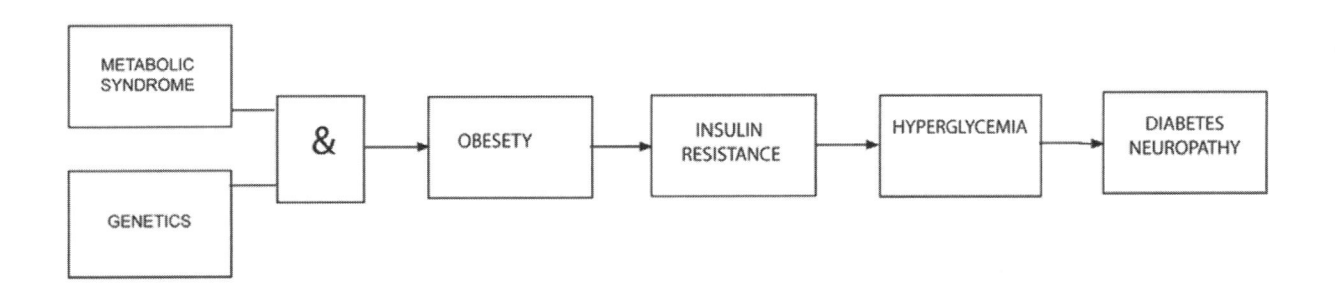

Figure 12.1 Hypothetical flowchart of events that occur in the development of type 2 diabetes neuropathy [293].

Generation of awareness of pathological pain also involves a cascade of parts of the central nervous system similar to many other disorders such as diabetes type 2 (Figure 12.1). An important question regarding pain involves which of the steps in such a cascade should be the target for treatment. Treating the structures that are malfunctioning may cure the disorder and thereby, eliminate the pain. This is the ideal situation, which, unfortunately, is rarely obtainable.

Treating structures that receive abnormal input may ameliorate symptoms during the treatment, but will not eliminate the problems and require continued treatment. Treating the wrong structure or correcting something that may appear abnormal, but which does not contribute to the pain, naturally provides no benefit to the patient. On the contrary, the treatment may cause side effects or it may worsen the pain. Unfortunately, this is a common result of an incorrect diagnosis where coincidence (correlation of abnormalities) does not cause the pain; examples are many, such as low back pain.

# Which components of pain should be aimed at treatment?

Most forms of pain have two components, the perception (awareness) and an adverse effect on a person. Little attention has been paid to the adverse effects (decrease in quality of life), which includes difficulties to sleep, difficulties to concentrate on intellectual tasks, and it may involve affective symptoms such as depression. The adverse effects are not always directly related to the perceived severity of the pain. This means that the analog scale representation of pain may not completely describe the severity of the pain.

Management of pain to a level that decreases the quality of life the least is important. It is more important to decrease the effect the pain has on a person than to decrease the perception (of the strength) of the pain. These two qualities of pain are often not affected by the same treatment.

Some treatments may decrease the effect pain has on a person more than the perception of the strength of the pain. For monitoring of the success of treatment, it is important to differentiate between these two different qualities of pain and it is important to ask the patients appropriate questions. Just asking a patient if the pain has changed is not sufficient.

# Methods used for treatment of pain in general

The treatments that are in routine use for the common forms of pain are many and they differ mainly with regards to their side effects, costs, and the involvement of the person with pain that the individual methods require.

In general, the treatment for pain is dominated by medications that can be obtained without a prescription, but pain medications that require a prescription are also common. Some of these medications are also effective for pathological pain, but for some kinds of pathological pain, the effectiveness of common pain medications is less than what it is for physiological pain.

There are great ambiguities, however, about which methods should be used to treat many of the most common pain conditions such as low back pain and carpal tunnel syndrome. Surgery is effective as treatment for disorders such as the microvascular compression operation for trigeminal neuralgia (TGN) [24, 129, 286], glossopharyngeal neuralgia (GPN), and hemifacial spasm (HFS).

Surgery is also often performed to treat other nerve compression disorders such as low back pain, carpal tunnel syndrome [308, 435], ulnar nerve entrapment, etc., however, with varying benefit to the patient [49, 238, 239].

Improvement of the health-related quality of life for persons with back pain is, therefore, not improving despite the availability of many different treatments [358]. The enormous economic interest in surgical treatment of low back pain has clouded assessments of efficacy of the used methods, especially regarding surgical interventions [290].

Other surgery-like methods, such as epidural injections of various substances, are methods that are frequently used, but where the benefit to the patient is questionable. Again, these treatments are highly profitable for hospitals and surgeons.

Treatment of such forms of pain as CRPS 1 and 2 are other examples where many different treatments have been used with varying degrees of benefit to the patients.

# Drug treatments

Administration of drugs for treatment of severe pain is still the most common means for controlling severe pain although the mechanisms of action are not completely understood. We will discuss some treatments that have been especially important in bringing new light to the understanding of the various forms of pain including central neuropathic pain. Drugs that are effective treatments of physiological pain may not be equally effective in treatments of pathological pain such as central neuropathic pain.

The choice of what medication to use to treat pathological pain is more complicated and depends on the kind of pain, the person's other diseases, and his/her age [3]. While some forms of pathological pain may respond to conventional painkillers such as NSAID and opioids, chronic neuropathic pain other forms of pathological pain respond poorly to treatment with NSAID and opioids. Other drugs, such as drugs that have been associated with the treatment of depression (nortriptylin) and drugs such as gabapentin (Neurontin) and pregabalin (Lyrica), are often more effective when administered alone or in combination with traditional pain killers. Some sodium channel blockers are effective in treating neuropathic pain.

Some recent developments have provided new approaches and new drugs have been developed or are under development. It is believed that a combination of new drugs that have been thoroughly tested in clinical trials together with an increased understanding of the role of neuroplasticity will lead to an improvement in treatments and prevention of pathological pain [359].

# Mood active drugs

Drugs that have little or no analgesic effect on acute (physiological) pain have found use in treatment of chronic neuropathic pain either alone or together with other drugs. The efficacy of the different kinds is different for different kinds of pain. Examples are antidepressants such as imipramine, amitriptyline, nortriptylin [400]. Sodium channel blockers such as carbamazepine and Mexilitine were some of the least effective of these drugs. Selective serotonin reuptake inhibitors (SSRIs) were less effective than imipramine.

Studies of the effectiveness of antidepressants have indicated that the serotonin system is involved in central neuropathic pain but the fact the selective serotonin reuptake inhibitors are less effective than non-specific drugs such as imipramine and nortriptylin[400] may set that assumption in question and indicate a more complex relationship between chronic neuropathic pain and the serotonin system.

However one serotonin receptor, the NMDA receptor may be an exception. An inhibitor of the NMDA receptor, Ketamine, has shown interesting effects on some forms of pain [429].

The use of opioids in treatment of chronic neuropathic pain has been controversial. Results of short-term studies have not provided clear evidence of efficacy in reducing the intensity of neuropathic pain. Longer term studies have demonstrated significant efficacy compared with placebo, but the results of these results have been set in question because of small size, short duration, and potentially inadequate handling of dropouts[260].

The efficacy of opioids as treatment of chronic neuropathic pain is therefore unclear. An important side effect of opioids is suppression of respiration, which can lead to death. This is especially a problem when opioids are used to manage pain over a long time where tolerance makes it necessary to increase the dosage. In general overdose has become a problem that has caused increasing number of deaths. Naloxone that is an effective (immediate) remedy that can reverse the effect of opioids is unfortunately not generally available.

There has recently been an interest in drugs such as Metformin for treatment of chronic pain. Metformin, which is in common use for treatment of diabetes type 2[430].

# Non-pharmacologic treatments

Treatment with natural substances such as Omega 3 [250] and cannabis [482]. Electrical stimulation of different kinds is in use to provide neuromodulation to change the function of neural structures in the spinal cord and the brain that are malfunctioning and causing pain. The different methods apply electrical stimulation to the skin (transdermal electrical stimulation, TENS) [461, 479], to the dorsal column of the spinal cord [276], and to the surface of the cerebral cortex [201, 275, 446] or in deep structures such as the thalamus (deep brain stimulation, DBS).

## Cannabis for pain management

It has been known for a long time that smoking cannabis could relieve pain. However, despite clinical evidence from studies in humans [2, 331, 353, 357] as well as experimental evidence from animal studies have shown evidence that cannabis and substances derived from cannabis are effective in relieving many forms of pain including central neuropathic pain with non-serious side effects.

The two main active components of cannabis, δ-9- tetrahydrocanabidiol (THC) and cannabidiol (CBD). Clinical studies have shown that especially CBD has good pain relieving effect in people experiencing neuropathic pain that persisted despite conventional treatment [482].

A cannabis-based medications such Nabiximols [213] a 1:1 mix of δ-9-tetrahydrocanabidiol (THC) together and cannabidiol (CBD) extract from cloned chemovars is licensed in the UK since 2010 (and Canada). It is recommended as the second or third line in treatment of central neuropathic pain [331]. These substances have also demonstrated efficacy in treatment of spasticity, neuropathic pain and bladder dysfunction [331]. Smoking cannabis has disadvantages such as side effects from the smoke and inaccuracy in administration of the active substances. Wilsey and coworkers (2012) suggested to use vaporized cannabis, which they showed had good therapeutically effect when inhaled by people with neuropathic pain, even drug resistant neuropathic pain [482]. [357]

Our understanding of the pharmacology of the active substance in the cannabis plants [357] and the basis for pain relief from administration of cannabis has increased rapidly. It seems likely that the beneficial effect from administration of substances from cannabis may be related to their effect on the affective qualities of pain. The receptors for these substances are located in the frontal part of the brain and in limbic structures. Recent studies using functional magnetic resonance imaging in healthy volunteers where pain was induced by application capsaicin have supported that hypothesis [228]. The intensity of pain and the hyperalgesia were diminished by THC and that effect correlated with right amygdala activity. The results also indicated that THC reduced the connectivity between the amygdala and sensory-motor areas. This emphasis the importance of using cannabis that is rich in CBD and poor in THC.

The side effects from pain treatment using cannabis are minimal. The risk of deaths from overdosage of cannabis substances is minimal compared with those of opioids; a death from overdosage of the conventional semi-synthetic opioids (prescription pain medication) in the US occurs every 19 minutes [69]. It is the second leading cause of accidental death (after car accidents).

# Neuromodulation

Neuromodulation refers to changes in the function of the nervous system by the nervous system itself or induced by external means, most often by electrical stimulation for therapeutic purposes for disorders of the nervous system. The stimulation may be applied to the skin (such as TENS), to the surface of the spinal cord or brain through implanted electrodes, or by electrodes placed deep in the brain (deep brain stimulation, DBS) such as in the basal ganglia for treating movement disorders such as Parkinson's disease.

The purpose of neuromodulation is often to reverse "bad" plastic changes that cause symptoms of disease such as pathological pain (or some forms of tinnitus). It is a general experience that such artificially induced neuromodulation can be very effective against several symptoms, but the beneficial effect is often limited to a certain time, often 5-10 years after which the symptoms return. The reason for that is assumed to be plastic changes that reverse the effect induced by the neuromodulation. Examples include DBS for movement disorders.

Electrical stimulation of the greater occipital nerve may offer some relief of the symptoms of fibromyalgia [330]. It is not known how this treatment can be beneficial for widespread bodily pain such as in fibromyalgia. Future research and growing clinical experience will show which of these pain conditions is the best candidate for peripheral nerve stimulation.

Vibration applied to the skin and acupuncture are all methods of neuromodulation that are effective in achieving relief from pain [157, 405]. Acupuncture is another treatment that uses electrical and other ways of activating receptors and nerves in the skin [157, 467]; the main function of which is neuromodulation.

The effectiveness of acupuncture in the treatment of pain is another indication that pathological pain can be modulated by activation of the peripheral nervous system (through activation of neuroplasticity). Electrical stimulation of the vagus nerve (VNS) is a more recent addition to the clinical use of neuromodulation [6].

Hypnosis is a form of neuromodulation that affects the function of the central nervous system, but not through electrical stimulation, rather through a person's own action [343]. Hypnosis is a learned strategy that involves achievement of an extreme level of relaxation.

Physical exercise has been shown to be beneficial for some forms of pain. Perhaps through a form of neuromodulation, it may affect the function of the central nervous system through increasing brain derived neurotrophic factors (BDNF) [144].

Peripheral nerve stimulation (PNS) is a form of neural modulation that has been used for the treatment of pathological pain for more than 40 years. Recently, there has been new interest in this technique and there is wider acceptance of neuromodulation in general as a treatment for individuals with refractory pain. Current indications and hardware choices that are in frequent use have been described by Slavin [405]. Published studies have shown that many forms of pathological pain can be relieved by forms of peripheral nerve stimulation.

The use of these techniques in the treatment of post-traumatic and postsurgical neuropathy, occipital neuralgia, and complex regional pain syndromes has been described. PNS in one form or another has also been described for new indications, such as migraines and daily headaches [34], cluster headaches, and fibromyalgia.

I form of peripheral nerve stimulation is what is known as transderm electrical nerve stimulation (TENS).

# Transdermal electrical nerve stimulation (TENS)

Transdermal electrical nerve stimulation (TENS) was invented for treatment of pain by Patrick Wall, neurologist-neurophysiologist, and William Sweet, neurosurgeon, on the basis of the gating hypothesis. The clinical use was described by Willer, 1988 [479]. TENS has, through its use during many years, shown it is an effective way of managing many forms of pain. It has essentially no side effects, but the fact that it requires active participation of the patient has severely limited its use. It has especially been used for the treatment of back pain.

Since TENS was developed on the basis of the gating hypothesis, it was primarily assumed to work by modulating the transmission of pain signals in the ascending spinal pain pathways. TENS has been assumed to work by activating $A\beta$ nerve fibers that have inhibitory influence on the pain circuits in lamina I and II of the spinal cord.

It has later been found to have a wider importance and there are indications that it can cause plastic changes in the spinal cord and brain and, thereby, reduce pain caused by activation of neuroplasticity. One may explain its action as reversing the bad plastic changes that cause pain.

TENS is effective for many kinds of pain such as deafferentation pain. It is not normally used for treating pain in the head, but it might have a similar effect by activating pain circuits in the caudal trigeminal nucleus. TENS has also been described as a way of relieving pain from pathological muscle contractions [479].

Vibration therapy, acupuncture, hypnosis, and biofeedback are other forms of therapy that may be used to treat various forms of pathological pain, including phantom pain. However, they are often of little help because they are not used in an optimal way, most likely because patients do not follow given instructions or perhaps because the instructions were not correct or not sufficiently detailed.

# Dorsal column stimulations

Spinal cord stimulation (SCS) can be an effective treatment for phantom pain. It uses stimulating electrodes placed closely (epidural) to the spinal cord and the patient only needs to switch it on and off [276, 398, 399]. Its action may be similar to that of TENS, but it has the advantage that the patient does not need to participate as is necessary for the use of TENS.

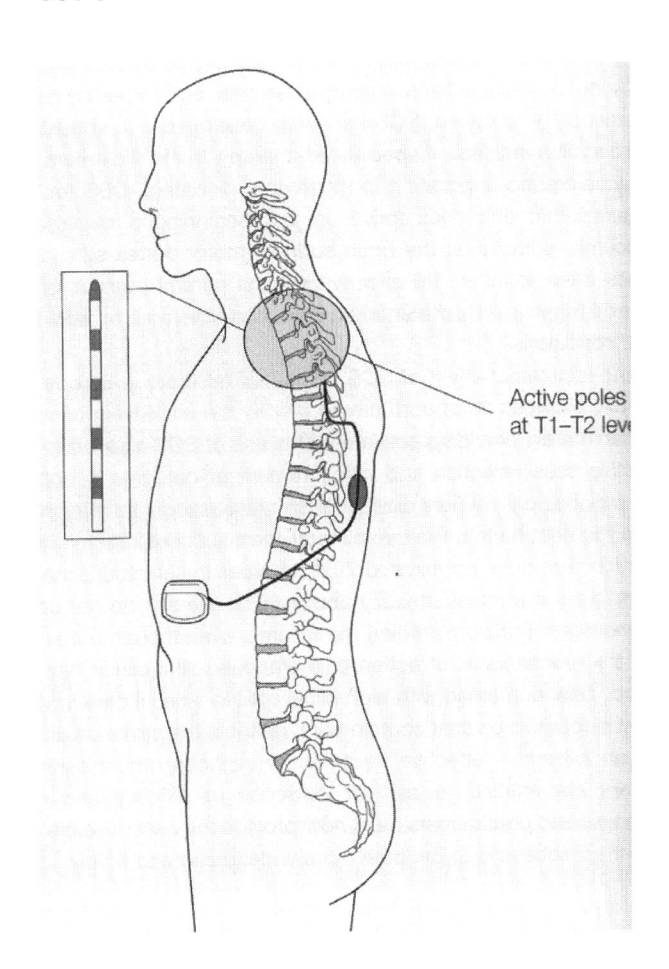

Figure 12.2 Placement of electrodes for dorsal column stimulation. (From Simpson, B.A., B.A. Meyerson, and B. Linderoth, Spinal cord and Brain Stimulation, in Wall and Melzack's Textbook of Pain, S.B. Mahon and M. Kolzenburg, Editors. 2006, Elsevier: Amsterdam. p. 563-582. [399]). (Artwork by Monica Javidnia.)

It has been hypothesized that the mechanism of central pain suppression from spinal cord stimulation involves activation of dorsal column fibers that orthodromically give rise to paresthesia and antidromically activation causing increased release of the inhibitory neurotransmitter GABA from dorsal horn interneurons that receive collaterals from the dorsal column fibers. This, in turn, is assumed to decrease the release of excitatory amino acids (EAA), glutamate, and aspartate following electrical stimulation of the dorsal column. [399].

# Electrical Stimulation of the prefrontal and motor cortices

It has been shown that electrical stimulation of premotor areas (PMA) and supplementary motor areas (SMA) [275, 446] can reduce pain, suggesting involvement of motor areas in pain perception (see Chapter 7). This is an indication that these regions of the cerebral cortex are involved in at least some forms of pain and other regions of the motor system may also be involved in generating the neural activity that causes pain. The thalamic projections to somatosensory area 3a, which is anatomically close to the premotor areas, may explain why electrical stimulation of the premotor areas can suppress pain.

Electrical stimulation of the somatosensory cortex has been used for the treatment of severe pain with bothersome allodynia [98]. A patient with a complex pain disorder that included a perception that her right eye was displaced was treated successfully for the pain by electrical stimulation of her cerebral cortex [97] (see Chapter 8).

The use of electrical stimulation of the motor cortices or the prefrontal cortex for control of neuropathic pain that is resistant to other treatments has recently been studied by many investigators[63, 201, 275, 314]. Stimulation of the motor cortex has also been found to reduce the pain elicited by stimulation of nociceptors[116]. The exact mechanisms for the beneficial effect of such stimulation are not known. Connections from the prefrontal motor cortex to the amygdala and other limbic structures could be responsible for the beneficial effect of electrical stimulation in pain but other connections to limbic structures could mediate the beneficial effect. Connections from the prefrontal motor cortex could activate the descending PAG pathways.

The fact that stimulation of the prefrontal cortex has a beneficial effect on some forms of pain has likewise increased our knowledge regarding the pathophysiology of neuropathic pain. The beneficial effect of motor cortex stimulation[63] decreases with time of use, as is the case for many other treatments of neuropathic pain.

The use of electrical stimulation of central nervous system structures for pain and motor disorders may induce changes in the organization and function of parts of the nervous system. These changes may be responsible for some of the side effects of such treatment. Some form of neuroplasticity may be responsible for the deterioration of the beneficial effect of making lesions in central nervous system structures or the use of deep brain stimulation (DBS).

The reduced efficacy of such intervention may thus be yet another example of expression of neuroplasticity, which counteract the anticipated effects of treatment.

# Use of repetitive transcranial magnetic stimulation

Some investigators [230] have used repetitive transcranial magnetic stimulation (rTMS) of the motor cortex for chronic pathological pain. Such stimulation induces electrical currents in the brain.

When applied to the surface of the brain, it activates cells and fibers in the superficial parts of the brain (mainly the cerebral cortex).

The study [230] showed that rTMS applied at 10 Hz and to an intensity that is above the threshold of sensation significantly lowered pain scores and thermal sensory thresholds in the painful zone, but did not lower mechanical sensory thresholds.

This study comprised 46 patients with chronic pathological pain. Ongoing pain level was scored before and after rTMS. Three types of rTMS sessions, performed at 1 Hz or 10 Hz using an active coil, or at 10 Hz using a sham coil, were compared. The relationships between rTMS-induced changes in sensory thresholds and in pain scores were studied.

These investigators of the above mentioned study [230] concluded on the basis of their study that the neural circuits that relay temperature sensations are potentially dysfunctional in chronic pathological pain secondary to sensitization or deafferentation-induced disinhibition. By acting on these structures, motor cortex stimulation seems to relieve pain and concomitantly improve innocuous thermal sensory discrimination.

# The role of the vagus nerve in pain

The vagus nerve (Latin meaning the wandering nerve) can activate the cholinergic system of the brain and promote plastic changes, thus similar to that of the basal nucleus of Meynert [16]. The afferent fibers of the vagus nerve also influence the immune system and it can affect many other systems of the brain. Studies in cats and monkeys have shown that electrical stimulation of the vagus nerve can attenuate the response from neurons in the dorsal horn to many different types of both harmful and innocuous stimuli [72].

Animal (rat) experiments have shown that activity in vagal afferents that innervate structures located under the diaphragm can modulate somatic pain impulses such as mechanical hyperalgesia [182]. At least some of the effect has been shown to be induced by endocrine signals released from the adrenal medulla. It was concluded that the brain in that way can control the sensitivity of pain receptors all over the body, even when the effect is elicited from an anatomically far distance. Illness responses (and hyperalgesia and pain) is mediated by the vagus nerve may be elicited by pathogenic stimuli in the viscera and mediated by the vagus nerve to the nucleus of the solitary tract, NST (nucleus tractus solitarii).

While somatic and visceral pain are mainly processed in the spinal cord and the trigeminal nucleus, there is some evidence that some forms of pain may be mediated by the vagus nerve and carried directly through that nerve to the brain, bypassing the spinal cord. An example is ischemia of the heart muscle (heart attack) that can present with pain that is referred to several places on the body and it may not give pain at all, but instead, give other sensations such as feeling ill. This is a typical sensation mediated by the vagus nerve.

The complexity of both the descending pathways and modulation of central pain impulses may explain some paradoxical effects. For example, benzodiazepines that are effective in treating pain caused by muscle contractions may enhance other forms of pain (for a review, see Møller 2006 p 226 [288]). This response is probably mediated by the vagus nerve to the nucleus of the solitary tract causing hyperalgesia and pain through descending pathways via nucleus raphe magnus, possibly involving the hypothalamus-pituitary-adrenal axis (HPA) system.

The involvement of the vagus nerve in sexual functions especially in women has been the focus of a few studies that seem to show that the vagus nerve supplies sensory input to the brain that bypasses the spinal cord[217, 475, 476]. There are indications that the vagus nerve provide some sensory input to the brain from the lower abdomen (genitalia) and that such activation may decrease pain perception[91].

# Electrical stimulation of the vagus nerve

Vagus nerve stimulation (VNS) is in clinical use for the treatment of refractory epilepsy (approved by FDA, 2005) [6, 209, 302, 367] and depression. It has been shown that VNS stimulation can control some forms of pain [209]. That electrical stimulation of the vagus nerve is beneficial in treatment of pain[58, 209] was surprising when first introduced. It was discovered in connection with the use of electrical stimulation of the vagus nerve in controlling epileptic seizures.

While the mechanisms for its effect on pain are still incompletely understood the use of vagus stimulation in pain control has provided evidence that that the vagus nerve play an important role in endogenous pain[137].

Vagus nerve stimulation has been shown to suppress experimentally induced pain. It seems as vagus nerve stimulation (VNS) may suppress acute pain thus an analgesic effect but not able to affect chronic (pathological) pain[209, 302]. VNS can influence some dorsal horn neurons that mediate pain [137, 182] as discussed in chapter 7 but it is not completely understood how vagus stimulation can control chronic neuropathic pain. The afferent fibers of the vagus nerve project to the NTS, which connects to many different parts of the brain (see Figure 3.13) and that may explain how the vagus nerve can influence chronic neuropathic pain.

Studies have shown indications that the vagus nerve may be involved in opioid induced analgesia. Studies in rats have shown that after severing of the vagus nerve, the analgesic effect of morphine decreases [137]. This means that intact functioning of the vagus nerve is important for the full analgesic effect of morphine and other opioids.

VNS appears to affect pain perception in depressed adults; a possible role of VNS in the treatment of severe refractory headaches, intractable chronic migraines, and cluster headaches has also been suggested. VNS for treatment of pain [302] is based on experimental studies that have shown that electrical stimulation of the vagus nerve can inhibit spinal pain reflexes and transmission of neural activity elicited by painful stimulations. Some of these studies found that VNS has a clear pain relieving effect on acute or inflammatory pain.

However, the results of other studies are partly contradictory, probably because the VNS effects depend on the stimulation parameters [209, 302]. Some studies in animals [6] used different stimulation protocols, including the one used in epileptic patients. In these studies, immunocytochemical tests showed that VNS changed spinal trigeminal nucleus neurons that could explain the VNS-induced pain relief.

Some clinical studies suggest the potential of VNS for treating individuals with chronic headaches, but the most adequate stimulation protocols must be established before it can be a routine clinical method for the treatment of pain [191, 192]. Clinical data have been collected from VNS-implanted epileptic patients in whom pain thresholds were measured and the VNS effect on co-existing headaches was assessed. In addition, in two pilot studies of a few patients, VNS was used to treat resistant, chronic headaches and migraines. Taken together, these clinical studies tend to confirm the pain relieving effect of VNS and to suggest its potential utility in chronic headache patients.

More recently, VNS has also been used for the treatment of tinnitus, depression, and eating disorders (leading to obesity). For more details about vagus nerve stimulation and pain, see Chapter 4.

# Anatomical basis for vagus nerve control of pain

As seen from Figure 3.13, the NTS projects to premotor systems and the autonomic systems. It also has heavy projections to limbic structures (behavioral and emotional structures) and endocrine systems controlling hormonal systems.

Specifically, the NTS projects to the parabrachial nucleus (PBN), the locus coeruleus (LC), and the dorsal raphe nucleus (DRN). The PBN projects to the thalamus, the amygdala, the insular cortex, the infralimbic cortex (ILC), the amygdala, and the hypothalamus. The locus coeruleus projects to the same structures. The DRN also projects to these same structures.

# Acupuncture for relieving pain

Understanding how acupuncture causes pain relief has improved during the recent decades. When acupuncture is used to treat chronic pain, the needles are inserted into the specific "acupuncture points" (acupoints) on the patient's body [502]. Manual acupuncture (MA) involves insertion of an acupuncture needle into an acupoint followed by the twisting of the needle up and down by hand.

Acupuncture [340] is based on insertion of fine needles into specific points of the body for treating various diseases or for alleviating symptoms such as pain. (The term acupuncture comes from Latin where the words 'acus' means needle and 'punctura' means to puncture). Acupuncture has been practiced in the Far East for at least 3000 years, but it is only in the last 30 years that interest has developed in the West. Now, acupuncture is probably the most popular alternative therapy practiced in the United States, Europe, and many Asian countries.

The scientific basis for the various effects of using acupuncture has been studied intensively during the recent decades. Many scientific studies have concerned understanding its effect to control pain [208, 340] as was discussed in Chapter 8. Acupuncture makes use of stimulation (electrically or mechanically) of receptors or nerve endings in the skin. In that way, it has similarities with electrical stimulation of peripheral nerves such as TENS, but the effect of acupuncture is wider and more complex.

Pain relief seems to occur only after a feeling of soreness, numbness, heaviness, and distension from the acupuncture manipulation. In MA, all types of afferent fibers ($A\beta$, $A\delta$, and C) are activated. In electrical acupuncture (EA), electrical currents are delivered to acupoints at a strength that can activate $A\beta$ and some $A\delta$ fibers. This means that somatosensory and pain circuits in the spinal cord and the brain are activated and many structures in the brain that are normally involved in pain are also activated. Thus, pain relief from acupuncture may be caused by activation of many different parts of the central nervous system.

In addition to the pain relieving effect of acupuncture, an increasing number of studies have demonstrated that acupuncture treatment can control some autonomic nervous system functions such as blood pressure regulation, relaxation of various sphincters, and other autonomic functions. There is increasing evidence that electrical acupuncture (EA) treatment is effective for various immunological diseases including allergic disorders, infections, autoimmune diseases, and immunodeficiency-syndromes [208]. One of the main contemporary uses of acupuncture is for the treatment of musculoskeletal pain [208, 340].

# Hypothesis for the action of acupuncture

Studies of neural mechanisms underlying acupuncture pain relief have focused on cellular and molecular processes and on changes detected by the use of functional brain imaging techniques. It has been found that many different signaling molecules are involved in mediating the pain relief from acupuncture; these include opioid peptides (μ, δ, and κ receptors), glutamate (NMDA and AMPA/KA receptors), 5-HT (serotonin), and cholecystokinin (CCK). The opioid peptides and their receptors in the PAG-RVM-spinal dorsal horn pathway play important roles in the ability of acupuncture to provide pain relief.

Electroacupuncture uses a stimulus with frequencies of 2 and 100 Hz, producing the release of enkephalin and dynorphin in the spinal cord, respectively. CCK acts against the pain relieving effect of acupuncture. It has been suggested that the individual differences in the efficacy of acupuncture in relieving pain is dependent on the density of CCK receptors [502].

The effect of electroacupuncture (acupuncture using electrical stimulation, EA) has similarities with that of TENS in that it activates Aβ fibers, which have an inhibitory effect on neural transmission in the dorsal horn. Acupuncture has other effects because the activation of Aβ fibers would not explain acupuncture's effect on chronic pain.

The pain relieving effect is probably mediated by stimulation of Aδ and, perhaps, C-fibers as well [467]. Figure 12.3 shows some hypotheses for the action of acupuncture stimulation of sensory afferents in skin and muscles.

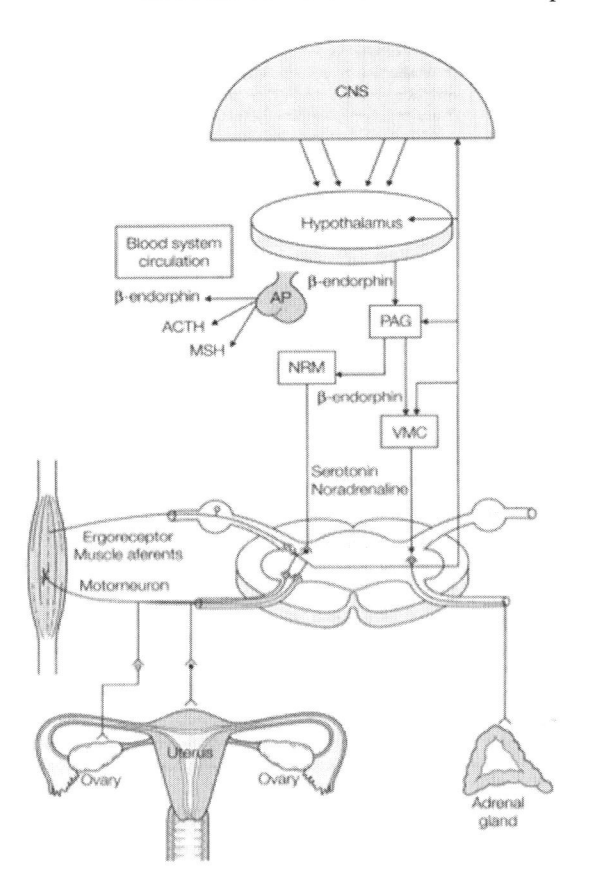

Figure 12.3 Illustration of hypotheses for the use of acupuncture in the treatment of pain. AP: Anterior pituitary, NRM: Nucleus raphe magnus, MSH: Melanocyte stimulating hormone, VMC: Vasomotor centers. (From Barlas, P. and T. Lundeberg, Transcutaneous electrical nerve stimulation and acupuncture, in Wall and Melzack's Textbook of Pain, S.B. McMahon and M. Koltzenburg, Editors. 2006, Elsevier: Amsterdam. p. 583-590 [26] after Sterner-Victorin 2000). Reprinted with the permission of Elsevier.

Animal studies (rat) that compared the effect of acupuncture and TENS [467] have shown that both methods caused similar elevations of withdrawal latencies of a tail flick. The analgesic effects of both methods have a slow onset and lasted after termination of the stimulations. Systemic administration of naloxone hydrochloride (2 mg/kg) (an antagonist to opioid receptors) partially antagonized the effect, indicating that some of the effects were caused by the liberation of endogenous opioids.

When stimulated at 2 and 15 Hz, the analgesia from both methods had indications of being mediated by endogenous opiates (since the effect could be abolished by administration of Naloxone), whereas the effect of stimulation at a high rate (100 Hz) could not be abolished by administration of naloxone, thus, it was assumed to be mediated by effects other than endogenous opiates [467].

# Hypnosis

Hypnosis is a practical method for managing pain [193]. It has its effects by providing an extreme level of relaxation and reduced monitoring and censoring of mental activity, including suspension of usual orientation. Hypnotic relaxation changes regional blood flow in the brain in many structures, including those that are involved in pathological pain. Increases in hypnotic relaxation are associated with increases in regional blood flow in the occipital cortex and with decreases in the mesencephalic tegmentum of the brain stem and right parietal lobule.

In contrast, mental absorption that is reported by an individual during hypnosis is associated with increases in regional cerebral blood flow within a network of brain structures including the pontomesencephalic brain stem, the medial thalamus, and the anterior cingulate cortex, as well as the inferior frontal and parietal lobule right hemisphere that are coordinated with each other.

Mental absorption is also associated with decreases in regional blood flow in the medial parietal cortex [343]. Changes in blood flow are assumed to be associated with (a sign of) changes in neural activity although the relationship may be less clear than often assumed.

Processing of painful stimulations in individuals who have chronic pain was investigated recently and the effect of hypnosis was evaluated [1]. Changes in brain activity evoked by painful repetitive pinprick stimulations of the left mental nerve region in individuals with chronic painful temporo-mandibular disorders (TMD) were studied with the use of fMRI.

In the control condition without hypnotic influence, the painful stimulation caused activation of the right posterior insula, primary somatosensory cortex (SI), Brodman area 21 (BA21) (middle temporal gyrus, see Appendix B), BA6 (premotor area), left BA40 (supramarginal gyrus, part of Wernicke's area) and BA4 (primary motor area) [1].

During hypnotic hyperalgesia, the same stimulation was associated with increased activity in the right posterior insula, BA6, and left BA40 whereas hypnotic hypoalgesia only was associated with activity in the right posterior insula. Activation of the primary somatosensory cortex decreased significantly during hypnotic hyperalgesia. During hypnotic hypoalgesia, activation of the right posterior insula, BA21, and left BA40 was observed.

The considerable involvement of parts of the insula is important and is another sign that more attention should be directed to the insula in attempts to understand the brain mechanisms in pathological pain. It is particularly interesting that the activity of the primary somatosensory area decreases during hyperalgesia.

Hypnosis can modulate pain perception both up and down (causing hyper- or hypo-algesia). When a person with chronic pain experiences an additional painful stimulation, the changes that occur in the activation of different structures from hypnosis that causes hypo-algesia are different from the structures that are affected by hypnosis in individuals with hyperalgesia.

These two kinds of reactions to hypnosis affect different brain structures differently as assessed by fMRI. This supports the results of other studies that have indicated that the primary somatosensory cortex may not be involved in pain, but that it is the secondary cortex that is involved with pain.

# Physical exercise

Physical exercise increases brain derived neurotrophic factor (BDNF) [144] and it has many known different (beneficial) effects, including relief of pain [271], an antidepressant effect, and it enhances the sense of well-being in general.

Another reason for the beneficial effect of physical exercise may be the reduction of body fat it causes. Fat cells secrete many different neuroactive substances that may affect the functions of parts of the nervous system. Physical exercise has been shown to have beneficial effects on underlying diseases such as diabetes, low back pain, etc.

# Administration of treatments

Poor results of medical treatment of pathological pain are often caused by incorrect selections of the drug that is used, the amount given may be too small and, in particular, the way it is administrated may be wrong. Correct administration of medication used for treating pathological pain is more complex than just taking a pill whenever it hurts. It is, therefore, important that the patients follow the instructions given by their physicians.

However, such instructions are normally given orally by a physician, a nurse, or a physician's assistant. The patients may either not understand the instructions or forget what they were told. The same problems apply to non-drug treatments including transdermal electrical nerve stimulation (TENS), acupuncture, hypnosis, and other relaxation therapies, thus whenever the patient administers the treatment. Suboptimal results are often caused by the way patients administrate their medications.

# Administration of pain medication

It was pointed out in Chapter 7 that taking sufficient amounts of pain medication is important for the treatment of acute pain. This is even more important for the treatment of pathological pain. Chronic pain is likely to recur when the effect of treatment abates. First of all, sufficient amounts of medication to eliminate the pain should be taken. Chronic pain should not be treated by taking medication when the pain occurs. Instead, medication should be taken before the pain occurs. A person with chronic pain knows the length of time the medication he/she takes keeps the pain away and can plan to take the medication again before the pain reoccurs. This is important because pain begets pain and pain can only be effectively treated by keeping it from recurring.

This is difficult to get patients to understand because people are used to taking medications to treat pain when the pain appears and not to keep it from occurring. It is also against the general philosophy in medicine that medications are for treatment and not for prevention. However, if pain medications are taken on a regular basis, the results are better than when taken in a haphazard fashion or when the pain appears.

Many people are afraid of taking pain medication in sufficiently large amounts and many people will only take so much that they can stand the pain. Unfortunately, this is supported by many physicians who tell their patients to "only take as much as necessary" without defining what they mean by "necessary".

Taking too little will often prolong the pain while treating pain with sufficient amounts of an effective pain reliever so that the pain is eliminated often keeps the pain from recurring after the effect of the pain medication has worn out. However, it may not always be possible to treat the pain in such a way that the pain disappears and the side effects of common pain medications may be an obstacle.

# Surgical treatment of pain

Pathological pain is, per definition, not caused by stimulation of pain receptors, but rather by changes in the function of the central nervous system (spinal cord or brain). Therefore, there is no surgical treatment for pathological pain.

Only a few kinds of surgical operations for chronic pain, such as those for microvascular decompression (MVD) for trigeminal and glossopharyngeal neuralgia, have a high rate of total relief of the pain [24]. This is in sharp contrast to the results of operations, such as those widely used to treat low back pain, which offer little chance of benefit to the patients.

Many individuals with pain have been persuaded to have various kinds of surgical operations to correct the problems that cause the pain "to get it over with", however, often with disappointing results. In most incidences, the benefits are questionable at best and these operations often cause more pain and severe complications may occur [238, 239]. Conventional treatment of pain, such as low back pain, often involves surgery or epidural injections, which may even make the situation worse. Surgery could be effective if it corrected a condition that would cause activation of plastic changes in the nervous system. The pain that is to be eliminated by an operation may, in fact, become worse after an operation and there may be some additional pain from the trauma caused by the operation [49].

Most people understand that an automobile salesman has an economic interest in selling you a car. Few understand that many surgeons have an economic interest in selling you an operation. Uncritical trust and belief in a person because he or she has a medical license has resulted in many disappointments. The fact that operations cannot be reversed just makes mistakes even worse. In the USA, there are federal regulations about declarations of risks in many forms of investment. While the pharmaceutical industry is obligated to provide information about side effects and beneficial effects of their products, similar regulations are missing for surgical operations.

# Treatment of specific pain disorders

There are specific pain disorders where different methods are used to treat the pain than those used to treat pain in general. Neuralgia, typically shooting pain localized to the distribution of one or more peripheral or cranial nerves, is an example where different kinds of treatments are effective.

Trigeminal neuralgia, glossopharyngeal neuralgia, and geniculate neuralgia are distinctly different from other kinds of neuralgias. Virus induced neuralgias constitute a group of their own. Examples are post-herpes neuralgia (PHN) and shingles.

A different group of neuralgias, diabetes and alcohol related peripheral neuralgias, also require different treatments than general pain conditions. Painful diabetic neuropathy (PDN) is getting more and more common as the prevalence of overweight and diabetes type 2 increases. Disorders where the sympathetic nervous system is assumed to play an important role (CRPS 1 and 2) also require specific treatments.

Virus induced neuralgias are common and post-herpetic neuralgia (PHN) is a common example of causes of peripheral neuropathic pain. Relief of pain from these conditions requires specific treatments.

Deafferentation pain is another form of pain that requires different treatment than general pain conditions.

# Treatment of neuralgia

A commonly used treatment for neuralgias is by medications that are also used for treating depression, such as second-generation tricyclic antidepressants (i.e. nortriptylin). Other drugs, such as gabapentin (Neurontin) or its follower, pregabalin (Lyrica), are also effective [195]. Pregabalin is an anti epileptic drug that reduces the synaptic release of several neurotransmitters[431]. More modern similar drugs, such as duloxetine (Cymbalta) are now in use. Often, a combination of drugs is used. Similar treatment is used for post-herpetic neuralgia (PHN), a sequel of herpes virus infections [506]. Medications, such as amitriptyline, imipramine, and desimipramin, may be helpful for persistent pain from herpes zoster oticus (post-herpetic neuralgia). Often, several drugs are used at the same time. Administration of vitamins, such as vitamin $B_1$ and $B_{12}$, can treat some forms of metabolic related peripheral neuralgia such as PDN and alcohol related neuralgia. It may also reduce the inflammation that is often involved in creating neuralgia pain.

Tegretol (carbamazepine, a sodium channel blocker) and Baclofen (a $GABA_B$ agonist) are also commonly used medications to treat painful neuralgias.

# Treatment of trigeminal neuralgia

Trigeminal neuralgia (TGN) can be effectively treated by three different treatments, namely two kinds of surgical operations, one consisting of causing a small lesion in the nerve root [426], the other by moving a blood vessel off the root of the trigeminal nerve (known as microvascular decompression, MVD) [24, 133, 185]. A slightly different surgical method consists of injecting glycerol around the trigeminal ganglion [153].

The pathophysiology of these so-called microvascular compression diseases has been studied extensively (for a review see [284, 286] ). The term microvascular compression assumes that the symptoms (pain or spasm that affects one side of the face, respectively) are caused by the "pounding of an artery into the nerve root" [185], until it was shown that veins could also cause the same symptoms as arteries [186].

The third method for treating TGN uses medications such as carbamazepine (Tegretol) or phenytoin (Dilantin). These drugs are sodium channel blockers and are commonly used in the treatment of epilepsy. Baclofen and gabapentin have also been used in the treatment of TGN [127]. All three methods have a high degree of success and the selection of which method to use to treat TGN depends, to a great extent, on the side effects and risks of complications.

MVD operations for TGN and glossopharyngeal neuralgia (GPN) are exceptionally effective [24] with success rates around 85 percent with a low risk of recurrence (after 15 years, pain recurred in 50 percent of individuals who had MVD operations). Treatments with medications have slightly less success and it depends on which drug is used and on the dosage [127].

Partial sectioning of the trigeminal nerve root can cause a very serious complication, anesthesia dolorosa, which means numbness and a constant burning pain that is resistive to most forms of treatment. Because of that, partial sectioning of the trigeminal nerve root is rarely performed anymore and it has been replaced by MVD operations (for a review, see [286]). MVD operations can have serious complications, but in the hands of surgeons skilled in the operation, the likelihood for such complications is small. Carbamazepine in high dosages has several side effects including drowsiness, vomiting, and unsteadiness, but it has also more serious side effects such a hair loss, anemia, and bleedings.

# Treatment of virus induced neuralgias

Pain from herpes zoster (chicken pox virus) nerve infection (shingles) can be reduced by immediate treatment with antiviral agents, such as acyclovir or famvir, that help reduce the duration of the rash and reduce the risk of subsequent chronic pain.

A vaccination for shingles reduces the risk by about 50 percent [380].

Serotonin noradrenalin reuptake inhibitors (SNRI), such as venlafaxine and duloxetine, are also promising drugs for the treatment of PDN with fewer adverse effects than tricyclic antidepressants (TCA). Several studies of the effect of selective serotonin reuptake inhibitors (SSRI) have shown conflicting results regarding the efficacy in relieving PDN-related pain. Carbamazepine, phenytoin, and valproic acid were shown to be effective in ameliorating PDN-related pain. Gabapentin and pregabalin have been proven to be effective for the treatment of PHN and PDN in a number of large placebo-controlled trials. These drugs are useful not only in relieving pain, but also in restoring quality of life.

Of the opioids, oxycodone, hydromorphone, and tramadol seem to be superior to placebos for the treatment of PHN and PDN. Topical agents, such as lidocaine 5 percent patches and topical capsaicin, are useful in ameliorating pain in patients with PHN, but these agents are unsatisfactory for the use as a sole agent. For many patients, combinations of drugs are necessary to produce adequate pain relief.

# Metabolic related peripheral nerve neuropathies

Metabolic related peripheral nerve neuropathies are characterized by burning pain that usually starts in the feet. Such peripheral neuropathies are typically complications to diabetes (painful diabetes neuropathy, PDN) and may accompany high alcohol intake (alcohol neuropathy). Individuals with these conditions have deficits regarding B vitamins especially; for alcohol neuropathies, probably because of general poor nutrition.

Peripheral neuropathies, such as diabetes or alcohol related neuropathies can often be effectively treated by administration of Vitamin B. Vitamin $B_1$ and $B_{12}$ are most effective, but other B vitamins are also beneficial. Treatment with B vitamins can reverse the disease and thereby, often provide total relief of the pain. This is unlike most forms of treatments used (described above), which provide (symptomatic) relief of the pain.

Vitamins are usually not regarded as drugs, and treatment with vitamins has not been viewed with the same respect as treatment with pharmaceutical drugs. Modern drugs especially have been regarded as having the ability to cure diseases. However, well executed studies have shown that administration of B vitamins, especially vitamin $B_{12}$, has a beneficial effect on pathological pain [65, 427] of various kinds including low back pain [256].

Administration of B vitamins can, in fact, eliminate or reduce some forms of pathological pain by reversing some of the disease processes, but the vitamins have to be taken in sufficient amount. The contents of these vitamins in commonly available multivitamins are not sufficient for such treatment.

In a double blind, randomized, placebo-controlled study, it was found that administrations of $B_{12}$ vitamins (Cyanocobalaminum 1000 mcg) showed a statistically significant difference in the efficacy of the active treatment both for visual analog scales (VAS) and for disability questionnaires (DQ) ($p < 0.0001$ and $p < 0.0002$, respectively). Consumption of paracetamol proved significantly higher in the placebo group than in the active treatment ($p < 0.0001$) [256]. The commonly available $B_{12}$ (cyanocoblamin) must be converted in the liver to become the active methylcobalamium.

Even better results might have been obtained using methylcobalamium, which does not need to be converted in the liver, as cyanocobalaminum requires. Methylcyanobalamin is available as a tablet that should not be swallowed but dissolved in the mouth. In other studies, animal experiments (rats) support the efficacy of vitamins $B_1$ (thiamine), $B_6$ (pyridoxine), and $B_{12}$ (cyanocobalaminum) together with dexamethasone were effective in reducing allodynia pain from spinal nerve ligations [65].

It has been suggested that increased levels of vitamin D may reduce pain because it reduces immune reactions either of the body or of the nervous system [169].

Vitamin D is a secosteroid. The active form 1,25-(OH)2-Vitamin D3, has hormone activities and most cells and tissues have vitamin D receptors. Studies have shown that Vitamin D can have a beneficial effect on numerous diseases, including osteoporosis, chronic musculoskeletal pain, diabetes (types 1 and 2), multiple sclerosis, cardiovascular disease, and cancers of the breast, prostate, and colon [150].

It has also been shown that there is a worldwide vitamin D deficiency, but various populations are affected differently. Vitamin D is normally synthesized in the skin, but it requires exposure to sunlight. The common use of sunscreen to reduce the risk of skin cancer has caused vitamin D deficit in many individuals.

Vitamin D also comes from the food supply, but vitamin D in normal food is limited (easily supplied as supplements) and most often inadequate to prevent deficiencies. Supplemental vitamin D is likely necessary to avoid deficiency, especially in winter months and when sunscreen is used in the summer.

The estimated cost saving effect of improving vitamin D status in Germany might be as much as 37.5 billion Euros annually. In view of the absence of side effects, administration of vitamins seems to be a "gentle" and inexpensive way of treating a serious condition [507].

# Low back pain

Low back pain is a common disorder that is treated in many different ways. The pain is often a combination of pathological and physiological pain [126] and in addition, muscle pain often occurs. Back pain has many forms. The aching, poorly defined pain and shooting pain that are often known as sciatica have different causes. Aching pain is generally assumed to involve small diameter nerve fibers, but it can also be pathological pain caused by changes in the function of the central nervous system.

The shooting pain is likely to involve large nerve fibers and these are subjected to compression of spinal nerves and their roots, while small diameter fibers such as unmyelinated (C-fibers) and small myelinated (A$\delta$) are not noticeably affected by mechanical compression. This means that only when back pain is of the shooting type and associated with weakness in the legs can it be concluded that the pain is caused by mechanical compression of spinal nerve roots.

# Surgical treatment of low back pain

Surgical operations for low back pain often aim at decompressing spinal nerve roots that are visibly compressed (on MRI) and such operations may include fusion of two or more vertebrae [238, 239].

Surgical treatment of uncomplicated, classical, aching low back pain has a poor prognosis regarding pain control and it carries several side effects [397]. In view of the poor results of surgery as treatment of the common forms of low back pain, several surgeons have stated that surgery should not be recommended as a general treatment [239, 451], and not done on the indications of pain, but only considered when the symptoms are muscle weakness and numbness [238, 239].

Such "root compression" was commonly regarded as a cause of pain such as that experienced with low back pain, carpal tunnel syndrome, ulnar compression syndrome, etc. This has resulted in many surgical treatments that have not provided benefits to the patients and some operations have caused serious complications. It is well-documented that surgical operations for low back pain that aim at correcting compression of spinal nerve roots in disorders, such as spinal stenosis, normally have little benefit to the patients [239, 319, 452, 472]; on the contrary, such operations often cause side effects in the form of (more) pain.

It is possible that nerve root compression from the rupture of a vertebral disk may cause the initial pain that is experienced in sciatica. Such events may activate neuroplasticity causing changes in the function of the spinal cord and possibly the brain, and that may be what causes the long-term (chronic) pain. Why the pain often varies and why it is referred to different parts of the body, such as various parts of the legs, may be explained by the fact that the pain is caused by changes in the function of parts of the central nervous system. It is not always possible to distinguish between radicular pain and referred pain.

In decisions about treatment, the risks of complications from surgery should not be overlooked. The fact that practically all forms of surgery result in postoperative pain should be taken into consideration when deciding about which form of therapy (if any) is to be used [239].

Pain from surgical trauma to bone occurs frequently [49], typically lasting for periods of weeks to many months and it is sometimes lifelong. Severe complications occur infrequently, but must be taken into account when selecting treatment. This means that the decision about surgery for low back pain must be considered carefully as stated by surgeons with a lifelong experience of treating back pain of various kinds [238, 239].

There is good evidence that discectomy is effective in the short term and particularly for sciatica types of back pain, but in the long term, it is not more effective than prolonged conservative care. There is a general consensus that treatment of acute low back pain should be conservative in the first 6-8 weeks [239, 451]. Patient information is important and it should emphasize advice to stay active, have physical therapy and physical exercise and, if overweight, lose weight. Administration of sufficient amounts of pain relievers, such as non-steroidal anti-inflammatory drugs (NSAID) or opioids, depending on the severity of the pain is important. NSAID should always be a part of the treatment because inflammation is an important component of the cause of most forms of back pain (see Chapter 8).

A few placebo-controlled trials did not support the use of TENS in the routine management of chronic low back pain. A study [104] found that individuals who had low back pain for a long time (medial duration of 4.1 years) had no benefit from TENS, but pain and other symptoms were improved after physical exercise.

# Epidural injections

Epidural corticosteroid injections and transforaminal peri-radicular injections of corticosteroids are in common use, but their efficacy in reducing pain long term has been questioned. Studies have shown little beneficial effects with common chronic low back pain [418].

Judgment about how to treat low back pain has been clouded by the enormous economic interests in specific treatments, especially surgical treatment, but also for epidural injections. These factors have masked and possibly distorted the results of assessments of efficacy of the used methods, which have shown poor outcomes for these kinds of treatment.

# Sciatica

An entity known as sciatica [200, 451], often described as a form of low back pain, is characterized by acute onset of shooting pain in the leg. However, the term is often used for less well-defined forms of low back pain. Sciatica is typically elicited by a specific event. Surgical treatment (discectomy) for back pain is effective in relieving the pain short term, but surgery is not more effective than conservative care for the relief of long term pain [239, 451].

Pain after spinal cord traumatic injuries requires specific treatment.

# Carpal tunnel syndrome

Carpal tunnel syndrome (CTS) is the most common entrapment neuropathy, with a reported prevalence of 3.72 percent in the United States [308]. There is evidence that pain and other symptoms of carpal tunnel syndrome are due to plastic changes, meaning that it may be a plasticity disorder and that the pain is pathological pain. Both fMRI studies [308] and studies using recordings of somatosensory evoked potentials [435] have shown evidence of increased excitability of the somatosensory cortex on the affected side.

Like for back pain, there is evidence that the immune system is involved in the pain from carpal tunnel syndrome, emphasizing the importance of using treatment with drugs that reduce inflammation (such as NSAID or perhaps steroids).

# Deafferentation pain

Deafferentation pain (central neuropathic pain) is pain caused by functional changes in the central nervous system (spinal cord and brain) brought about by activation of neuroplasticity. The pain is debilitating and the pain, a form of central neuropathic pain, responds poorly to treatment with conventional methods including strong pain relievers.

There is evidence that deafferentation pain is associated with reorganization of the primary somatosensory cortex and the degree of reorganization is related to the intensity of the deafferentation pain [201, 314, 333].

One of these studies [98] revealed that relief of severe deafferentation pain could be achieved by reversing the cortical reorganization by transcranial magnetic stimulation (TMS), which can modulate cortical activity by inducing an electrical current in the target regions of the brain. Other investigators have used stimulation of the motor cortex for treating deafferentation pain [369]. This study showed that stimulation of the primary motor cortex (M1) is an effective treatment for intractable deafferentation pain.

The treatment of pain by stimulation of the primary motor cortex [369] started in 1990 and the results of many studies (involving 271 participants) have been reported. The patients who were treated had suffered from post-stroke pain (59 percent), trigeminal neuropathic pain, brachial plexus injury, spinal cord injury, peripheral nerve injury, and phantom-limb pain. The stimulation was applied through electrodes placed epidural over the primary motor cortex, subdural, or within the central sulcus (thus, between motor and sensory cortices). Overall, the studies found that electrical stimulation of M1 is a very promising technique; nearly 60 percent of the treated patients improved with a higher than 50 percent pain relief after several months of follow-up and sometimes after a few years in most reports.

Similar benefit is obtained by the implantation of epidural stimulating electrodes over the area of electrophysiological signal abnormality in the primary somatosensory cortex [97]. Tsubokawa and Meyerson [275, 446] have described the use of electrical stimulation of pre-motor areas for the treatment of deafferentation pain. Improvement in sensory detection thresholds was found to be associated with pathological pain relief produced by epidural motor cortex stimulation with surgically implanted electrodes.

# Treatment of amputation pain

It has been described in case studies that TENS can relieve amputation pain [140], but no randomized controlled trials (RCT) have been published on which to judge the effectiveness of TENS for the management of phantom pain and stump pain [303].

There are many reasons why pain and other sensations referred to an amputated limb may persist after amputation. The main reason is that the brain still keeps a map of the amputated limb. This may cause pain and other sensations referred to the amputated limb. The pain may be treated by various methods as described below. The map of the amputated limb in the brain may also cause a distorted body image where the amputated limb may be stuck in an unpleasant position with its owner unable to move it. The mirror treatment described below may solve the problems including the pain.

Cutting peripheral nerves, such as always occurs in amputations, causes deprivation of sensory input, which activates neuroplasticity and that, may contribute to the pain that is experienced after amputations (deafferentation pain). This means that at least some part of the amputation pain is a form of deafferentation pain.

Another reason for pain after amputations is that a neuroma forms at the location where a nerve was severed when a limb is amputated. Neuromas are benign (non-cancerous) growths consisting of axon sprouts that form at the end of a cut nerve. Formations of axon sprouts are the body's attempts to re-innervate the limb. Since there is no place for the nerves to go, the sprouts pile up and form the neuroma, which is pain sensitive and may generate pain spontaneously. Unfortunately, surgical removal of a neuroma rarely solves the problem, but the risk of occurrence of a neuroma may be reduced by proper surgical procedures.

It is generally agreed that aggressive pain management immediately after the amputation decreases the risks of developing phantom limb pain [277]. Blockage of pain transmission in the spinal cord for 72 hours before the amputation (by lumbar epidural blockade, (LEB) has a beneficial long term effect on the development of amputation pain [14].

Seven days after the operation, three patients in the LEB group and nine patients in the control group had phantom limb pain (p less than 0.10). After 6 months, all patients in the LEB group were pain-free, whilst 5 patients in the control group had pain (p less than 0.05). After 1 year, all the patients in the LEB group were still pain-free, and 3 patients in the control group had phantom limb pain (p less than 0.20) [14].

# Correcting distorted body image

After amputation, a person's body image is often distorted, resulting in various kinds of phantom perceptions. We have described some of these in Chapter 8. Here we show some ways to correct distorted body images.

## Use of mirrors

It was mentioned in Chapter 8 that phantom sensations including pain often occur after amputations of a body part such as a limb. In addition to sensations referred to specific locations on the limb that the person no longer has, there are often other unpleasant phenomena such as perception of the limb in an awkward position, which the person is unable to change.

It is known that body perception (part of the perception of "self") is normally being updated constantly. The signals that cause updating of these maps come from receptors in the body parts in question together with other sensory input, especially vision. This means that updating body perceptions to a great extent relies on tactile input from the body. After an amputation, this can no longer occur and the body perception is stuck in the perception that existed before the amputation.

This has inspired a novel treatment for phantom limb pain using a mirror. A study by Pons et.al (1991) [333] showed that loss of input (through deafferentation) could change the maps of the body that exist on the surface of the somatosensory cerebral cortex to a much greater extent than earlier believed.

This inspired Vilayanur Ramachandran, a neurologist, to find a cure for phantom limb symptoms. Using the hypothesis that the body image is closely related to how the body looks, thus depending on visual observation of the body, Ramachandran [346] developed a mirror technique to correct the misrepresentation of an amputated body part such as a limb. He drew the conclusion that the symptoms amputees had were caused by re-organization of the cortical map of the amputated body part [346] and that it was caused by the absence of sensory input that normally maintained and updated these maps.

Using very simple means consisting of a set of mirrors, Ramachandran and his co-workers [346, 347] were able to eliminate the phantom limb symptoms in many amputees by correcting these maps with visual input. Often, a phantom limb is painful because it is felt to be stuck in an uncomfortable or unnatural position, and the patient feels they cannot move it. The purpose of the mirror box (Figure 12.4) is to retrain the brain and thereby, eliminate the learned paralysis.

Through the use of artificial visual feedback, it becomes possible for the patient to "move" the phantom limb and to unclench, for example, a hand from potentially painful positions. The correction of the body image will also relieve other symptoms of the amputation including pain. Repeated training using such visual feedback has led to long term improvements in some individuals with phantom limb symptoms.

# The mirror box

The mirror box has two holes and a patient with an amputated arm inserts his/her hand into one hole, and the "phantom" is pretended to be inserted into the other. The patient with an amputated left arm places the good arm (right arm) into one side of the box. By the means of the mirror, the patient sees a reflection of the good hand where the missing limb would be (indicated in lower contrast, in Figure 12.4).

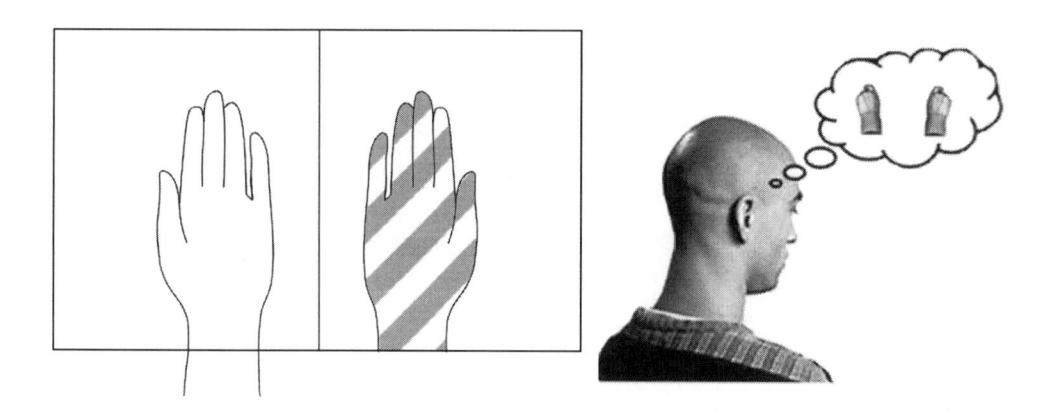

Figure 12.4 Mirror box: A patient inserts their hand into one hole, and their "phantom" limb into the other. When viewed from an angle, the brain is tricked into seeing two complete hands. From: Ramachandran, V.S., Plasticity and functional recovery in neurology. Clin Med., 2005. 5(4): p. 368-73. [346]. Artwork by Monica Javidnia.

The patient looks into the mirror on the side with the good limb and makes "mirror symmetric" movements, as a symphony conductor might or as we do when we clap our hands. Because the patient who is being treated sees the reflected image of the good hand moving, it appears as if the phantom limb is also moving. When the patient moves his/her good arm, it looks like the amputated arm is moving as well.

Thus, the patient receives artificial visual feedback that the "resurrected" limb is now moving when he/she moves the good arm. Through the use of this artificial visual feedback, it becomes possible for the patient to "move" the phantom limb, and to unclench it from potentially painful positions. Because this visual feedback elicits sensations that are related to the movement of a limb, Ramachandran and Rogers-Ramachandran [350] called this kind of treatment synesthesia, although this is true only in the broadest sense of the term.

The success of the mirror method inspired a team of researchers at the University of Pool, UK [79] and the University of Manchester [304] in England to experiment with a technology called "immersive virtual reality" to combat the discomfort that is a part of phantom limb syndrome [304]. The researchers reported that with this technique, phantom limb pain could be relieved by attaching the sufferer's real limb to an interface that allows them to see two limbs moving in a computer-generated simulation. This works on the same principle as the mirror box technique in that it "tricks" the somatosensory cortex by the illusion, except that the computer created illusion is thought to be stronger. This kind of development of treatment for phantom sensations inspired by the original work by Ramachandran is in steady progress in many laboratories and clinics [79].

The mirror box is also of use in the rehabilitation of patients with hemiparesis (paralysis on one side of the body) due to stroke [4].

# Neurophysiological basis for the phantom limb syndrome

Herta Flor and her colleagues have studied neural reorganization that leads to phantom limb pain using neuroelectric source imaging techniques [122, 123]. They find that telescoping phantoms (the phantom limb is perceived to be getting shorter) can lead to increased cortical reorganization (and associated pain) [199], while use of the mirror reverses these changes and thereby, leads to a reduction in pain [123]. For example, in phantom limbs due to arm amputation, Flor and her colleagues found that the distance the representation of the limb has been displaced predicts the degree of pain.

However, with the mirror box, the representation of the limb is no longer displaced relative to its counterpart in the other (non-affected) hemisphere. That is, use of the mirror box can eliminate the remapping associated with phantom limb pain.

# Treatment of pain from muscle spasms

Massages [342] or applications of heat are efficient as treatments for muscle spasms. The massage of tendons that activate the Golgi tendon organs is especially effective in reducing muscle spasms because of the direct inhibitory influence from these receptors on $\alpha$ motoneurons [84]. Golgi tendon receptors sense the tension of muscles and provide inhibitory input to $\alpha$ motoneurons. Administration of central muscle relaxants, such as benzodiazepines (for example Valium), is effective in treating painful muscle spasm such as often occurs in connection with low back pain.

# Cancer pain

Cancer pain has been regarded to be a separate form of pain and treatment of cancer pain has, at least in the past, been regarded to have some special features that warrant separate considerations from general pain conditions.

As our understanding of these pain conditions improves, cancer pain seems more and more similar to general pain conditions and similar treatments are effective. Cancer pain can, therefore, for the most part be treated in similar ways as pain that has other causes.

The view that cancer and non-cancer pain are different entities has resulted in the assumption that treatment with opioids would have different outcomes. Treatments of non-cancer pain have involved fear that opioid treatment may lead to addiction, dependence, and ineffective relief. Now, treatment of cancer does not have that fear and liberal administration of opioids can be made for the treatment of terminal cancer.

# Treatment of pain related to autonomic nervous system disorders

Many pathological pain syndromes [415] have been regarded to be a form of sympathetically maintained pain (SMP) and that has led to treatments that interrupt or reduce the activity of the sympathetic nervous system [27].

Pain conditions that can be related to the autonomic nervous system are mainly Complex Regional Pain Syndromes type 1 and 2 (CRPS 1 and CRPS 2), earlier known as Reflex Sympathetic Dystrophy (RSD) and Causalgia, respectively.

The term SMP is used to describe pain that is believed to be caused by a malfunction of the sympathetic nervous system. It is, however, often difficult to establish proof for the existence of such a relationship between pain and malfunction of the sympathetic nervous systems. Tests using intravenous administration of phentolamine have been regarded to be effective in identifying patients with SMP, but the results of studies of the involvement of the sympathetic nervous system using such methods have varied [27].

Sympathectomy, surgically or chemically, has been tried when there is evidence of involvement of the sympathetic nervous system in an individual with pain, but agreement among clinicians about the efficacy is lacking. Different methods, such as chemical sympathectomy employing alcohol or phenol injections to destroy ganglia, surgical ablation, heath or laser interruption of the sympathetic chain, have been described.

It is an understatement to claim that currently available treatments of sympathetic nervous system disorders are unsatisfactory. To that, comes the poor understanding of disorders of the sympathetic nervous system in general and the fact that few physicians have experience in treating such disorders.

Malfunction of the sympathetic nervous system is not only involved in some forms of pain (especially CRPS), but it also is the cause of symptoms such as excessive sweating as often occurs in women at the beginning of menopause. These symptoms are often treated by clonidine, which is an $\alpha_2$ adrenergic receptor agonist. This receptor senses the level of circulating adrenaline in the blood and controls the production of adrenaline in the adrenal glands.

Increased sensitivity of these receptors reduces circulating adrenaline (epinephrine). Administration of clonidine also reduces blood pressure (antihypertensive) and it counteracts the effect of drugs such as amphetamine.

Administration of clonidine has been tried as treatment for CRPS 1 and 2 [95]. Some reports find that clonidine delivered through the skin using a transdermal patch placed on the skin at a location where light touch causes pain (allodynia) could eliminate or substantially reduce allodynia. Hyperalgesia to mechanical and cold stimuli was also reduced. It was confirmed that the effect was not caused by a local anesthetic effect. In this study, the effect was only observed in 4 out of 6 patients studied [95]. The observations in this study suggested that SMP is mediated via $\alpha_1$-adrenergic receptors located in the affected tissue.

Individuals with CRPS 1 or CRPS 2 characteristically have ongoing pain and pain to light touch (allodynia). Some individuals with signs of increased sympathetic activity obtain pain relief following interruption of sympathetic function to the affected area and that is taken as a confirmation that they have sympathetically maintained pain (SMP) [95].

However, only one randomized, double blind, placebo or active controlled study assessing the effects of sympathectomy for pathological pain and CRPS has been published [419]. Thus, treatment directed to the sympathetic nervous system for pathological pain and CRPS is based on very little high quality evidence. Increased sympathetic activity has also been suspected to be involved in other pain conditions such as fibromyalgia and chronic pain syndrome [252].

Many different kinds of treatment are in use for CRPS and the opinions and evidence of their efficacy varies. However, it seems to be agreed upon that treatment, whatever it is, should be instituted without delay. Aggressive pain management and reduced motion of affected body parts are important for the recovery from these kinds of pain disorders [27]. It also seems to be generally accepted that physical therapy is beneficial. Surgical sympathectomy is sometimes done when tests show substantial benefit from blocking sympathetic transmission in specific ganglia and if oral administration of appropriate medications (sympatholytica) fails [327].

# Stress and pain

Stress of various kinds is associated with increased sympathetic activity and some of the poorly defined pain syndromes may, therefore, be related to stress of some kind. Stress also affects the immune system, including that of the central nervous system, indicating the existence of yet another link between stress and pain. This perhaps also explains why a change in life style, including physical exercise that reduces stress, has shown beneficial effects on disorders such as pathological pain of various kinds. Similar observations have been made in relation to various forms of mood disorders such as depression, which also benefits from physical exercise [27]. Administration of vitamins, and especially of Omega-3, has also been shown to have beneficial effects on some forms of pathological pain [492] and on depression [323].

# Placebo effect

The placebo effect is benefit from the belief that a treatment is effective although the treatment has no active components [149, 233]. The beneficial effect is caused solely by the patient believing that he/she has received a treatment that is beneficial. The positive effect of non-active treatment (placebo) confirms that there is a strong relationship between pain and the mind.

Most treatments have placebo effects, but the effect is especially pronounced regarding pain. However, placebo effects are short term effects. It has been suggested that the placebo effect could be caused by endogenous opioids that were produced and one study of postoperative pain in surgical patients [233] supported that hypothesis.

The participants in the study who responded positively to non-active treatment had increased pain after the administration of naloxone that blocks opioid receptors. Those who did not respond to the first administration of the placebo did not respond to naloxone either.

More recent studies have revealed a far more complex cause of the placebo effect, involving many different brain areas such as the anterior cingulate cortex, anterior insula, prefrontal cortex, and periaqueductal grey [218].

# Examples of attempts to develop new methods for pain control

The increased knowledge about many forms of pain achieved through recent extensive research efforts has made it possible to develop new methods for treatment of different kinds of pain. Increased knowledge about the role of the NMDA receptors has inspired new efforts to find ways of manipulating this receptor. The beneficial effect of administration of common substances such as Omega 3 and vitamins has come into focus. We discussed the use of cannabis for pain control and the development of new methods for neuromodulation above, especially the possibility of controlling neuropathic pain through electrical stimulation of the vagus nerve in connection with somatosensory stimulation that is now under extensive studies.

## NMDA receptors

It has been known for a long time that N-methyl-D-aspartate (NMDA) receptors and neurokinin receptors are involved in central neuropathic pain [491] (see Chapter 1). It has been suggested that NMDA receptor antagonists, such as the experimental drug MK 801 from the pharmaceutical company Merck, would be effective in the treatment of central neuropathic pain. So far, however, attempts to modulate or affect the effect of glutamate that is found throughout the central nervous system have had little clinical success.

The NMDA receptor antagonist, MK 801, has been available for many years, but the success in using it in the practical treatment of pain has not materialized, mainly because of the severe side effects such as liver toxicity.

Ketamine, another NMDA receptor antagonist administrated intravenously, has been shown to have some beneficial effect on pathological pain [413, 414]. However, this drug also has considerable side effects (including psychiatric symptoms) that have prevented its introduction in clinical medicine. The abundance of glutamate and the presence of glutamate receptors in so many parts of the central nervous systems have prevented the development of practically useful drugs that manipulate glutamate or its receptors in a way that can be used to safely treat such specific medical conditions as pain.

Many of the drugs developed, such as those for manipulating the NMDA receptor, have failed because of their side effects, which are also problems with commonly used drugs such as NSAID and opioids. Despite its bad reputation, Thalidomide is still in clinical use for treatment of certain pain conditions [7]. Thalidomide reduces the production of the tumor necrosis factor-alpha (TNF-$\alpha$) from macrophages and administration of thalidomide has been shown to reduce thermal hyperalgesia [410].

A drug, etanercept (trade name Enbrel), is used to treat autoimmune diseases by inhibiting TNF-$\alpha$. The drug might also be used to treat severe pain. It is under FDA investigation for approval. Other possible drugs may come from carrageenan (a family of linear sulfated polysaccharides that is extracted from red seaweed) that induces hyperalgesia [93] and can be reduced by knocking out TNF-$\alpha$ receptors.

A study using $GABA_A$-receptor point-mutated knock-in mice in which specific $GABA_A$ receptor subtypes have been selectively rendered insensitive to benzodiazepine-site ligands has shown that pronounced analgesia can be achieved by specifically targeting spinal $GABA_A$ receptors containing the $\alpha_2$ and/or $\alpha_3$ subunits [214]. A non-sedative ('$\alpha_1$-sparing') benzodiazepine-site ligand, L-838,417, is an experimental drug developed by pharmaceutical company Merck, Sharp and Dohme. While it has similar, but more specific effects than benzodiazepines, it is classed as a non-benzodiazepine anxiolytic. It has been shown to be highly effective against inflammatory and pathological pain, yet devoid of unwanted sedation, motor impairment, and tolerance development [214]. L-838,417 not only diminished the pain input to the brain, but also reduced the activity of brain areas related to the associative-emotional components of pain, as shown by functional magnetic resonance imaging in rats. The development of such subtype-selective GABAergic drugs is an example of the new developments in the treatment of chronic pain that is often refractory to classical pain relievers.

# Vitamins

Vitamins, such as vitamins $B_1$ and $B_{12}$, are effective for treatment of many forms of peripheral neuropathy. Vitamin D (D3) has also [28, 150] favorable effects in management of some forms of pain. Vitamins in norm food are probably sufficient to avoid symptoms of deficit but the amounts of many common vitamins are too small to achieve optimal effects.

Vitamins as supplements are available in many forms. Different kinds of multivitamin tablets contain most of the important vitamins but in too small amounts to achieve the optimal effects.

# Omega-3

The importance of Omega-3 fatty acids for well-being is well-known, but these fatty acids can also be useful in the treatment of diseases as is beginning to become known, although it is slow to win the approval by the medical community. Omega-3 fatty acids can affect the immune system and it has been shown that administration of Omega-3 has beneficial effects on diseases where the immune system is involved such as rheumatoid arthritis [365].

Administration of Omega-3 has potentials for management of many forms of pain and these fatty acids may even have similar pain relieving effect as NSAID. While Omega-3 and vitamins have the advantages that they are essentially free of side effects, they are not used to the extent of their benefit. The fact that they are common substances may be a psychological disadvantage because many people, including health professionals, seem to favor new and sophisticated (and expensive) pharmaceutical products.

Omega-3 and vitamins are generally beneficial and they are inexpensive, especially for people who do not eat adequately. Omega-3 fatty acids are available in normal food items such as fish, especially salmon, but generally in too small amounts to have any noticeable effect in treatment. Eating large quantities of salmon also implies a risk from the mercury that is present in salmon. Omega-3 has been recommended as a dietary supplement for some time. More recently, it has been specifically recommended for treatment of disorders such as depression and pain. The beneficial effects on pain from administration of Omega-3 as a dietary supplement has been demonstrated recently [250].

This study using a questionnaire sent to 250 patients, 125 of whom returned the questionnaire. The participants had taken fish oil that has high contents of Omega-3 for an average of 75 days; 85 percent took 1200 mg and 22 percent took 2400 mg of EFAs (eicosapentaenoic acid and decosahexaenoic acid). Fifty-nine percent of those who had returned their questionnaires discontinued their prescription NSAID medications for pain and 60 percent of the participants stated that their overall pain was improved after having taken fish oil; 80 percent stated they were satisfied with their improvement, and 88 percent stated they would continue to take the fish oil. No significant side effects were reported [250].

There are two omega fatty acids that are of particular interest, Omega-3 and Omega-6, which in many ways compete. The complex actions of these fatty acids especially on prostaglandins have been studied for many years, but only recently have they found clinical interest [13].

The first members of the prostaglandin family were discovered in the 1930s by Ulf von Euler, and some of these substances were synthesized in the 1960s by Sune Bergstrom. In 1971, it was found that aspirin inhibited synthesis of prostaglandins. The group of prostaglandin E is synthesized in the cyclooxygenase (COX) pathway.

The effects of Omega-3 and 6 are through prostaglandins. Omega-3 and 6 involves mainly two of the prostaglandins, namely $PGE_2$ and $PGE_3$, but in different ways. $PGE_3$ has anti-inflammatory effects and it reduces pain while $PGE_2$ promotes inflammatory action. Omega-3 increases that anti-inflammatory effect of prostaglandin $E_3$ ($PGE_3$) while suppressing prostaglandin $E_2$ ($PGE_2$) that has inflammatory and pain producing actions (NSAID suppress synthesis of $PGE_2$).

Since many of the effects of Omega-3 and Omega-6 are opposite, the final effect is determined by the ratio between Omega-3 and Omega-6. Prostaglandin $E_2$ ($PGE_2$) and $E_3$ ($PGE_3$) both use the enzymes cyclooxygenase (COX 1 and COX 2), but the pathways are different [250] (Figure 12.5).

Thus, the more EPA from fish oil (x-3 EFA), the less COX (cyclooxygenase) and LOX (lipooxygenase) are available for the arachidonic pathway. This COX pathway also produces other prostaglandins such as thromboxane and prostaglandins D and F.

## Omega-3 Fatty Acid Pathway

Alpha-Linolenic Acid (ALA)
↓ delta-6 desaturase
Steridonic Acid
↓ elongase
Eicosatraenoic Acid
↓ delta-5 desaturase
Eicosapentaenoic Acid (EPA) <-> Decosahexanic Acid (DHA)
↓ COX → PGE3
↓ LOX → LTB5

3-Series of anti-inflammatory prostaglandins and 5-Series of anti-inflammatory leukotrienes

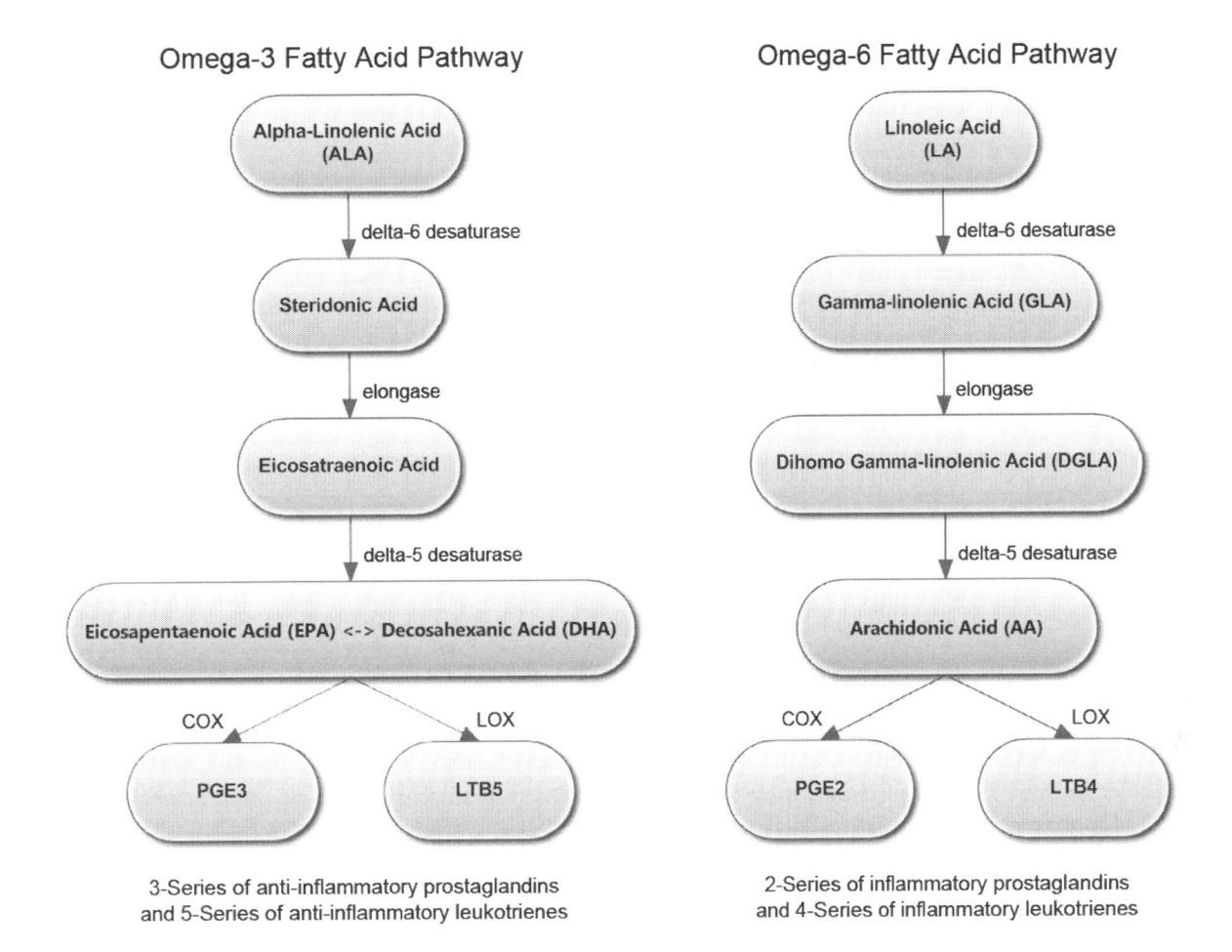

## Omega-6 Fatty Acid Pathway

Linoleic Acid (LA)
↓ delta-6 desaturase
Gamma-linolenic Acid (GLA)
↓ elongase
Dihomo Gamma-linolenic Acid (DGLA)
↓ delta-5 desaturase
Arachidonic Acid (AA)
↓ COX → PGE2
↓ LOX → LTB4

2-Series of inflammatory prostaglandins and 4-Series of inflammatory leukotrienes

Figure 12.5. The two pathways for synthesis of $PGE_2$ and $PGE_3$ using COX and LOX as the enzymes for conversion. (From: Maroon, J., C. and J. W. Bost (2006). "Omega-3 fatty acids (fish oil) as an anti-inflammatory: an alternative to nonsteroidal anti-inflammatory drugs for discogenic pain." Surg Neurol. 65(4): 326-331. [250]). Artwork by Monica Javidnia.

It has been shown that administration of Omega-3 has a pain relieving effect that is similar as that of the NSAID Aspirin and without the side effects [250]. Since Aspirin and other NSAID inhibit synthesis of prostaglandins, their effect somehow neutralizes the effect of Omega-3. Administration of NSAID should, therefore, be terminated when Omega-3 is administrated to treat pain.

# Immune reactions and pain

The immune system of the central nervous system (microglia and astrocytes) is involved in many kinds of pain (see Chapter 10). This is one reason why anti-inflammatory medications can control pathological pain. There is considerable evidence that glia cells, particularly microglia and astrocytes, play an important role in central sensitization [130]. It is also known that when microglia cells are activated, they produce several chemicals that regulate synaptic transmissions in the central nervous system and that may be one of the reasons why microglia are involved in pathological pain.

The findings that the central nervous system has its own immune system and that this immune system is involved in many forms of pain may open new avenues for treatment of pathological pain [478] including reduction of opioid tolerance [468, 474].

Tolerance is especially a problem for long-term use of opioids because of the loss of drug effects or the necessity for escalating doses to produce pain relief. There is evidence that immune systems are involved in creating tolerance to opioids. Opioids are effective in relieving many forms of pathological pain, but concerns of misuse, abuse, and tolerance severely influence their clinical use.

It, therefore, seems likely that we may see treatments that are aimed at glia cells as therapies in addition to those that are now in use and which are aimed at the nerve cells and their transmitter substances (see Chapter 8). It has already been shown that there is a link between activation of microglia cells as a neuroimmune reaction and the pain relieving action of morphine [176, 278].

It is already known that substances such as propentofylline, pentoxifylline, fluorocitrate, and minocycline decrease microglial activation and inhibit proinflammatory cytokines that can decrease pathological pain. Control of microglial activity may, therefore, open ways to activate anti-inflammatory cytokines like IL-10, which are shown to reduce allodynia and hyperalgesia.

There are, therefore, many reasons why microglia especially, but also astrocytes, may be a valid target for the treatment of pathological pain. Some safe and clinically well-tolerated inhibitors of glia activation are potential useful agents for the treatment of pathological pain [278]. Minocycline is especially likely to be a good candidate for use in management of chronic pain. Minocycline, as discussed above, can potently inhibit microglial activation and proliferation when activated. Microglia are usually only active for a short period while astrocytes are activated for a much longer period.

Astrocytes make close contacts with synapses and their reactions after nerve injuries, arthritis, and tumor growth is more persistent than microglial reactions and their reactions are better correlated with chronic pain behaviors.

Astrocytes that are activated communicate with other cells through many different signaling molecules that can have different effects on chronic pain conditions. There is considerable evidence that when activated astrocytes release substances (see Table 12.1), such as pro-inflammatory cytokines, such as interleukin IL-1β and chemokine, such as monocyte chemo attractant protein-1 MCP-1/also called CCL2, persistent pain states in the spinal cord are enhanced and prolonged . Other substances, such as the interleukins (IL)1β, are powerful modulators of synaptic transmission in the spinal cord where they enhance excitatory synaptic transmission and suppress inhibitory synaptic transmission.

## Table 12.1

| Signaling molecule | Changes in chronic pain conditions | Role in chronic pain |
|---|---|---|
| ALXR | Up-regulation | Inhibition |
| bFGF | Up-regulation | Facilitation |
| CCL2/MCP-1 | Up-regulation | Facilitation |
| Connexin-43 | Up-regulation | Not tested |
| Endothelin receptor-B | Up-regulation | Not tested |
| ERK | Up-regulation | Facilitation |
| GLAST | Down-regulation | Not tested |
| GLT-1 | Down-regulation | Inhibition |
| IL-18 receptor | Up-regulation | Facilitation |
| Interleukin 1β | Up-regulation | Facilitation |
| MMP-2 | Up-regulation | Facilitation |
| Neurokinin-2 receptor | Not tested | Facilitation |
| pJNK | Up-regulation | Facilitation |
| pJNK1 | Up-regulation | Facilitation |
| p-c-jun | Up-regulation | Not tested |
| TAK1 | Up-regulation | Facilitation |
| TNF-α | Up-regulation | Facilitation |
| TPA | Up-regulation | Facilitation |

Table 12.1 Signaling molecules in astrocytes. Abbreviations: ALXR: lipoxin A4 receptor; GLT-1: glutamate transporter-1; MMP-2: matrix metalloproteinase-2; TAK1: transforming growth factor-activated kinase 1; TPA: tissue type plasminogen activator. Data from Gao, Y.J. and R.R. Ji, Targeting astrocyte signaling for chronic pain. Neurotherapeutics, 2010. 7(4): p. 482-93.

Almost all cells have both inhibitory and excitatory functions and it is the balance between these two opposite functions that determine how a cell will react to input signals. Other substances secreted from activated astrocytes, such as the MCP-1, increase pain sensitivity through direct activation of NMDA receptors in neurons in the dorsal horn of the spinal cord.

There seem to be ample possibilities for pharmacological manipulation of the actions of astrocytes; for example, it seems possible to affect the inhibition caused by the IL-1β, c-Jun N-terminal kinase, and MCP-1. Interventions in specific signaling pathways in astrocytes may offer new approaches for the management of chronic pain. The metalloprotease-2 signaling via spinal administration has already been shown to attenuate inflammatory, pathological, or cancer pain [130].

In general, it seems possible to improve treatment of pathological pain by using drugs that decrease inflammation [498]. Since vitamin D (D3) can reduce immune reactions, it has been suggested that increased levels of vitamin D may reduce pain when affected by immune reactions either of the body or of the nervous system [169].

# Minocycline

A recent study emphasized the beneficial effects of administration of minocycline, an inhibitor of microglial activation, together with administration of morphine for the treatment of pain; minocycline suppresses morphine-induced respiratory depression, suppresses morphine-induced reward, and enhances systemic morphine-induced relief of pain [175]. There is recent evidence that minocycline attenuates morphine tolerance related to its effect on microglia. Combined with morphine, minocycline has a synergetic effect. On the basis of these findings, it has been hypothesized that the combination of morphine and minocycline may produce a dual effect with morphine as a pain reliever and minocycline selectively inhibits the activation of microglia [76].

Due to the modulating effect of minocycline on some of the effects of morphine, minocycline may offer an improved treatment of pain disorders such as intractable postherpetic neuralgia (PHN) when administrated together with morphine [76]. Treatment of PHN with traditional pharmaceutical agents has often lead to intolerable side effects at dosages below the efficient dose.

Other studies have shown beneficial effects of administration of an inhibitor of microglial activation, minocycline, on burn pain [73]. Burn pain is assumed to have strong central components and it is difficult to treat because of poor responses to common pain relievers. When administrated at the same time as the burn injury occurred and for 1 week thereafter, minocycline has long-lasting effects on the pain by decreasing hyper responsiveness of cells in the dorsal horns and reducing allodynia for at least 1 month [73].

Better understanding of the immune system of the central nervous system and how it is involved in pathologies such as some forms of pain will most likely open opportunities for different kinds of treatment of many kinds of pain.

# Reducing the risk of pain

Actions to prevent pain have received little attention and this is similar to the lack of serious efforts to prevent other diseases. Few treatments that serve to reduce the risk of pain have been described. Thus, this is another area of pain management that awaits development.

Surgical operations almost always cause more or less persistent pain after the operation, which may last weeks, months, or even years. For example, it is known that after orthopedic operations, the prevalence of complex regional pain syndrome (CRPS), phantom limb pain can be high. For example, persistent pain following total joint arthroplasty affects an alarmingly high number of people [355].

As we have discussed in several places in this book, activation of neuroplasticity can cause the development of central neuropathic pain. Manipulations of nerves in the anesthetized patient result in massive and abnormal neural activity arriving at the spinal cord and brain before it becomes blocked by the anesthesia. This abnormal neural activity has a large potential to cause activation of bad neuroplasticity that can cause persistent pain after the operation. The remedy would be to block the neural activity that is caused by the surgical manipulations before it reaches the spinal cord [261].

This can be done easily by local anesthetics applied to the nerves before the surgical manipulations begin. Other methods would be to use anesthetic regiments that are aimed at more peripheral structures of the nervous system.

Using several different pharmacological agents together to achieve freedom of pain during operations allows a reduction in the doses of individual drugs and that may reduce postoperative pain.

The lower prevalence of opioid-related adverse events is another beneficial effect [355]. This means that modifications of anesthesia regiments may be effective in reducing pain after some kinds of operations. Earlier, development of anesthesia regiments focused on lowering the risk of death with little emphasis on pain and other adverse effects that manifest after an operation, such as cognitive deficits resulting in a lowered quality of life.

# Reducing the risk of amputation pain

Avoiding surgical operations that have no benefit is perhaps the most effective way of preventing pain.

As mentioned above, pain often occurs after amputations where large nerves have been cut and subsequently develop neuroma. There are several ways that the risk of phantom pain after an amputation can be reduced. It was mentioned in Chapter 8 that the risk of developing phantom limb pain depends on an individual's pain before the amputation. The risk of postoperative phantom pain can be reduced by aggressively treating existing pain before an amputation is performed because there is evidence that pain before amputations may persist after the amputation. Epidural anesthesia could, therefore, possibly reduce the risk of postoperative pain after amputations [473]. The efficacy of such treatment supports the hypothesis that neuroplasticity is a factor in amputation pain. The risk of postoperative pain can be reduced by applying a local anesthetic to block neural conduction in the nerves that are going to be severed. The risk can be reduced by a simple procedure that reduces the risk of sprouting of axons at the site where a nerve is cut.

Surgical treatments of the nerve stump have been explored in an effort to minimize pain. These treatments can be broadly divided into two methods. One is to shorten the nerve stump. The other method consists of covering the proximal nerve stump by burying it into adjacent tissues or inserting it into a vein or tube. It is generally thought that the mechanism of reduction of pain from covering the proximal nerve stump protects the nerve stump from scar tissue or prevents nerve regeneration, although the details remain unclear [321].

Animal experiments [321] have shown that covering the proximal nerve stump can reduce the risk of neuroma formation after severing a peripheral nerve, but it is not known exactly how that is achieved. The results were based on an animal model (rat) where the proximal nerve stump of the sciatic nerve was introduced into a silicone tube while the control rats had no tube. The score of autotomy (self amputation) observed in the tube group was lower than that in the control group at 3 days to 2 weeks after surgery indicating that the silicone tube had decreased the pain.

Toluidine blue staining showed that the increase in the number of mast cells was inhibited at 1, 2, and 4 weeks after surgery and in the number of lymphocytes at 1 and 2 weeks after surgery in the tube group.

It was believed that blocking the infiltration of inflammatory cells into the proximal nerve stump by the silicone tube was the cause of the decreased signs of pain. Examination of the expression of nerve growth factor (NGF) by inflammatory cells and of the NGF receptor TrkA in the proximal nerve stump and the dorsal root ganglion showed that the NGF immunoreactivity, (NGF-IR) decreased at 1, 2, and 4 weeks after surgery in the tube group, suggesting that this might be one of the reasons for reduced pain from the proximal stump [321].

There is evidence that overstimulation that occurs during a surgical operation to amputate a limb is involved in one of the causes of phantom limb syndrome. Studies have shown that the risk of pain and other phantom limb symptoms can be reduced by applying local anesthetics to the peripheral nerve before surgery [14]. However, the results of other studies have set that in doubt [261]. Anyhow, experience shows that it is difficult to get surgeons to take actions such as making local blocks of peripheral nerves before an operation. One reason may be that surgeons in their postoperative assessment are focused on the outcome of the operation regarding the therapeutically goal to a lesser extent than on side effects such as pain, which is regarded unavoidable.

# Importance of a person's life style

In general, there is no doubt that the risk of acquiring some forms of pain depends on life style. Low back pain, carpal tunnel syndrome, and other occupation related disorders are clear examples. For low back pain, there is no doubt that many factors influence the risk of getting low back pain. The risk is clearly related to body weight which has been confirmed by studies that have shown that a high body mass index (BMI) is associated with higher levels of back pain intensity [450].

Higher levels of pain intensity were positively associated with total fat mass and with lower limb fat mass. Similar relationships were observed with trunk, android, and gynoid fat mass. After adjusting for confounders, no measures of lean tissue mass were associated with higher pain intensity or disability ($p>0.10$). Thus, these studies show that greater fat, but not lean tissue mass, is associated with high levels of low back pain intensity and disability [450].

Since low back pain occurs more frequently in people who are overweight or obese, the general increase in body weight of people that has occurred during the last decade or two is one reason for the increase in the occurrence of low back pain. The lack of physical exercise is another likely reason [358].

The choice of life style, including good nutrition, keeping a normal body weight, physical exercise, etc., no doubt plays an important role in coping with pain and probably also in the severity of pain, at least for some kinds of pain. Adequate intake of nutrients including vitamins, absence of alcohol and smoking of cigarettes are no doubt important, but the importance is probably underestimated because few studies have addressed the importance of lifestyle.

Diabetes type 2 is a disease that is closely related to lifestyle and especially being overweight or obese increases the risk of acquiring diabetes type 2 dramatically. Diabetes is associated with several unpleasant symptoms such as pain, especially peripheral neuropathy (painful diabetic neuropathy, PDN). It is treatable and the risk of acquiring diabetes type 2 can be reduced considerably by maintaining a normal life style, especially regarding eating the right kinds of food and eating in moderation. A similar disorder is alcohol related peripheral neuropathy, which naturally can be avoided by not drinking alcohol (in excess).

However, the promotion of even the simplest changes in life style meet resistance because the general public sentiment is that if (when) disease strikes, there will be a treatment available that can restore health. Experience does not support that hypothesis [290].

# Appendix A
# Neuroplasticity

# Introduction

There is evidence that the symptoms of central neuropathic pain are caused by changes in the function of the spinal cord and the brain and many of these changes in function are caused by activation of neuroplasticity. Central neuropathic pain is, therefore, a plasticity disorder similar to other disorders that are caused by plastic changes in the central nervous system (spinal cord and brain) such as some forms of tinnitus, some forms of muscle spasm, and spasticity.

The changes in the function and in the organization of the dorsal horns of the spinal cord and in structures in the brain that normally process pain signals from the periphery of the nervous system are now believed to play an important role in the cause of several forms of pain and its accompanying symptoms, allodynia and hyperpathia. Loss or reduction of normal inhibition in the spinal cord is an important contribution to the abnormal function that causes central neuropathic pain [214]. Plasticity diseases that are caused by changes in the function of the brain and the spinal cord have received much less attention than they deserve. One reason is that no tests have yet been designed that can detect and measure the changes in the brain that cause plasticity diseases such as pain, tinnitus, and phantom limb symptoms. Much research has been driven by what could be seen and what could be measured, and that is also so for the diagnosis of diseases. Diseases that cannot be studied by tests are given much less attention than diseases where there is what are called objective signs that can be measured or visualized. There are no tests that can monitor progress in the treatment of most plasticity diseases. Because plasticity diseases have no detectable physical signs, diagnosis of these diseases must rely on the patients' description of their symptoms.

This Appendix will discuss the basics of neuroplasticity and its role in different kinds of pain disorders.

# What is neuroplasticity?

Neuroplasticity is a general term that covers aspects of the nervous system being plastic, or malleable which means that it can change its function. Neuroplasticity involves changes in the function and to some extent the structure of neural circuits in the spinal cord and the brain. This means that the nervous system is not hard-wired and the way it functions is not fixed, but can change.

Neuroplasticity is a property of the central nervous system (spinal cord and brain) that is apparent only when activated, thus similar to genes. The fact that the spinal cord and the brain are plastic has important effects on many of the different functions of the nervous system, including the processing of pain signals from receptors (physiological pain) and on the creation of pathological pain.

There are two kinds of neuroplasticity, one is beneficial and one has harmful effects causing signs of diseases [292]. The beneficial plasticity makes it possible to adapt to changing demands and to redirect tasks from parts of the brain that were damaged such as from strokes to functional parts. Activation of neuroplasticity is necessary for normal childhood development.

Harmful plasticity can cause diseases that are called plasticity disorders in this book. Central neuropathic pain is an example of a plasticity disorder. Others are severe tinnitus, spasm, and spasticity. Neuroplasticity is involved in creating the symptoms of other diseases such as low back pain, fibromyalgia, and probably also diseases such as chronic fatigue syndrome.

A change in the processing of pain signals that occurs in the spinal cord and the caudal trigeminal nucleus can create different abnormal states of the neural circuits in these structures including re-routing (change in connectivity) of information.

Plasticity is a property of the nervous system that is only apparent when activated. Plastic changes in the function of the nervous system have similarities with learning, but also important differences. What is learned must be recalled voluntarily, but the skills learned through activation of neuroplasticity are always available. Plastic changes occur without conscious awareness.

Acquiring the ability to pronounce an unfamiliar word is a skill that is always available, like the ability to do physical tasks such as bicycling, which when learned, is always available. What is learned, on the other hand, must always be recalled and it can be forgotten.

The brain can change the way it functions at any time during life, but this ability to change its function is greater in young individual than in adults. The period where it is easiest to induce plastic changes is known as the critical period. The experience with cochlear implants shows that the critical period for hearing is probably 3-4 years. For vision in humans, it is probably 2-3 years, with different aspects of vision having different critical periods.

## Implications of plastic changes

Plastic changes in the spinal cord and the brain can cause a wide range of changes in function. Plastic changes can increase excitability and re-route information, which in turn can cause improvements of performance or hyperactivity that may be regarded as harmful. It can improve motor performance by extending the regions of the brain that are devoted to a specific task that is done often. The opposite is also the case. Thus, studies have indicated that if a part of the cerebral cortex of one sense (for example, the auditory cortex) does not receive signals during the critical period, it may be taken over by other senses such as vision [172].

Re-routing of information can direct tasks to different parts of the brain in case some parts have lost function through damage. Activation of neuroplasticity makes it possible to learn new skills.

After injury to the brain or spinal cord, neural signals can be redirected to functional regions of the central nervous system through activation of neuroplasticity. Plasticity of the spinal cord and the brain can make can it possible to regain function after injuries, such as trauma, strokes, etc., which have destroyed neural tissue.

Activation of neuroplasticity can change the way specific parts of the spinal cord and the brain compensate for lost functions such as may occur from trauma to the brain including strokes. Reduced functions may be improved by increasing the gain in neural circuits in sensory and motor systems of the brain and the spinal cord. Such changes in the gain can be overdone causing hyperactive disorders.

This is one way that neuroplasticity can become harmful. This is a form of maladaptation. When activation of neuroplasticity goes wrong, it can cause diseases such as forms of chronic pain and some forms of tinnitus (ringing in the ears).

The unwanted effects of expression of neuroplasticity (or more correctly, the effects that are of no benefit to the individuals or are harmful) are hyperactivity, such as tinnitus, tremor, spasticity, and pain such as central neuropathic pain, phantom limb symptoms, and spasticity after spinal cord trauma, etc. (Section III discusses such diseases in more detail).

Activation of neuroplasticity is absolutely necessary for the development of the nervous system that occurs during the first 2 years of life for the organization of the nervous system that was laid down before birth and guided by inheritance. Neuroplasticity can correct or modify genetic programs for development and it can change the developments of the nervous system in individual persons. This is in addition to the programmed development that is controlled by genes and caused by what is known as epigenetic (above or over genetics).

There are many forms of plasticity diseases that have in common that they may be regarded as a misdirected change in function of the central nervous system that are elicited by the expression of neuroplasticity. The most common plasticity diseases are some forms of pain (central neuropathic pain) and some forms of tinnitus. Some forms of muscle spasm (and spasticity) are also plasticity diseases.

There are other diseases where activation of neuroplasticity plays a role such as movement diseases. For example, neuroplasticity plays an important role in many forms of spasm and spasticity. These diseases do indeed have visible signs, but the changes in the function of the nervous system that cause spasm or spasticity are difficult to study. Often, other causes are suggested for such diseases because their causes are not easy to detect.

# Nature of plastic changes

A change in synaptic efficacy is the main way that changes in function are accomplished, but elimination and creation of new synapses are also parts of the repertoire of neuroplasticity, which also includes the elimination of entire cells through programmed cell death. Activation of neuroplasticity can change the balance between inhibition and excitation in cells.

A change in synthesis of proteins in nerve cells is also a part of plastic changes [394]. Most cells have both excitatory and inhibitory input. Plastic changes often occur in the relationship between excitation and inhibition, most often shifting towards excitation.

While most plastic changes involve changes in synaptic efficacy and thus, are reversible, changes caused by activation of neuroplasticity may in fact also cause structural changes in the brain. Hebb (1949) postulated that when many neurons fire at the same time, it may change the morphology in such a way that the neurons will connect morphologically together. This principle later became known as "neurons that fire together, wire together". This is a form of activity dependent synaptic plasticity. It is also important to understand that changes in the function of the nervous system that are caused by the expression of neuroplasticity can become permanent. Long term potentiation (LTP) and long-term depression (LTD), that are associated with many functions of the brain, especially memory, are associated with neuroplasticity. High-frequency trains of nerve impulses are effective in inducing LTP.

This means that activation of neuroplasticity can create a bistable condition where neural circuits have two different stable modes of function, one normal and one pathologic mode. This means that temporary and reversible plastic changes can be made permanent by such morphological changes.

The elimination or creation of new connections and altered synaptic efficacy cannot be measured. It is, therefore, difficult to study the biological phenomena of the expression of neuroplasticity. Often, only the effect of such changes can be observed and rarely can the effects be quantified.

One of the first scientists to show that the function of the brain could be changed due to plasticity was Goddard. Goddard showed that impulses of electrical current that were passed through the amygdala in rats every day first gave no visible reactions in the rats. However, after doing it every day for 4-6 weeks, the electrical current began to evoke epileptic seizures [141]. Goddard likened it with lighting a fire and he called it "kindling". Similar reactions have later been shown to occur in many other parts of the brain [457]. For example, neuroplasticity (or kindling) was assumed to be the cause of the involuntary muscle contractions in a disease known as hemifacial spasm [297], a rare disease that causes attacks of involuntary contractions of muscles in one side of the face.

These studies indicated that malfunctioning of the facial motonucleus (that controls the "mimic" muscles of the face) was the cause of the symptoms [284].

Other studies showed that similar signs as occur in people with hemifacial spasm could be created in animals by passing electrical impulses through the facial nerve in rats [385], thus a further indication of the involvement of neuroplasticity in creating the symptoms of hemifacial spasm.

# What can activate neuroplasticity?

Signals coming from outside and entering the brain through our senses or from inside the body can activate neuroplasticity as can events that occur in the spinal cord or the brain. Deprivation of sensory input is a strong activator of neuroplasticity, as is frequent stimulation with the same stimuli. Both cause functional changes, but are different. Frequent use of motor systems and reflexes activate neuroplasticity that makes reflexes stronger and easier to activate.

Studies in animals have shown that activation of neuroplasticity, such as may occur when signals from the body to one segment is cut off, can unmask connections to nerve cells in one segment so that signals from distant segments can activate neurons in the segment that has been deprived of signals from the body [460]. These studies illustrate the great power of deprivation of input, which often occurs after trauma, including amputations.

Deprivation of sensory input, such as in deaf people, causes some parts of the brain to be unused. If that occurs before or just after birth, other senses may invade the unused parts of the auditory cortex and paradoxically, these cells that are anatomically located in the auditory cortex will respond to light. The nerve fibers that normally carry information from peripheral vision take over regions of the auditory cerebral cortex.

There are systems in the brain that facilitate plastic changes, making it easier for sensory stimulation to cause functional changes. One system is the basal nucleus (nucleus of Meynert). Stimulating that nucleus at the same time that the stimulus aimed at eliciting plastic changes is presented enhances the induced plastic changes [16, 205]. It was later shown that electrical stimulation of the vagus nerve have similar effects as stimulation of the nucleus basalis [114]. Such "pairing" of stimuli is now being developed for clinical use.

Stimulation of the vagus nerve has similar effects and is a more attractive method to use because the electrodes for stimulation of the vagus nerve can be placed where the nerve travels in the neck, thus requiring minimal surgical exploration.

# Appendix B
## Brodmann's areas of the cerebral cortex

### Lateral surface of the brain

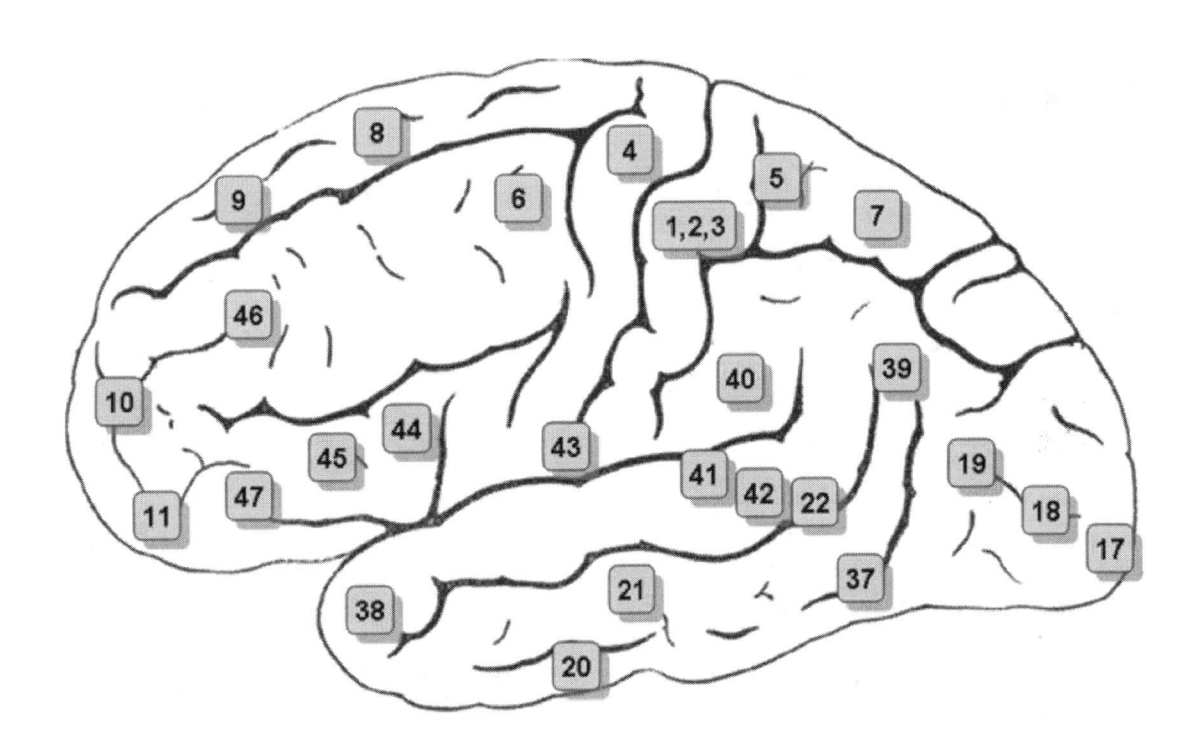

## Medial surface

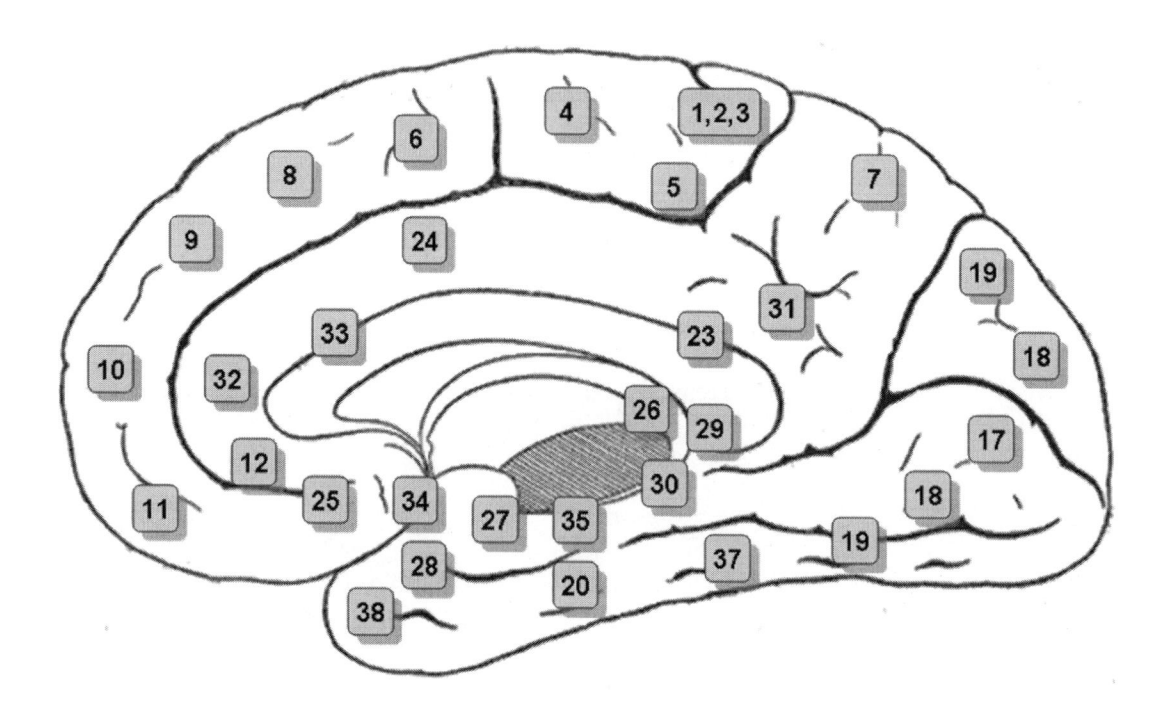

Areas 1, 2, & 3 - Primary somatosensory cortex (frequently referred to as Areas 3, 1, 2 by convention)

Area 4 - Primary motor cortex

Area 5 - Somatosensory association cortex

Area 6 - Pre-motor and supplementary motor cortex (secondary motor cortex)

Area 7 - Somatosensory association cortex

Area 8 - Includes frontal eye fields

Area 9 - Dorsolateral prefrontal cortex

Area 10 - Frontopolar area (most rostral part of superior and middle frontal gyri)

Area 11 - Orbitofrontal area (orbital and rectus gyri, plus part of the rostral part of the superior frontal gyrus)

Area 12 - Orbitofrontal area (used to be part of BA11, refers to the area between the superior frontal gyrus and the inferior rostral sulcus)

Area 13 and Area 14* - Insular cortex

Area 15* - Anterior temporal lobe

Area 17 - Primary visual cortex (V1)

Area 18 - Visual association cortex (V2)

Area 19 - V3

Area 20 - Inferior temporal gyrus

Area 21 - Middle temporal gyrus

Area 22 - Superior temporal gyrus, of which the rostral part participates with Wernicke's area

Area 23 - Ventral posterior cingulate cortex

Area 24 - Ventral anterior cingulate cortex

Area 25 - Subgenual cortex

Area 26 - Ectosplenial area

Area 28 - Posterior entorhinal cortex

Area 29 - Retrosplenial cingular cortex

Area 30 - Part of cingular cortex

Area 31 - Dorsal posterior cingular cortex

Area 32 - Dorsal anterior cingulate cortex

Area 34 - Anterior entorhinal cortex (on the parahippocampal gyrus)

Area 35 - Perirhinal cortex (on the parahippocampal gyrus)

Area 36 - Parahippocampal cortex (on the parahippocampal gyrus)

Area 37 - Fusiform gyrus

Area 38 - Temporopolar area (most rostral part of the superior and middle temporal gyri)

Area 39 - Angular gyrus, part of Wernicke's area

Area 40 - Supramarginal gyrus, part of Wernicke's area

Areas 41 & 42 - Primary and auditory association cortex

Area 43 - Subcentral area (between insula and post/precentral gyrus)

Area 44 - Pars opercularis, part of Broca's area

Area 45 - Pars triangularis Broca's area

Area 46 - Dorsolateral prefrontal cortex

Area 47 - Inferior prefrontal gyrus

Area 48 - Retrosubicular area (a small part of the medial surface of the temporal lobe)

Area 52 - Parainsular area (at the junction of the temporal lobe and the insula)

# References

1. Abrahamsen, R., M. Dietz, S. Lodahl, A. Roepstorff, et al., *Effect of hypnotic pain modulation on brain activity in patients with temporomandibular disorder pain.* Pain., 2010. 151(3): p. 825-33.
2. Aggarwal, S., *Cannabinergic pain medicine: a concise clinical primer and survey of randomized-controlled trial results.* Clin J Pain., 2013. 29(2): p. 162-71.
3. Ahmad, M. and C.R. Goucke, *Management strategies for the treatment of neuropathic pain in the elderly.* Drugs Aging, 2002. 19(12): p. 929-45.
4. Altschuler, E.L., S.B. Wisdom, L. Stone, C. Foster, et al., *Rehabilitation of hemiparesis after stroke with a mirror.* Lancet., 1999. 353(9169): p. 2035-6.
5. Andrew, D. and A.D. Craig, *Spinothalamic lamina I neurons sensitive to histamine: a central pathway for itch.* Nat. Neurosci., 2001. 4(1): p. 72-7.
6. Ansari, S., K. Chaudhri, and K. Al Moutaery, *Vagus nerve stimulation: Indications and limitations.* Acta Neuroschir. Suppl, 2007. 97(2): p. 281-286.
7. Apfel, S., C. and D.W. Zochodne, *Thalidomide neuropathy: too much or too long?* Neurology., 2004. 62(12): p. 2158-9.
8. Apkarian, A., J. Hashmi, and M. Baliki, *Pain and the brain: specificity and plasticity of the brain in clinical chronic pain.* Pain, 2010. 152(3 Suppl): p. 49-64.
9. Apkarian, A.V., *Human Brain Imaging Studies of Chronic Pain: Translational Opportunities.*, in *SourceTranslational Pain Research: From Mouse to Man*, L. Kruger and A.R. Light, Editors. 2010, CRC Press: Boca Raton, FL.
10. Apkarian, A.V., M.N. Baliki, and P.Y. Geha, *Towards a theory of chronic pain.* Prog Neurobiol., 2009. 87(2): p. 81-97.
11. Apkarian, A.V., M.C. Bushnell, R.D. Treede, and J.K. Zubieta, *Human brain mechanisms of pain perception and regulation in health and disease.* Eur J Pain., 2005. 9(4): p. 463-84.
12. Arle, J.E. and J. Shils, *Motor cortex stimulation for pain and movement disorders.* Neurotherapeutics, 2008. 5(1): p. 37-49.
13. Ausman, J.I., *Why omega-3 fatty acids are important to neurosurgeons.* Surg Neurol., 2006. 65: p. 325.
14. Bach, S., M.F. Noreng, and N.U. Tjellden, *Phantom limb pain in amputees during the first 12 months following limb amputation, after preoperative lumbar epidural blockade.* Pain, 1988. 33: p. 297-301.
15. Badoer, E., *Microglia: activation in acute and chronic inflammatory states and in response to cardiovascular dysfunction.* Int J Biochem Cell Biol., 2010. 42(10): p. 1580-5.
16. Bakin, J.S. and N.M. Weinberger, *Induction of a physiological memory in the cerebral cortex by stimulation of the nucleus basalis.* Proc. Natl. Acad. Sci. USA, 1996. 93(20): p. 11219-24.
17. Baliki, M., B. Petre, S. Torbey, K. Herrmann, et al., *Corticostriatal functional connectivity predicts transition to chronic back pain.* Nat Neurosci., 2012. 15(8).
18. Baliki, M., T. Schnitzer, W. Baue, and A. Apkarian, *Brain morphological signatures for chronic pain.* PLoS One, 2011. 6(10).
19. Baliki, M.N., P.Y. Geha, and A.V. Apkarian, *Parsing pain perception between nociceptive representation and magnitude estimation.* Neurophysiol., 2009. 101(2): p. 875–87.
20. Baliki, M.N., P.Y. Geha, A.V. Apkarian, and D.R. Chialvo, *Chronic pain hurts the brain, disrupting the default-mode network dynamics.* J Neurosci., 2008. 28: p. 1398-1403.
21. Bano, D., M. Agostini, G. Melino, and P. Nicotera, *Ageing, neuronal connectivity and brain disorders: an unsolved ripple effect.* Mol Neurobiol., 2011. 43(2).
22. Barberá, J. and R. Albert-Pampló, *Centrocentral anastomosis of the proximal nerve stump in the treatment of painful amputation neuromas of major nerves.* J Neurosurg., 1993. 79(3): p. 331-4.
23. Barker, A.T., R. Jalinous, and I.L. Freeston, *Non-invasive magnetic stimulation of the human motor cortex.* Lancet, 1985: p. 1106-1107.

24. Barker, F.G., P.J. Jannetta, D.J. Bissonette, M.V. Larkins, et al., *The long-term outcome of microvascular decompression for trigeminal neuralgia.* N. Eng. J. Med., 1996. 334: p. 1077-1083.
25. Barker, F.G., P.J. Jannetta, D.J. Bissonette, P.T. Shields, et al., *Microvascular Decompression for Hemifacial Spasm.* J. Neurosurg., 1995. 82: p. 201-210.
26. Barlas, P. and T. Lundeberg, *Transcutaneous electrical nerve stimualtion and acupunture,* in *Wall and Melzack's Textbook of Pain,* S.B. McMahon and M. Koltzenburg, Editors. 2006, Elsevier: Amsterdam. p. 583-590.
27. Baron, R., *Complex regional pain syndromes,* in *Wall and Melzack's Textbook of Pain,* S.B. McMahon and M. Koltzenburg, Editors. 2006, Elsevier: Amsterdam. p. 1011-1027.
28. Bartley, J., *Post herpetic neuralgia, schwann cell activation and vitamin D.* Med Hypotheses., 2009. 73(6): p. 927-9.
29. Basbaum, A.I., C.H. Clanton, and H.L. Fields, *Three bulbospinal pathways from the rostral medulla of the cat: and autoradiographic study of pain modulating systems.* J. Comp. Neurol., 1978. 178: p. 209-224.
30. Benedetti, F., H.S. Mayberg, T.D. Wager, C.S. Stohler, et al., *Neurobiological mechanisms of the placebo effect.* J Neurosci., 2005. 25: p. 10390–10402.
31. Bennett, R.M., *Fibromyalgia,* in *Handbook of Pain,* P.D. Wall and R. Melzack, Editors. 1999, Churchill Livingstone: Edinburgh. p. 579-601.
32. Berthoud, H.R. and W.L. Neuhuber, *Functional and chemical anatomy of the afferent vagal system.* Autonomic Neurosci., 2000. 85(1-3): p. 1-17.
33. Bielefeldt, K. and G.F. Gebhart, *Visceral pain: basic mechanisms,* in *Textbook of Pain,* S.B. McMahon and M. Koltzenburg, Editors. 2006, Elsevier: Amsterdam. p. 721-736.
34. Bigal, M.E. and R.B. Lipton, *Headache,* in *Wall and Melzack's Textbook of Pain,* S.B. Mahon and M. Kolzenburg, Editors. 2006, Elsevier: Amsterdam. p. 837-850.
35. Bingel, U. and I. Tracey, *Imaging CNS Modulation of Pain in Humans.* Physiology 2008. 23: p. 371-380.
36. Blackburn-Munro, G. and R.E. Blackburn-Munro, *Chronic pain, chronic stress and depression: coincidence or consequence?* J Neuroendocrinol, 2001. 13(12): p. 1009-23.
37. Blomqvist, A., E.T. Zhang, and A.D. Craig, *Cytoarchitectonic and immunohistochemical characterization of a specific pain and temperature relay, the posterior portion of the ventral medial nucleus, in the human thalamus.* Brain, 2000. 123(3): p. 601-19.
38. Boivie, J., *Central pain,* in *Textbook of Pain,* P.D. Wall and R. Melzack, Editors. 1999, Churchill Livingstone: Edinburgh. p. 879-914.
39. Bolay, H. and M.A. Moskowitz, *Mechanisms of pain modulation in chronic syndromes.* Neurology, 2002. 59(5 Suppl. 2): p. S2-7.
40. Bonica, J.J., *Introduction: semantic, epidemiologic, and educational issues,* in *Pain and central nervous system disease: the central pain syndromes,* K.L. Casey, Editor. 1991, Raven Press: New York. p. 13-29.
41. Borg-Stein, J. and S.A. Simon, *Focused review: myofascial pain.* Arch. Phys. Med. Rehab., 2002. 83(3): p. S40-7, S48-9.
42. Borsook, D., J. Upadhyay, E.H. Chudler, and L. Becerra, *A key role of the basal ganglia in pain and analgesia--insights gained through human functional imaging.* Mol Pain, 2010. 6(27).
43. Boscan, P., A.E. Pickering, and J.F. Paton, *The nucleus of the solitary tract: an integrating station for nociceptive and cardiorespiratory afferents.* Exp. Physiol, 2002. 87: p. 259–266.
44. Bove, G.M. and A.R. Light, *The nervi nervorum: missing link for neuropathic pain?* J. Pain, 1997. 6(3).
45. Braz, J.M., M.A. Nassar, J.N. Wood, and A.I. Basbaum, *Parallel "pain" pathways arise from subpopulations of primary afferent nociceptor.* Neuron., 2005 47(6): p. 787-93.
46. Breivik, H., P.C. Borchgrevink, S.M. Allen, L.A. Rosseland, et al., *Assessment of pain.* British journal of anaesthesia, 2008. 101(1): p. 17–24.
47. Breivik, H., B. Collett, V. Ventafridda, R. Cohen, et al., *Survey of chronic pain in Europe: prevalence, impact on daily life, and treatment.* Eur J Pain, 2006. 10(4): p. 287-333.

48. Brierley, S.M., R.C. Jones, G. Gebhart, F., and L.A. Blackshaw, *Splanchnic and pelvic mechanosensory afferents signal different qualities of colonic stimuli in mice.* Gastroenterology., 2004. 127(1): p. 166-78.
49. Brisby, H., *Pathology and possible mechanisms of nervous system response to disc degeneration.* J. Bone and Joint Surg., 2006. 88A Suppl. 2(Suppl. 2): p. 68-71.
50. Brodal, P., *The central nervous system.* 1998, New York: Oxford Press.
51. Brodal, P., *The central nervous system.* 3rd ed. 2004, New York: Oxford Press.
52. Brown, J.A., *Motor cortex stimulation.* Neurosurg Focus., 2001. 11(3): p. E5.
53. Bruce, T.O., *Comorbid depression in rheumatoid arthritis: pathophysiology and clinical implications.* Curr Psychiatry Rep., 2008. 10(3): p. 258-64.
54. Brüggemann, J., V. Galhardo, and A. Apkarian, *Immediate reorganization of the rat somatosensory thalamus after partial ligation of sciatic nerve.* J. Pain, 2001. 2(4): p. 220-8.
55. Brumovsky, P.R. and G.F. Gebhart, *Visceral organ cross-sensitization - an integrated perspective.* Auton Neurosci., 2010. 153(1-2): p. 106-15.
56. Brune, K. and H.U. Zeilhofer, *Antipyretic amalgesics: basic aspects,* in *Wall and Melzak's Textbook of Pain,* S.B. McMahon and M. Koltzenburg, Editors. 2006, Elsevier, Churchill, Livingstone: Amsterdam. p. 459-69.
57. Buchwald, J.S. and C.M. Huang, *Far field acoustic response: Origins in the cat.* Science, 1975. 189: p. 382-384.
58. Busch, V., F. Zeman, A. Heckel, F. Menne, et al., *The effect of transcutaneous vagus nerve stimulation on pain perception--an experimental study.* Brain Stimul., 2013. 6(2): p. 202-9.
59. Bushnell, M.C. and A.V. Apkarian, *Representation of pain in the brain,* in *Wall and Melzak's Textbook of Pain,* S.B. McMahon and M. Koltzenburg, Editors. 2006, Elsevier: Amsterdam. p. 107-124.
60. Bushnell, M.C., G.H. Duncan, R.K. Hofbauer, B. Ha, et al., *Pain perception: is there a role for primary somatosensory cortex?* Proc Natl Acad Sci U S A, 1999. 96(14): p. 7705-9.
61. Buskila, D. and P. Sarzi-Puttini, *Fibromyalgia and Autoimmune Diseases: the Pain behind Autoimmunity.* IMAJ, 2008. 10: p. 77-78.
62. Cacace, A.T., J.P. Cousins, S.M. Parnes, D.J. McFarland, et al., *Cutaneous-evoked tinnitus. II: Review of neuroanatomical, physiological and functional imaging studies.* Audiol. Neurotol., 1999. 4(5): p. 258-268.
63. Canavero, S., V. Bonicalzi, M. Dotta, S. Vighetti, et al., *Low-rate repetitive TMS allays central pain.* Neurol. Res., 2003. 25: p. 151-152.
64. Candiotti, K.A. and M.C. Gitlin, *Review of the effect of opioid-related side effects on the undertreatment of moderate to severe chronic non-cancer pain: tapentadol, a step toward a solution?* Curr Med Res Opin., 2010. 26(7): p. 1677-84.
65. Caram-Salas, N.L., G. Reyes-García, R. Medina-Santillán, and V. Granados-Soto, *Thiamine and cyanocobalamin relieve neuropathic pain in rats: synergy with dexamethasone.* Pharmacology 2006. 77(2): p. 53-62.
66. Carstens, E., *Altered spinal processing in animal models of radicular and neuropathic pain,* in *Nervous system plasticity and chronic pain,* J. Sandkühler, B. Bromm, and G.F. Gebhart, Editors. 2000, Elsevier: Amsterdam.
67. Casey, K., J. Lorenz, and S. Minoshima, *Insights into the pathophysiology of neuropathic pain through functional brain imaging.* Exp Neurol., 2003. 184: p. S80-8.
68. Casoli, T., G. Di Stefano, M. Balietti, M. Solazzi, et al., *Peripheral inflammatory biomarkers of Alzheimer's disease: the role of platelets.* Biogerontology., 2010. 11(5): p. 627-33.
69. CDC, *CDC grand rounds: prescription drug overdoses - a U.S. epidemic.* MMWR Morb Mortal Wkly Rep., 2012. 61: p. 10.
70. Cervero, F., *Sensory innervation of the viscera: peripheral basis of visceral pain.* Physiol. Rev., 1994. 74: p. 95-138.
71. Chan, B.L., R. Witt, A.P. Charrow, A. Magee, et al., *Mirror therapy for phantom limb pain.* N Engl J Med., 2007. 357(21): p. 2206-7.

72. Chandler, M.J., S.F. Hobbs, D.C. Bolser, and R.D. Foreman, *Effects of vagal afferent stimulation on cervical spinothalamic tract neurons in monkeys.* Pain, 1991. 44: p. 81-87.
73. Chang, Y.W. and S.G. Waxman, *Minocycline attenuates mechanical allodynia and central sensitization following peripheral second-degree burn injury.* J Pain, 2010. 11(11): p. 1146-54.
74. Chen, A.L., T.J. Chen, R.L. Waite, J. Reinking, et al., *Hypothesizing that brain reward circuitry genes are genetic antecedents of pain sensitivity and critical diagnostic and pharmacogenomic treatment targets for chronic pain conditions.* Med Hypotheses., 2009 72(1): p. 14-22.
75. Chen, H., T.J. Lamer, R.H. Rho, K.A. Marshall, et al., *Contemporary management of neuropathic pain for the primary care physician.* Mayo Clin Proc., 2004. 79(12): p. 1533-45.
76. Chen, S., H. Hui, D. Zhang, and Y. Xue, *The combination of morphine and minocycline may be a good treatment for intractable post-herpetic neuralgia.* Med Hypotheses., 2010 75(6): p.:663-5.
77. Clauw, D.J. and L.J. Crofford, *Chronic widespread pain and fibromyalgia: what we know, and what we need to know.* Clin. Reumatology, 2003. 17: p. 685-701.
78. Cohen, A.D., R. Masalha, E. Medvedovsky, and D.A. Vardy, *Brachioradial pruritus : a symptom of neuropathy.* J. Am. Acad. Dermatol., 2003. 48(6): p. 825-8.
79. Cole, J., S. Crowle, G. Austwick, and D.H. Slater, *Exploratory findings with virtual reality for phantom limb pain; from stump motion to agency and analgesia.* Disabil Rehabil., 2009. 31(10): p. 846-54.
80. Cole, L.J., M.J. Farrell, E.P. Duff, J.B. Barber, et al., *Pain sensitivity and fMRI pain-related brain activity in Alzheimer's disease.* Brain Behav Immun., 2006. 129: p. 2957-65.
81. Cousins, M. and I. Power, *Acute and postoperative pain*, in *Textbook of Pain*, P.D. Wall and R. Melzack, Editors. 1999, Churchill Livingstone: Edinburgh. p. 447-491.
82. Cousins, M.J. and P.O. Bridenbbaugh, *Neural blockade in clinical anesthesia and management of pain.* 3rd ed. 1998, Philadelphia: Lippingcott-Raven.
83. Cousins, M.J. and G.D. Philips, *Acute Pain Management. Clinics in critical care medicine.* 1986, Edinburgh: Churchill Livingstone.
84. Crago, A., J.C. Houk, and W.Z. Rymer, *Sampling of total muscle force by tendon organs.* J. Neurophys., 1982. 47: p. 1069-1083.
85. Craig, A.D., *How do you feel? Interoception: the sense of the physiological condition of the body.* Nat Rev Neurosci., 2002. 3(8): p. 655-66.
86. Craig, A.D. and E.T. Zhang, *Anterior cingulate projection from MDvc (a lamina I spinothalamic target in the medial thalamus of the monkey).* Soc. Neurosci.Abstr., 1996. 22: p. 111.
87. Craig, A.D. and E.T. Zhang, *Retrograde analyses of spinothalamic projections in the macaque monkey: input to posterolateral thalamus.* J Comp Neurol, 2006. 499(6): p. 953-64.
88. Critchley, H.D., S. Wiens, P. Rotshtein, A. Ohman, et al., *Neural systems supporting interoceptive awareness.* Nat. Neurosci., 2004. 7(2): p. 189–95.
89. Crofford, L.J., *Pain management in fibromyalgia.* Curr Opin Rheumatol, 2008. 20(3): p. 246-50.
90. Crook, J., E. Rideout, and G. Browne, *The prevalence of Pain Complaints in a General Population.* Pain, 1984. 18: p. 299-314.
91. Crowley, W.R., J.F. Rodriguez-Sierra, and B.R. Komisaruk, *Analgesia induced by vagina stimulation in rats is apparently independent of a morphine-sensitive process.* Psychopharmacology, 1977. 54(3): p. 223-5.
92. Cuellar, J.M. and E. Carstens, *Electrophysiological evidence of enhanced nociceptive transmission in response to dorsal root exposure to nucleus pulposus*, in *Immune and glial regulation of pain*, J.A. DeLeo, L.S. Sorkin, and L.R. Watkins, Editors. 2007: Seattle. p. 143-154.
93. Cunha, T.M., W.A.J. Verri, J.S. Silva, S. Poole, et al., *A cascade of cytokines mediates mechanical inflammatory hypernociception in mice.* Proc Natl Acad Sci U S A., 2005. 102(5): p. 1755-60.
94. Davidson, S. and G.J. Giesler, *he multiple pathways for itch and their interactions with pain.* Trends Neurosci., 2010. 33(12): p. 550-8.
95. Davis, K.D., R.D. Treede, S.N. Raja, R.A. Meyer, et al., *Topical application of clonidine relieves hyperalgesia in patients with sympathetically maintained pain.* Pain., 1991. 47(3): p. 309-17.

96. De Ridder, D., *A heuristic Model of Tinnitus*, in *Textbook of Tinnitus*, A.R. Møller, et al., Editors. 2010, Springer: New York. p. 171-198.
97. De Ridder, D., G. De Mulder, T. Menovsky, S. Sunaert, et al., *Electrical stimulation of auditory and somatosensory cortices for treatment of tinnitus and pain.* Tinnitus: Pathophysiology and Treatment, Progress in Brain Research, 2007. 166: p. 377-388.
98. De Ridder, D., G. De Mulder, E. Verstraeten, S. Sunaert, et al., *Somatosensory cortex stimulation for deafferentation pain.* Acta Neurochir, 2007. 97(Suppl. Pt. 2): p. 67-74.
99. De Ridder, D., A.B. Elgoyhen, R. Romo, and B. Langguth, *Phantom percepts: tinnitus and pain as persisting aversive memory networks.* Proc Natl Acad Sci U S A, 2011. 108(20): p. 8075-80.
100. DeJongste, M.J.L., R.A. Tio, and R.D. Foreman, *Chronic therapeutically refractory angina pectoris.* Heart, 2004. 90(2).
101. del Rey, A., H. Yau, A. Randolf, M. Centeno, et al., *Chronic neuropathic pain-like behavior correlates with IL-1β expression and disrupts cytokine interactions in the hippocampus.* Pain, 2011. 152(12): p. 2827-35.
102. Devor, M., *The pathophysiology of damaged peripheral nerves*, in *Textbook of pain*, P.D. Wall and R. Melzack, Editors. 1994, Churchill Livingstone: Edinburgh. p. 79-100.
103. Devor, M. and Z. Seltzer, *Pathophysiology of damaged nerves in relation to chronic pain*, in *Textbook of Pain*, P.D. Wall and R. Melzack, Editors. 1999, Churchill Livingstone: Edinburgh. p. 129-164.
104. Deyo, R.A., N.E. Walsh, D.C. Martin, L.S. Schoenfeld, et al., *A controlled trial of transcutaneous electrical nerve stimulation (TENS) and exercise for chronic low back pain.* N Engl J Med., 1990. 322(23): p. 1627-34.
105. Dickenson, A.H., *NMDA receptors antagonists as an analgesic.* Prog. in Pain Res. and Management, 1994. 1: p. 173-187.
106. Dickinson, B.D., C.A. Head, S. Gitlow, and A.J.r. Osbahr, *Maldynia: pathophysiology and management of neuropathic and maladaptive pain--a report of the AMA Council on Science and Public Health.* Pain Med., 2010. 11(11): p. 1635-53.
107. Dobashi, T., S. Tanabe, H. Jin, T. Nishino, et al., *Valproate attenuates the development of morphine antinociceptive tolerance.* Neurosci Lett., 2010. 485(2): p. 125-8.
108. Dostrovsky, J.O. and A.D. Craig, *Ascending projection systems*, in *Wall and Melzak's Textbook of Pain*, S.B. McMahon and M. Koltzenburg, Editors. 2006, Elsevier: Amsterdam. p. 187-203.
109. Doubell, T.P., R.J. Mannion, and C.J. Woolf, *The dorsal horn: state-dependent sensory processing, plasticity and the generation of pain*, in *Handbook of Pain*, P.D. Wall and R. Melzack, Editors. 1999, Churchill Livingstone: Edinburgh. p. 165-181.
110. Drzezga, A., U. Darsow, R.D. Treede, H. Siebner, et al., *Central activation by histamine-induced itch: Analogies to pain processing: a correlational analysis of O-15 H2O positron emission tomography studies.* Pain, 2001. 92(1-2): p. 295-305.
111. Dum, R.P., D.J. Levinthal, and P.L. Strick, *The spinothalamic system targets motor and sensory areas in the cerebral cortex of monkeys.* J Neurosci., 2009. 29(45): p. 14223-35.
112. DuPen, A., D. Shen, and M. Ersek, *Mechanisms of Opioid-Induced Tolerance and Hyperalgesia.* Pain Manag Nurs., 2007. 8(3).
113. Elbert, T., C. Pantev, C. Wienbruch, B. Rockstroh, et al., *Increased cortical representation of the fingers of the left hand in string players.* Science, 1995. 270(5234): p. 305-7.
114. Engineer, N.D., J.R. Riley, J.D. Seale, W.A. Vrana, et al., *Reversing pathological neural activity using targeted plasticity.* Nature, 2011. 470(7332): p. 101-4.
115. Esteban, A. and P. Molina-Negro, *Primary hemifacial spasm: a neurophysiological study.* J. Neurol. Neurosurg. Psych., 1986. 49: p. 58-63.
116. Farina, S., M. Tinazzi, D. Pera le, and M. Valeriani, *Pain-related modulation of the human motor cortex.* Neurol. Res., 2003. 25: p. 130-142.
117. Farmer, M.A., M.N. Baliki, and A.V. Apkarian, *A dynamic Network perspective of chronic pain.* Neurosci Lett, 2012. 520(2): p. 197-203.

118. Fields, H.L., *Pain modulation: expectation, opioid analgesia and virtual pain.* Prog Brain Res., 2000. 122: p. 245–253.
119. Fields, H.L. and A.I. Basbaum, *Central nervous system mechanism of pain modulation*, in *Textbook of Pain*, P.D. Wall and R. Melzack, Editors. 1999, Churchill Livingstone: Edinburgh. p. 309-329.
120. Fields, H.L., A.I. Basbaum, and M.M. Heinricher, *Central nervous system mechanisms of pain modulation*, in *Wall and Melzak's Textbook of Pain*, S.B. McMahon and M. Koltzenburg, Editors. 2006, Elsevier: Amsterdam. p. 125-142.
121. Fields, R.D., *New culprits in chronic pain.* Scientific American, 2009. Nov: p. 50-57.
122. Flor, H., T. Elbert, S. Knecht, C. Wienbruch, et al., *Phantom-limb pain as a perceptual correlate of cortical reorganization following arm amputation.* Nature, 1995. 375(6531): p. 482-4.
123. Flor, H., L. Nikolajsen, and T. Staehelin Jensen, *Phantom limb pain: a case of maladaptive CNS plasticity?* Nat Rev Neurosci., 2006. 7(11): p. 873-81.
124. Ford, B., *Pain in Parkinson's disease.* Mov Disord., 2010. 25(Suppl 1): p. S98-103.
125. Forsythe, L.P., B. Thorn, M. Day, and G. Shelby, *Race and Sex Differences in Primary Appraisals, Catastrophizing, and Experimental Pain Outcomes.* J Pain. , 2011.
126. Freynhagen, R. and R. Baron, *The evaluation of neuropathic components in low back pain.* Curr Pain Headache Rep. , 2009. 13(3): p. 185-90.
127. Fromm, G., *Medical treatment of patients with trigeminal neuralgia*, in *Fromm G.H and Sessle B.J. Trigeminal Neuralgia*. 1991, Butterworth-Heinemann: Boston. p. 133-144.
128. Fromm, G.H., *Pathophysiology of trigeminal neuralgia*, in *Trigeminal Neuralgia*, G.H. Fromm and B.J. Sessle, Editors. 1991, Butterworth-Heinemann: Boston. p. 105-130.
129. Fromm, G.H. and B.J. Sessle, *Trigeminal Neuralgia.* 1991, Boston: Butterworth-Heinemann.
130. Gao , Y.J. and R.R. Ji, *Chemokines, neuronal-glial interactions, and central processing of neuropathic pain.* Pharmacol Ther., 2010. 126(1): p. 56-68.
131. García-Larrea, L., R. Peyron, P. Mertens, B. Laurent, et al., *Functional imaging and neurophysiological assessment of spinal and brain therapeutic modulation in humans.* Arch Med Res., 2000. 31(3): p. 248-57.
132. Gardner, W., *Crosstalk -- The paradoxical transmission of a nerve impulse.* Arch. Neurol., 1966. 14: p. 149-156.
133. Gardner, W. and M. Miklos, *Response of trigeminal neuralgia to "decompression" of sensory root.* JAMA, 1959(170): p. 1773-1776.
134. Gardner, W.J., *Concerning the mechanism of trigeminal neuralgia and hemifacial spasm.* J. Neurosurg., 1962(19): p. 947-958.
135. Gardner, W.J. and G.A. Sava, *Hemifacial spasm -- a reversible pathophysiologic state.* J. Neurosurg., 1962(19): p. 240-247.
136. Gauriau, C. and J.F. Bernard, *Pain pathways and parabrachial circuits in the rat.* Exp. Physiol, 2002. 87: p. 752-61.
137. Gebhart, G.F. and A. Randich, *Vagal modulation of nociception.* Am. Pain Soc. J., 1992. 1: p. 26-32.
138. Geha, P., M. Baliki, R. Harden, W. Bauer, et al., *The brain in chronic CRPS pain: abnormal gray-white matter interactions in emotional and autonomic regions.* Neuron., 2008. 60(4): p. 570-81.
139. Giesler, G.J., R.P. Yezierski, K.D. Gerhart, and W.D. Willis, *Spinothalamic tract neurons that project to medial and/or lateral thalamic nuclei: evidence for a physiologically novel population of spinal cord neurons.* J Neurophysiol. , 1981. 46(6): p. 1285-308.
140. Giuffrida, O., L. Simpson, and P.W. Halligan, *Contralateral stimulation, using TENS, of phantom limb pain: two confirmatory cases.* Pain Med. , 2010. 11(1): p. 133-41.
141. Goddard, G.V., *Amygdaloid stimulation and learning in the rat.* J. Comp. Physiol. Psychol., 1964. 58: p. 23-30.
142. Goehler, L.E., R.P. Gaykema, M.K. Hansen, K. Anderson, et al., *Vagal immune-to-brain communication: a visceral chemosensory pathway.* Auton Neurosci, 2000. 85(1-3): p. 49-59.

143. Goldenberg, D.L., *Pain/Depression dyad: a key to a better understanding and treatment of functional somatic syndromes.* Am J Med., 2010. 123(8): p. 675-82.
144. Gómez-Pinilla, F., Z. Ying, R.R. Roy, R. Molteni, et al., *Voluntary exercise induces a BDNF-mediated mechanism that promotes neuroplasticity.* J Neurophysiol., 2002. 88(5): p. 2187-95.
145. Gouda, J.J. and J.A. Brown, *Atypical facial pain and other pain syndromes.* Neurosurgery Clinics of North America, 1997. 8(1): p. 87-100.
146. Goupille, P., M. Jayson, J. Valat, and A. Freemont, *The role of inflammation in disk herniation-associated radiculopathy.* Semin Arthritis Rheum., 1998. 28(1): p. 60-71.
147. Graeber, M.B. and W.J. Streit, *Microglia: biology and pathology.* Acta Neuropathol., 2010. 119: p. 89-105.
148. Graven-Nielsen, T. and S. Mense, *The peripheral apparatus of muscle pain: evidence from animal and human studies.* Clin. J. Pain., 2001. 17(1): p. 2-10.
149. Grevert, P., L.H. Albert, and A. Goldstein, *Partial antagonism of placebo analgesia by naloxone.* Pain, 1983. 16: p. 129-143.
150. Gröber, U., *Vitamin D--an old vitamin in a new perspective.* Med Monatsschr Pharm, 2010. 33(10): p. 376-83.
151. Gybels, J.M. and R.R. Tasker, *Central neurosurgery,* in *Textbook of Pain,* P.D. Wall and R. Melzack, Editors. 1999, Churchill Levingstone: Edinburgh. p. 1307-1339.
152. Hadjipavlou, G., P. Dunckley, T.E. Behrens, and I. Tracey, *Determining anatomical connectivities between cortical and brainstem pain processing regions in humans: a diffusion tensor imaging study in healthy controls.* Pain 2006. 123: p. 169–178.
153. Hakanson, S., *Trigeminal neuralgia treated by injection of glycerol into the trigeminal cistern.* Neurosurgery, 1981(9): p. 638-646.
154. Hameed, H., M. Hameed, and P.J. Christo, *The effect of morphine on glial cells as a potential therapeutic target for pharmacological development of analgesic drugs.* Curr Pain Headache Rep., 2010. 14(2): p. 96-104.
155. Hanagasi, H.A., S. Akat, H. Gurvit, J. Yazici, et al., *Pain is common in Parkinson's disease.* Clin Neurol Neurosurg, 2010.
156. Handwerker, H.O., W. Magerl, F. Klemm, and R.A. Westerman, *Quantitative evaluation of itch sensation,* in *Fine Afferent Nerve Fibers and Pain,* R.F. Schmidt, H.-G. Schaible, and C. Vahle-Hinz, Editors. 1987, VCH Verlagsgesellschaft: Germany. p. 462-473.
157. Hansson, P. and T. Lundeberg, *Transcutaneous electrical nerve stimulation, vibration and acupuncture as pain-relieving measures,* in *Textbook of Pain,* P.D. Wall and R. Melzack, Editors. 1999, Churchill Livingstone: Edinburgh. p. 1341-1351.
158. Hashmi, J., M. Baliki, L. Huang, A. Baria, et al., *Shape shifting pain: chronification of back pain shifts brain representation from nociceptive to emotional circuits.* Brain, 2013. 136(9): p. 2751-68.
159. Hassanzadeh, K., B. Habibi-asl, S. Farajnia, and L. Roshangar, *Minocycline prevents morphine-induced apoptosis in rat cerebral cortex and lumbar spinal cord: a possible mechanism for attenuating morphine tolerance.* Neurotox Res., 2011. 19(4): p. 649-59.
160. Hassenbusch, S.J., P.K. Pillay, and G.H. Barnett, *Radiofrequency cingulotomy for intractable cancer pain using stereotaxis guided by magnetic resonance imaging.* Neurosurg., 1990. 27(2): p. 220-3.
161. Hathway, G.J., D. Vega-Avelaira, A. Moss, R. Ingram, et al., *Brief, low frequency stimulation of rat peripheral C-fibres evokes prolonged microglial-induced central sensitization in adults but not in neonates.* Pain., 2009. 144: p. 110-8.
162. Hawkey, C.J., *COX-2 inhibitors.* Lancet, 1999. 353: p. 307-314.
163. Heinricher, M.M., I. Tavares, J.L. Leith, and B.M. Lumb, *Descending control of nociception: Specificity, recruitment and plasticity.* Brain Res. Rev., 2009. 60: p. 214–225.
164. Helme, R.D. and S.J. Gibson, *The epidemiology of pain in elderly people.* Clin Geriatr Med., 2001. 17(3): p. 417-31.

165. Hikosaka, O., E. Bromberg-Martin, S. Hong, and M. Matsumoto, *New insights on the subcortical representation of reward.* Curr Opin Neurobiol., 2008. 18(2): p. 203-8.
166. Hippisley-Cox, J. and C. Coupland, *Risk of myocardial infarction in patients taking cyclo-oxygenase-2 inhibitors or conventional non-steroidal anti-inflammatory drugs: population based nested case-control analysis.* BMJ, 2005. 330(7504): p. 1366.
167. Hirsh, A.T., S.Z. George, J.E. Bialosky, and M.E. Robinson, *Fear of Pain, Pain Catastrophizing, and Acute Pain Perception: Relative Prediction and Timing of Assessment.* J. Pain, 2008. 9(9): p. 806-812.
168. Hitzelberger, W.E. and R.M. Witten, *Abnormal myelograms in asymptomatic patients.* J. Neurosurg., 1968. 28: p. 204-6.
169. Holick, M.F., *Sunlight and vitamin D for bone health and prevention of autoimmune diseases, cancers, and cardiovascular disease.* Am J Clin Nutr., 2004. 80(6): p. 1678S-88S.
170. Hong, C.Z., *Pathophysiology of myofascial trigger point.* Journal of the Formosan Medical Association, 1996. 95(2): p. 93-104.
171. Hong, C.Z. and D.G. Simons, *Pathophysiologic and electrophysiologic mechanisms of myofascial trigger points.* Arch Phys. Med. Rehab., 1998. 79(7): p. 863-72.
172. Horng, S.H. and M. Sur, *Visual activity and cortical rewiring: Activity-dependent plasticity of cortical networks*, in *Reprogramming the brain, Progress in Brain Research*, A.R. Møller, Editor. 2006, Elsevier: Amsterdam. p. 3-11.
173. Hróbjartsson, A. and P.C. Gøtzsche, *Is the placebo powerless? An analysis of clinical trials comparing placebo with no treatment.* New England Journal of Medicine, 2001. 344(21): p. 1594–1602.
174. Hubbard, D.R. and G.M. Berkoff, *Myofascial trigger points show spontaneous needle EMG activity.* Spine, 1993. 18(13): p. 1803-7.
175. Hutchinson, M.R., A.L. Northcutt, L.W. Chao, J.J. Kearney, et al., *Minocycline suppresses morphine-induced respiratory depression, suppresses morphine-induced reward, and enhances systemic morphine-induced analgesia.* Brain Behav Immun., 2008. 22(8): p. 1248-56.
176. Inoue, K. and M. Tsuda, *Microglia and neuropathic pain.* Glia, 2009. 57(14): p. 1469-79.
177. Inui, K., D.T. Tran, M. Qiu, X. Wang, et al., *Pain-related magnetic fields evoked by intra-epidermal electrical stimulation in humans.* Clin. Neurophysiol., 2002. 113: p. 298-304.
178. Jänig, W., *Neurobiology of visceral afferent neurons: neuroanatomy, functions, organ regulations and sensations.* Biol Psychol., 1996. 42(1-2): p. 29-51.
179. Jänig, W., *The puzzle of "reflex sympathetic dystrophy": mechanisms, hypotheses, open questions*, in *Reflex sympathetic dystrophy: a reappraisal*, W. Jänig and M. Stanton-Hicks, Editors. 1996, IASP Press: Seattle. p. 1-24.
180. Jänig, W. and H.J. Häbler, *Sympathetic nervous system: contribution to chronic pain.* Prog. Brain Res., 2000. 129: p. 451-68.
181. Jänig, W., S.G. Khasar, J.D. Levine, and F.J. Miao, *The role of vagal visceral afferents in the control of nociception.* Prog Brain Res., 2000. 122: p. 273-87.
182. Jänig, W., S.G. Khasar, J.D. Levine, and F.J.-P. Miao, *The role of vagal visceral afferents in the control of nociception. The biological basis for mind body interaction.* Prog. Brain Res., 2000. 122: p. 271-285.
183. Jänig, W. and J.D. Levine, *Autonomic-endocrine-immune interactions in acute and chronic pain*, S.B. McMahon and M. Koltzenburg, Editors. 2006, Elsevier: Amsterdam. p. 205-218.
184. Jänig, W. and M. Stanton-Hicks, *Reflex sympathetic dystrophy -- a reapraisal.* 1996, Seattle: ISAP.
185. Jannetta, P.J., *Arterial compression of the trigeminal nerve at the pons in patients with trigeminal neuralgia.* J. Neurosurg., 1967. 26: p. 169-162.
186. Jannetta, P.J., *Hemifacial spasm caused by a venule: Case report.* Neurosurgery, 1984. 14: p. 89-92.
187. Jansen, P.H., R.G. Lecluse, and A.L. Verbeek, *Past and current understanding of the pathophysiology of muscle cramps: why treatment of varicose veins does not relieve leg cramps.* J Eur Acad Dermatol Venereol., 1999. 12(3): p. 222-9.

188. Jastreboff, P.J., *Phantom auditory perception (tinnitus): Mechanisms of generation and perception.* Neurosci. Res., 1990. 8: p. 221-254.
189. Jastreboff, P.J., *Tinnitus Retraining Therapy*, in *Textbook of Tinnitus*, A.R. Møller, et al., Editors. 2010, Springer: New York. p. 575-596.
190. Jastreboff, P.J. and M.M. Jastreboff, *Tinnitus Retraining Therapy (TRT) as a method for treatment of tinnitus and hyperacusis patients.* J. Am. Acad. Audiol., 2000. 11(3): p. 162-77.
191. Jenkins, B. and S.J. Tepper, *Neurostimulation for Primary Headache Disorders, Part 1: Pathophysiology and Anatomy, History of Neuromodulation in Headache Treatment, and Review of Peripheral Neuromodulation in Primary Headaches.* Headache, 2011.
192. Jenkins, B. and S.J. Tepper, *Neurostimulation for Primary Headache Disorders: Part 2, Review of Central Neurostimulators for Primary Headache, Overall Therapeutic Efficacy, Safety, Cost, Patient Selection, and Future Research in Headache Neuromodulation.* Headache, 2011.
193. Jensen, M. and D.R. Patterson, *Hypnotic treatment of chronic pain.* J Behav Med, 2006. 29(1): p. 95–124.
194. Jinks, S.L. and E. Carstens, *Responses of superficial dorsal horn neurons to intradermal serotonin and other irritants: comparison with scratching behavior.* J. Neurophys., 2002. 87(3): p. 1280-9.
195. Johnson, R.W., G. Wasner, P. Saddier, and R. Baron, *Postherpetic neuralgia: epidemiology, pathophysiology and management.* Expert Rev Neurother., 2007. 7(11): p. 1581-95.
196. Jones, R.C., L. Xu, and G.F. Gebhart, *The mechanosensitivity of mouse colon afferent fibers and their sensitization by inflammatory mediators require transient receptor potential vanilloid 1 and acid-sensing ion channel 3.* J. Neurosci, 2005. 25: p. 10981–10989.
197. Kakigi, R., T. Diep, Y. Qiu, X. Wang, et al., *Cerebral responses following stimulation of unmyelinated C-fibers in humans: eletro- and magneto-encephalographic study.* Neurosci. Res., 2003.
198. Kannel, W.B. and R.D. Abbott, *Incidence and prognosis of unrecognized myocardial infarction.* N. Eng. J. Med., 1984. 311: p. 1144-1147.
199. Karl, A., W. Mühlnickel, R. Kurth, and H. Flor, *Neuroelectric source imaging of steady-state movement-related cortical potentials in human upper extremity amputees with and without phantom limb pain.* Pain, 2004. 110(90–102).
200. Karppinen, J., *New perspectives on sciatica*, in *Immune and glial regulation of pain*, J.A. DeLeo, L.S. Sorkin, and L.R. Watkins, Editors. 2007, IASP Press: Seattle. p. 385-406.
201. Katayama, Y., T. Tsubokawa, and T. Yamamoto, *Chronic motor cortex stimulation for central deafferentation pain: experience with bulbar pain secondary to Wallenberg syndrome.* Stereotact. Funct. Neurosurg., 1995. 34: p. 42-48.
202. Katusic, S., C. Beard, E. Bergstralh, and L. Kurland, *Incidence and clinical features of trigeminal neuralgia, Rochester, Minnesota 1945-1984.* Ann Neurol, 1990(27): p. 89-95.
203. Keay, K.A., C.I. Clement, A. Depaulis, and R. Bandler, *Different representations of inescapable noxious stimuli in the periaqueductal gray and upper cervical spinal cord of freely moving rats.* Neurosci Lett, 2001. 313(1-2): p. 17-20.
204. Kidd, B.L. and L.A. Urban, *Mechanisms of inflammatory pain.* Br J Anaesth., 2001. 87(1): p. 3-11.
205. Kilgard, M.P. and M.M. Merzenich, *Cortical map reorganization enabled by nucleus basalis activity.* Science, 1998. 279: p. 1714-1718.
206. Kilgard, M.P. and M.M. Merzenich, *Plasticity of temporal information processing in the primary auditory cortex.* Nature Neurosci., 1998. 1: p. 727-731.
207. Kim, H.S. and Y.H. Suh, *Minocycline and neurodegenerative diseases.* Behav Brain Res., 2009. 196(2): p. 168-79.
208. Kim, S.K. and H. Bae, *Acupuncture and immune modulation.* Auton Neurosci., 2010. 157(1-2): p. 38-41.
209. Kirchner, A., F. Birklein, H. Stefan, and H.O. Handwerker, *Left vagus nerve stimulation suppresses experimentally induced pain.* Neurology, 2000. 55(8): p. 1167-71.
210. Kjellberg, F. and M.R. Tramer, *Pharmacological control of opioid-induced pruritus: a quantitative systematic review of randomized trials.* Europ. J. .Anaesthesiol., 2001. 18(6): p. 346-57.

211. Kleinjung, T., B. Langguth, and E. Khedr, *Transcranial magnetic stimulation*, in *Textbook of Tinnitus*, A.R. Møller, et al., Editors. 2010, Springer: New York. p. 697-710.
212. Klit, H., N.B. Finnerup, and T.S. Jensen, *Central post-stroke pain: clinical characteristics, pathophysiology, and management.* Lancet Neurol., 2009. 8(9): p. 857-68.
213. Klumpers, L., T. Beumer, J. van Hasselt, A. Lipplaa, et al., *Novel Δ(9) -tetrahydrocannabinol formulation Namisol® has beneficial pharmacokinetics and promising pharmacodynamic effects.* Br J Clin Pharmacol. , 2012. 74(1).
214. Knabl, J., R. Witschi, K. Hösl, H. Reinold, et al., *Reversal of pathological pain through specific spinal GABAA receptor subtypes.* Nature 451, 330-334 2008.
215. Knighton, R.S. and P.R. Dumke, *Pain*. 1966, Boston: Little Brown.
216. Koltzenburg, M. and S.B. McMahon, *The enigmatic role of the sympathetic nervous system in chronic pain.* Trends Pharmacol Sci., 1991. 12(11): p. 399-402.
217. Komisaruk, B.R., C.A. Gerdes, and B. Whipple, *'Complete' spinal cord injury does not block perceptual responses to genital self-stimulation in women.* Arch. Neurol., 1997. 54(12): p. 1513-20.
218. Kong, J., T.J. Kaptchuk, G. Polich, I. Kirsch, et al., *Placebo analgesia: findings from brain imaging studies and emerging hypotheses.* Rev Neurosci., 2007. 18(3-4): p. 173-90.
219. Konstantinou, K. and K.M. Dunn, *Sciatica: review of epidemiological studies and prevalence estimates.* Spine, 2008. 33(22): p. 2464-72.
220. Kugelberg, E., *Activation of human nerves by ischemia.* Arch. Neurol. Psychiat., 1948. 60: p. 140-152.
221. Kuijper, B., J.T. Tans, B.F. van der Kallen, F. Nollet, et al., *Root compression on MRI compared with clinical findings in patients with recent onset cervical radiculopathy.* J Neurol Neurosurg Psychiatry, 2010.
222. Kuraishi, Y., T. Yamaguchi, and T. Miyamoto, *Itch -scratch responses induced by opioids through central mu opioid receptors in mice.* 2000. 7(3): p. 248-52.
223. Kuroki, A. and A.R. Møller, *Facial nerve demyelination and vascular compression are both needed to induce facial hyperactivity: A study in rats.* Acta Neurochir. (Wien), 1994. 126: p. 149-157.
224. Langguth, B., M. Landgrebe, T. Kleinjung, G.P. Sand, et al., *Tinnitus and depression.* World J Biol Psychiatry, 2011.
225. Larson, A.M., J. Polson, R.J. Fontana, T.J. Davern, et al., *Acetaminophen-induced acute liver failure: results of a United States multicenter, prospective study.* Hepatology., 2005. 42(6): p. 1364-72.
226. Layzer, R.B., *Muscle Pain, Cramps, and Fatigue*, in *Myology, 2nd ed*, A.G. Engel and C. Franzini-Armstrong, Editors. 1994, McGraw-Hill: New York. p. 1754–1768.
227. LeDoux, J.E., *Brain mechanisms of emotion and emotional learning.* Curr. Opin. Neurobiol., 1992. 2: p. 191-197.
228. Lee, M., M. Ploner, K. Wiech, U. Bingel, et al., *Amygdala activity contributes to the dissociative effect of cannabis on pain perception.* J. Pain, 2013. 154(1): p. 124-134.
229. Lee, W.M., *Acetaminophen and the U.S. Acute Liver Failure Study Group: lowering the risks of hepatic failure.* Hepatology, 2004. 40(1): p. 6-9.
230. Lefaucheur, J.P., X. Drouot , I. Ménard-Lefaucheur, Y. Keravel, et al., *Motor cortex rTMS in chronic neuropathic pain: pain relief is associated with thermal sensory perception improvement.* J Neurol Neurosurg Psychiatry, 2008. 79(9): p. 1044-9.
231. Leone, M., A. Proietti Cecchini, E. Mea, V. Tullo, et al., *Neuroimaging and pain: a window on the autonomic nervous system.* Neurol Sci. , 2006. Suppl 2: p. 134-7.
232. Levine, J.D., N.C. Gordon, and H.I. Fields, *Naloxone dose dependently produces analgesia and hyperalgesia in postoperative pain.* Nature, 1979. 278: p. 740 - 741.
233. Levine, J.D., N.C. Gordon, and H.L. Fields, *The mechanism of placebo analgesia.* Lancet, 1978: p. 654-657.
234. Levine, J.D. and D.B. Reichling, *Fibromyalgia: the nerve of that disease.* J Rheumatol 2005. 75 Suppl: p. 29-37.

235. Li, H. and N. Mizuno, *Single neurons in the spinal trigeminal and dorsal column nuclei project to both the cochlear nucleus and the inferior colliculus by way of axon collaterals: a fluorescent retrograde double-labeling study in the rat.*. Neurosci Res, 1997. 29: p. 135-42.
236. Liang, C., H. Li, Y. Tao, C. Shen, et al., *New hypothesis of chronic back pain: low pH promotes nerve ingrowth into damaged intervertebral disks.* Acta Anaesthesiol Scand., 2013. 57(3): p. 271-7.
237. Llinas, R.R., U. Ribary, D. Jeanmonod, E. Kronberg, et al., *Thalamocortical dysrhythmia: A neurological and neuropsychiatric syndrome characterized by magnetoencephalography.* Proc Natl Acad Sci, 1999. 96(26): p. 15222-7.
238. Long, D., *Surgical treatment for back and neck pain*, in *Wall and Melzak's Textbook of Pain*, S.B. McMahon and M. Koltzenburg, Editors. 2006, Elsevier: Amsterdam. p. 683-97.
239. Long, D.M., *Chronic back pain*, in *Handbook of Pain*, P.D. Wall and R. Melzack, Editors. 1999, Churchill Livingstone: Edinburgh. p. 539-538.
240. Lumb, B.M., *Inescapable and escapable pain is represented in distinct hypothalamic-midbrain circuits: specific roles of Ad- and C-nociceptors.* Exp. Physiol., 2002. 87: p. 281-86.
241. Ma, C., K.W. Greenquist, and R.H. Lamotte, *Inflammatory mediators enhance the excitability of chronically compressed dorsal root ganglion neurons.* J Neurophysiol., 2006. 95(4): p. 2098-107.
242. Macfarlane, G.J., G.T. Jones, and J. McBeth, *Epidemiology of pain*, in *Wall and Melzack's Textbook of Pain*, S.B. McMahon and M. Koltzenburg, Editors. 2006, Elsevier: Amsterdam.
243. Malmberg, A.B., *Central changes*, in *Pain in Peripheral Nerve diseases. Pain Headache*, C. Sommer, Editor. 2001, Karger: Basel. p. 149-167.
244. Manchikanti, L., V. Singh, S. Datta, S.P. Cohen, et al., *Comprehensive review of epidemiology, scope, and impact of spinal pain.* Pain Physician., 2009. 12(4): p. E35-70.
245. ManiIa, M.N., *Leg cramps in relation to metabolic syndrome.* Georgian Med News., 2009. 166: p. 51-4.
246. Mansour, A., M. Baliki, L. Huang, S. Torbey, et al., *Brain white matter structural properties predict transition to chronic pain.* Pain, 2013. 154(10): p. 2160-8.
247. Mansour, A., M. Baliki, L. Huang, S. Torbey, et al., *Brain white matter structural properties predict transition to chronic pain.* Pain, 2013. 154(10): p. 2160-8.
248. Mansour, A., M. Farmer, M. Baliki, and A. Apkarian, *Chronic pain: The role of learning and brain plasticity.* Restor Neurol Neurosci, 2013.
249. Marchand, F., M. Perretti, and S.B. McMahon, *Role of the immune system in chronic pain.* Nat. Rev. Neurosci., 2005. 6(7): p. 521–32.
250. Maroon, J., C. and J.W. Bost, *Omega-3 fatty acids (fish oil) as an anti-inflammatory: an alternative to nonsteroidal anti-inflammatory drugs for discogenic pain.* Surg Neurol., 2006. 65(4): p. 326-31.
251. Marshall, B.J., *Helicobacter pylori: a primer for 1994.* Gastroenterologist., 1993. 1(4): p. 241-7.
252. Martinez-Lavin, M., *Fibromyalgia as a sympathetically maintained pain syndrome.* Curr Pain Headache Rep., 2004. 8(5): p. 385-9.
253. Massey, E.W. and J.M. Massey, *Forearm neuropathy and pruritus.* Southern Medical J., 1986. 79(10): p. 1259-1260.
254. Mathews, E.S. and S.J. Scrivani, *Percutaneous stereotactic radiofrequency thermal rhizotomy for the treatment of trigeminal neuralgia.* Mount Sinai J. Med., 2000. 67(4): p. 288-99.
255. Mäurer, M. and K. Reiners, *Mononeuropathies*, in *Pain in Peripheral Nerve diseases. Pain Headache*, C. Sommer, Editor. 2001, Karger: Basel. p. 37-52.
256. Mauro, G.L., Martorana. U, P. Cataldo, G. Brancato, et al., *Vitamin B12 in low back pain: a randomised, double-blind, placebo-controlled study.* Eur Rev Med Pharmacol Sci., 2000. 4(3): p. 53-8.
257. Maves, T.J., P.S. Pechman, G.F. Gebhart, and S.T. Meller, *Possible chemical contribution from chromic gut sutures produces disorders of pain sensation like those seen in man.* Pain, 1993. 54: p. 57-69.
258. McCabe, C.S., R.C. Haigh, N.G. Shenker, J. Lewis, et al., *Phantoms in rheumatology.* Novartis Found Symp., 2004. 260: p. 154-74.

259. McMahon, S.B., W.B. Cafferty, and F. Marchand, *Immune and glial cell factors as pain mediators and modulators.* Exp Neurol. , 2005. 192(2): p. 444-62.
260. McNicol, E., Midbari A, and E. E., *Opioids for neuropathic pain.* Cochrane Database Syst Rev. , 2013. 8(Aug 29).
261. McQuay, H., *Do preemptive treatments provide better pain control?*, in *Progr. Pain Res. Management*, G.F. Gebhart, D.L. Hammond, and T. Jensen, Editors. 1994, IASP Press: Seattle, WA. p. 709-723.
262. McQuay, H.J. and A. Moore, *NSAIDS and Coxibs: clinical use*, in *Wall and Melzack's Textbook of Pain*, S.B. Mahon and M. Kolzenburg, Editors. 2006, Elsevier: Amsterdam. p. 471-480.
263. Melzack, R. and K.I. Casey, *Sensory, motivational, and central control determinants of pain*, in *The skin senses*, D.R. Kenshalo, Editor. 1968, Thomas: Springfield. p. 423-443.
264. Melzack, R. and P.D. Wall, *Pain mechanisms: A new theory.* Science, 1965. 150: p. 971-979.
265. Melzack, R. and P.D. Wall, *The challenge of pain.* 2nd ed. 1996: Penguin.
266. Mendell, L.M., *Modifiability of spinal synapses.* Physiol Rev, 1984. 64: p. 260-324.
267. Mense, S., *Referral of muscle pain: new aspects.* Am. Pain Soc. J., 1994. 3: p. 1-9.
268. Mense, S. and M. H., *Bradykinin-induced modulation of the response behaviour of different types of feline group III and IV muscle receptors.* J. Physiol., 1988. 398: p. 49-63.
269. Mense, S.S., *Functional neuroanatomy for pain stimuli. Reception, transmission, and processing (In German).* Schmerz, 2004. 18(3): p. 225-37.
270. Mergenthaler, P., U. Dirnagl, and A. Meisel, *Pathophysiology of stroke: lessons from animal models.* Metab Brain Dis., 2004. 19(3-4): p. 151-67.
271. Merighi, A., C. Salio, A. Ghirri, L. Lossi, et al., *BDNF as a pain modulator.* Prog Neurobiol., 2008. 85(3): p. 297-317.
272. Merskey, H. and N. Bogduk, *Classification of chronic pain.* 1994, IASP Press: Seattle. p. 1-222.
273. Metz, A., H. Yau, M. Centeno, A. Apkarian, et al., *Morphological and functional reorganization of rat medial prefrontal cortex in neuropathic pain.* Proc Natl Acad Sci U S A, 2009. 106(7): p. 2423-8.
274. Meyer, R.A., M. Ringkamp, J.N. Campbell, and S.N. Raja, *Peripheral mechanisms of cutaneous nociception*, in *Wall and Melzak's Textbook of Pain*, S.B. McMahon and M. Koltzenburg, (Eds.), Editors. 2006, Elsevier: Amsterdam. p. 3-34.
275. Meyerson, B.A., U. Lindblom, B. Linderoth, and G. Lind, *Motor cortex stimulation as treatment of trigeminal neuropathic pain.* Acta Neurochir. - Supplementum, 1993. 58: p. 105-3.
276. Meyerson, B.A. and B. Linderoth, *Mechanism of spinal cord stimulation in neuropathic pain.* Neurol. Res., 2000. 22: p. 285-292.
277. Middleton, C., *The causes and treatments of phantom limb pain.* Nurs Times. , 2003 99(35): p. 30-3.
278. Mika, J., *Modulation of microglia can attenuate neuropathic pain symptoms and enhance morphine effectiveness.* Pharmacol Rep. , 2008. 60(3): p. 297-307.
279. Mika, J., A. Wawrzczak-Bargiela, ., M. Osikowicz, W. Makuch, et al., *Attenuation of morphine tolerance by minocycline and pentoxifylline in naive and neuropathic mice.* Brain Behav Immun., 2009. 23(1): p. 75-84.
280. Millan, M.J., *Descending control of pain.* Prog. Neurobiol, 2002. 66: p. 355–474.
281. Miwa, J.M., R. Freedman, and H.A. Lester, *Neural systems governed by nicotinic acetylcholine receptors: emerging hypotheses.* Neuron., 2011. 70: p. 20-33.
282. Mochizuki, H., N. Sadato, D.N. Saito, H. Toyoda, et al., *Neural correlates of perceptual difference between itching and pain: a human fMRI study.* Neuroimage, 2007 36(3): p. 706-17.
283. Møller, A.R., *Hemifacial spasm: Ephaptic transmission or hyperexcitability of the facial motor nucleus?* Exp. Neurol., 1987. 98: p. 110-119.
284. Møller, A.R., *Cranial nerve dysfunction syndromes: Pathophysiology of microvascular compression.*, in *Neurosurgical Topics Book 13, 'Surgery of Cranial Nerves of the Posterior Fossa,' Chapter 2*, D.L. Barrow, Editor. 1993, American Association of Neurological Surgeons: Park Ridge. IL. p. 105-129.
285. Møller, A.R., *Similarities Between Chronic Pain and Tinnitus.* Am. J. Otol., 1997. 18: p. 577-585.

286. Møller, A.R., *Vascular compression of cranial nerves. I: History of the microvascular decompression operation*. Neurol. Res., 1998. 20: p. 727-731.
287. Møller, A.R., *Sensory Systems: Anatomy and Physiology*. 2003, Amsterdam: Academic Press.
288. Møller, A.R., *Neural plasticity and disorders of the nervous system*. 2006, Cambridge: Cambridge University Press
289. Møller, A.R., *Neurophysiologic abnormalities in autism*, in *New Autism Research Developments*, B.S. Mesmere, Editor. 2007, Nova Science Publishers: New York.
290. Møller, A.R., *A new epidemic: Harm in Medicine*. 2007: Nova Science Publishers.
291. Møller, A.R., *Tinnitus and Pain*, in *Tinnitus: Pathophysiology and Treatment, Progress in Brain Research*, B. Langguth, et al., Editors. 2007, Elsevier: Amsterdam. p. 47-53.
292. Møller, A.R., *Neural Plasticity: For Good and Bad*. Progress of Theoretical Physics, 2008. Supplement No 173: p. 48-65.
293. Møller, A.R., *Plasticity diseases*. Neurol. Res., 2009. 31(10): p. 1023-30.
294. Møller, A.R., *Intraoperative Neurophysiological Monitoring. Intraoperative Neurophysiology*, 3rd ed. 2010, New York: Springer.
295. Møller, A.R., *Misophonia, phonophobia and "exploding head" syndrome*, in *Textbook of Tinnitus*, A.R. Møller, et al., Editors. 2010, Springer: New York. p. 25-27.
296. Møller, A.R., *Similarities between tinnitus and pain* in *Textbook of Tinnitus*, A.R. Møller, et al., Editors. 2010, Springer: New York. p. 113-120.
297. Møller, A.R. and P.J. Jannetta, *On the origin of synkinesis in hemifacial spasm: Results of intracranial recordings*. J. Neurosurg., 1984. 61: p. 569-576.
298. Møller, A.R. and P.J. Jannetta, *Blink reflex in patients with hemifacial spasm: Observations during microvascular decompression operations*. J. Neurol. Sci., 1986. 72: p. 171-182.
299. Møller, A.R., M.B. Møller, and M. Yokota, *Some forms of tinnitus may involve the extralemniscal auditory pathway*. Laryngoscope, 1992. 102: p. 1165-1171.
300. Møller, A.R. and T. Pinkerton, *Temporal integration of pain from electrical stimulation of the skin*. Neurol. Res, 1997. 19: p. 481-488.
301. Møller, A.R. and S. Shore, *Interaction between somatosensory and auditory systems*, in *Textbook of Tinnitus*, A.R. Møller, et al., Editors. 2010, Springer: New York. p. 69-76.
302. Multon, S. and J. Schoenen, *Pain control by vagus nerve stimulation: from animal to man...and back*. Acta Neurol Belg. , 2005. 105(2): p. 62-7.
303. Mulvey, M.R., A.M. Bagnall, M.I. Johnson, and P.R. Marchant, *Transcutaneous electrical nerve stimulation (TENS) for phantom pain and stump pain following amputation in adults*. Cochrane Database Syst Rev. , 2010. 12(5).
304. Murray, C.D., S. Pettifer, T. Howard, E.L. Patchick, et al., *The treatment of phantom limb pain using immersive virtual reality: three case studies*. Disabil Rehabil., 2007. 29(18): p. 1465-9.
305. Mutso, A., D. Radzicki, M. Baliki, L. Huang, et al., *Abnormalities in hippocampal functioning with persistent pain*. J Neurosci., 2012. 32(17): p. 2827-35.
306. Nagai, M., K. Kishi, and S. Kato, *Insular cortex and neuropsychiatric disorders: a review of recent literature*. Eur Psychiatry., 2007. 22(6): p. 387-94.
307. Nakai, O., S. Itagaki, and S. Saito, *Electromyographic analysis of spasmodic torticollis*. Tenth Meeting of the World Society for Stereotactic and Functional Neurosurgery. Abstract, 1989.
308. Napadow, V., J. Liu, M. Li, N. Kettner, et al., *Somatosensory cortical plasticity in carpal tunnel syndrome treated by acupuncture*. Hum Brain Mapp, 2007. 28: p. 159-71.
309. Narins, C.R., W. Zareba, A.J. Moss, R.E. Goldstein, et al., *Clinical implications of silent versus symptomatic exercise-induced myocardial ischemia in patients with stable coronary disease*. J. Am. Col. Cardiol., 1997. 29(4): p. 756-63.
310. Narumiya, S., *Prostanoids and inflammation: a new concept arising from receptor knockout mice*. J Mol Med (Berl). 2009. 87(10): p. 1015-22.

311. Neri Serneri, G.G., M. Boddi, L. Arata, C. Rostagno, et al., *Silent ischemia in unstable angina is related to an altered cardiac norepinephrine handling.* Circulation, 1993. 87(6): p. 1928-37.
312. Neugebauer, V., W. Li, G.C. Bird, and J.S. Han, *The amygdala and persistent pain.* Neuroscientist, 2004. 10(3): p. 221-34.
313. Newham, D.J. and K.R. Mills, *Muscles, tendons and ligaments*, in *Handbook of Pain*, P.D. Wall and R. Melzack, Editors. 1999, Churchill Livingstone: Edinburgh. p. 517-538.
314. Nguyen, J.P., Y. Keravel, A. Feve, T. Uchiyama, et al., *Treatment of deafferentation pain by chronic stimulation of the motor cortex. Report of a series of 20 cases.* Acta Neurochir. Suppl (Wien), 1997. 8(54-60).
315. Nielsen, V., *Pathophysiological aspects of hemifacial spasm. Part I. Evidence of ectopic excitation and ephaptic transmission.* Neurology, 1984. 34: p. 418-426.
316. Nieuwenhuys, R., J. Voogd, and C. van Huijzen, *The Human central nervous system.* 2008, New York: Springer.
317. Nikolajsen, L. and T.S. Jensen, *Phantom Limb*, in *Wall and Melzak's Textbook of Pain.*, S.B. McMahon and M. Koltzenburg, Editors. 2006, Elsevier: Amsterdam. p. 961-71.
318. Niv, D. and S. Kreitler, *Pain and quality of life.* Pain Pract. , 2001. 1(2): p. 150-61.
319. Nordin, M., F. Balague, and C. Cedraschi, *Nonspecific lower-back pain: surgical versus nonsurgical treatment.* Clin Orthop Relat Res, 2006. 443: p. 156-67.
320. Ohayon, M.M., *Specific characteristics of the pain/depression association in the general population.* J Clin Psychiatry. , 2004. 65(Suppl 12): p. 5-9.
321. Okuda, T., O. Ishida, Y. Fujimoto, N. Tanaka, et al., *The autotomy relief effect of a silicone tube covering the proximal nerve stump.* J Orthop Res., 2006. 24(7): p. 1427-37.
322. Okumus, M., E. Ceceli, F. Tuncay, S. Kocaoglu, et al., *The relationship between serum trace elements, vitamin B12, folic acid and clinical parameters in patients with myofascial pain syndrome.* Br J Nutr. , 2010. 106(5): p. 700-7.
323. Osher, Y. and R.H. Belmaker, *Omega-3 fatty acids in depression: a review of three studies.* CNS Neurosci Ther., 2009. 15(2): p. 128-33.
324. Padi, S.S. and S.K. Kulkarni, *Minocycline prevents the development of neuropathic pain, but not acute pain: possible anti-inflammatory and antioxidant mechanisms.* Eur J Pharmacol, 2008. 601: p. 79-87.
325. Pagni, C.A., M. Lanotte, and S. Canavero, *How frequent is anesthesia dolorosa following spinal posterior rhizotomy? A retrospective analysis of fifteen patients.* Pain, 1993. 54(3): p. 323-7.
326. Palecek, J., *The role of dorsal columns pathway in visceral pain.* Physiol Res., 2004. 53(Suppl 1): p. S125-30.
327. Patil, P.G. and J.N. Campbell, *Peripheral and central nervous system surgery for pain*, in *Wall and Melzack's Textbook of Pain*, S.B. McMahon and M. Koltzenburg, Editors. 2006, Elsevier: Amsterdam. p. 591-601.
328. Penfield, W. and T. Rasmussen, *The cerebral cortex of man: a clinical study of localization of function.* 1950, New York: Macmillan.
329. Pillay, P.K. and S.J. Hassenbusch, *Bilateral MRI-guided stereotactic cingulotomy for intractable pain.* Stereotact. Funct. Neurosurg., 1992. 59(1-4): p. 33-8.
330. Plazier, M., S. Vanneste, I. Dekelver, M. Thimineur, et al., *Peripheral nerve stimulation for fibromyalgia.* Prog Neurol Surg, 2011. 24: p. 133-46.
331. Podda, G. and C. Constantinescu, *Nabiximols in the treatment of spasticity, pain and urinary symptoms due to multiple sclerosis.* Expert Opin Biol Ther, 2012. 12(11): p. 1517-31.
332. Podivinsky, F., *Torticollis*, in *Handbook of Clinical Neurology, Diseases of the Basal Ganglia*, P.J. Vinken and G.W. Bruyn, Editors. 1968, North Holland Publishing Co: New York. p. 567-603.
333. Pons, T.P., P.E. Garraghty, A.K. Ommaya, J.H. Kaas, et al., *Massive cortical reorganization after sensory deafferentation in adult macaques.* Science, 1991. 252(1857-60).

334. Price, D.D., *Psychological and neural mechanisms of the affective dimension of pain.* Science, 2000. 288: p. 1769-1772.
335. Price, D.D., S. Long, and C. Huitt, *Sensory testing of pathophysiological mechanisms of pain in patients with reflex sympathetic dystrophy.* Pain, 1992. 49: p. 163-173.
336. Procacci, P., M. Zoppi, and M. Maresca, *Heart, vascular and haemopathic pain,* in *Textbook of Pain,* P.D. Wall and R. Melzack, Editors. 1999, Churchill Livingstone: Edinburgh. p. 621-639.
337. Procacci, P., M. Zoppi, L. Padeletti, and M. Maresca, *Myocardial infarction without pain. A study of the sensory function of the upper limbs.* Pain, 1976. 2: p. 309-313.
338. Procaccio, P. and M. Zoppi, *Pathophysiology and clinical aspects of visceral and referred pain,* in *Proceedings of the Third World Congress on Pain,* J.J. Bonica, U. Lindblom, and A. Iggo, Editors. 1983, Raven Press: New York. p. 643-658.
339. Puretic, M.B. and V. Demarin, *Neuroplasticity mechanisms in pathophysiology of chronic pain.* Acta Clin Croat, 2012. 51(3): p. 425-9.
340. Pyne, D. and N.G. Shenker, *Demystifying acupuncture.* Rheumatology, 2008. 47: p. 1132-6.
341. Quasthoff, S. and C. Sommer, *Peripheral mechanisms,* in *Pain in Peripheral Nerve diseases. Pain Headache,* C. Sommer, Editor. 2001, Karger: Basel. p. 110-148.
342. Quinn, C., C. Chandler, and A. Moraska, *Massage therapy and frequency of chronic tension headaches.* Am. J. Public Health, 2002. 92(10): p. 1657-61.
343. Rainville, P., R.K. Hofbauer, M.C. Bushnell, and e. al, *Hypnosis modulates activity in brain structures involved in the regulation of conciousness.* J. Cogn. Neurosci., 2002. 14: p. 887-901.
344. Raja, S.N., J.N. Campbell, and R.A. Meyer, *Evidence for different mechanisms of primary and secondary hyperalgesia following heat injury to the glabrous skin.* Brain, 1984. 107: p. 1791-1188.
345. Ralston, D., D. and H.J.r. Ralston, *The terminations of corticospinal tract axons in the macaque monkey.* J Comp Neurol., 1985 242(3): p. 325-37.
346. Ramachandran, V.S., *Plasticity and functional recovery in neurology.* Clin Med., 2005. 5(4): p. 368-73.
347. Ramachandran, V.S. and E.L. Altschuler, *The use of visual feedback, in particular mirror visual feedback, in restoring brain function.* Brain, 2009. 132(7)): p. 1693-710.
348. Ramachandran, V.S., E.L. Altschuler, L. Stone, M. Al-Aboudi, et al., *Can mirrors alleviate visual hemineglect?* Medical Hypotheses, 1999. 52 303–305(4): p. 303–305.
349. Ramachandran, V.S. and W. Hirstein, *The perception of phantom limbs. The D. O. Hebb lecture.* Brain, 1998. 121 ( Pt 9)(Pt 9): p. 1603-30.
350. Ramachandran, V.S., D. Rogers-Ramachandran, and M. Stewart, *Perceptual correlates of massive cortical reorganization. [letter; comment].* Science, 1992. 258: p. 1159-60.
351. Rapkin, A.J., *Chronic pelvic pain,* in *Textbook of pain,* P.D. Wall and R. Melzack, Editors. 1999, Churchill Livingstone: Edinburgh. p. 641-659.
352. Rasminsky, M., *Ephaptic transmission between single nerve fibers in the spinal nerve roots of dystrophic mice.* J. Physiol. (Lond.), 1980. 305: p. 151-169.
353. Reisfield, G., M., *Medical cannabis and chronic opioid therapy.* J Pain Palliat Care Pharmacother. , 2010. 24(4): p. 356-61.
354. Ren, K. and R. Dubner, *Descending modulation in persistent pain: an update.* Pain, 2002. 100(1-2): p. 1-6.
355. Reuben, S.S. and A. Buvanendran, *Preventing the development of chronic pain after orthopaedic surgery with preventive multimodal analgesic techniques.* J Bone Joint Surg Am. , 2007. 89(6): p. 1343-58.
356. Rexed, B.A., *Cytoarchitectonic atlas of the spinal cord.* J. Comp. Neurol., 1954. 100: p. 297-379.
357. Rice, A., *Cannabinoids and pain.* Curr Opin Investig Drugs., 2001. 2(3): p. 399-414.
358. Rivinoja, A.E., M.V. Paananen, S.P. Taimela, S. Solovieva, et al., *Sports, Smoking, and Overweight During Adolescence as Predictors of Sciatica in Adulthood: A 28-Year Follow-up Study of a Birth Cohort.* Am J Epidemiol., 2011.
359. Ro, L.S. and K.H. Chang, *Neuropathic pain: mechanisms and treatments.* Chang Gung Med J. , 2005. 28(9): p. 597-605.

360. Roberts, J., M.H. Ossipov, and F. Porreca, *Glial activation in the rostroventromedial medulla promotes descending facilitation to mediate inflammatory hypersensitivity.* Eur J Neurosci., 2009. 30(2): p. 229-41.
361. Robinson, D., R. and G.F. Gebhart, *Inside information: the unique features of visceral sensation.* Mol Interv, 2008. 8(5): p. 242-53.
362. Robinson, M.J., S.E. Edwards, S. Iyengar, F. Bymaste, et al., *Depression and pain.* Front Biosci., 2009. 14: p. 5031-51.
363. Rösler, K.M., *Transcranial magnetic brain stimulation: a tool to investigate central motor pathways.* News Physiol. Sci., 2001. 16: p. 297-302.
364. Ruch, T.C., *Pathophysiology of pain*, in *The brain and neural function*, T.C. Ruch and H.D. Patton, Editors. 1979, W.B.Saunders: Philadelphia. p. 272-324.
365. Ruggiero, C., F. Lattanzio, F. Lauretani, B. Gasperini, et al., *Omega-3 polyunsaturated fatty acids and immune-mediated diseases: inflammatory bowel disease and rheumatoid arthritis.* Curr Pharm Des, 2009. 15(36): p. 4135-48.
366. Russell, I.J. and C.S. Bieber, *Myofacial pain and fibromyalgia syndrome*, in *Wall and Melzak's Textbook of Pain.* , S.B. McMahon and M. Koltzenburg, Editors. 2006, Elsevier, Churchill, Livingstone: Amsterdam. p. 669-681.
367. Rutecki, P., *Anatomical, physiological, and theoretical basis for the antiepileptic effect of vagus nerve stimulation.* Eplepsia, 1990. 31 Suppl 2: p. S1-6.
368. Sacco, T. and B. Sacchetti, *Role of secondary sensory cortices in emotional memory storage and retrieval in rats.* Science. , 2010. 329(5992): p. 649-56.
369. Saitoh, Y. and T. Yoshimine, *Stimulation of primary motor cortex for intractable deafferentation pain.* Acta Neurochir Suppl., 2007. 97: p. 51-6.
370. Sakata, D., C. Yao, and S. Narumiya, *Emerging roles of prostanoids in T cell-mediated immunity.* IUBMB Life, 2010. 62(8): p. 591-6.
371. Sandkühler, J., *Models and mechanisms of hyperalgesia and allodynia.* Physiol. Rev, 2009. 89: p. 707-758.
372. Sandroni, P., *Central neuropathic itch: A new treatment option?* Neurology, 2002. 59: p. 778--780.
373. Sarlani, E., A.H. Schwartz, J.D. Greenspan, and E.G. Grace, *Facial pain as first manifestation of lung cancer: a case of lung cancer-related cluster headache and a review of the literature.* J Orofac Pain., 2003. 17(3): p. 262-7.
374. Sauro, M.D. and R.P. Greenberg, *Endogenous opiates and the placebo effect: a meta-analytic review.* J Psychosom Res, 2005. 58(2): p. 115-20.
375. Scadding, J.W., *Complex regional pain syndrome*, in *Textbook of pain*, P.D. Wall and R. Melzack, Editors. 1999, Churchill Livingstone: Edinburgh. p. 835-849.
376. Schäfers, M. and C. Sommer, *Polyneuropathies*, in *Pain in Peripheral Nerve diseases. Pain Headache*, C. Sommer, Editor. 2001, Karger: Basel. p. 53-108.
377. Schlee, W., V. Leirer, I.T. Kolassa, N. Weisz, et al., *Age-related changes in neural functional connectivity and its behavioral relevance.* BMC Neurosci., 2012. 13(1).
378. Schlee, W., V. Leirer, S. Kolassa, F. Thurm, et al., *Development of large-scale functional networks over the lifespan.* Neurobiol Aging, 2012.
379. Schlee, W., I. Lorenz, T. Hartmann, N. Müller, et al., *A Global Brain Model of Tinnitus*, in *Textbook of Tinnitus*, A.R. Møller, et al., Editors. 2010, Springer: New York. p. 161-170.
380. Schmader, K., J.W. Gnann, and C.P. Watson, *The epidemiological, clinical, and pathological rationale for the herpes zoster vaccine.* J Infect Dis., 2008 197(Suppl 2): p. S207-15.
381. Schmelz, M., *Itch—mediators and mechanisms.* J. Dermatol. Sci., 2002. 28: p. 91-96.
382. Schmelz, M., *Itch and pain.* Dermatol Ther., 2005. 18(4): p. 304-7.
383. Schmelz, M. and H.O. Handwerker, *Itch*, in *Textbook of Pain*, S.B. McMahon and M. Koltzenburg, Editors. 2006, Elsevier: Amsterdam. p. 219-227.
384. Schmidt, B.L., D.T. Hamamoto, D.A. Simone, and G.L. Wilcox, *Mechanism of cancer pain.* Mol Interv., 2010: p. 164-78.

385. Sen, C.N. and A.R. Møller, *Signs of hemifacial spasm created by chronic periodic stimulation of the facial nerve in the rat.* Exp. Neurol., 1987. 98: p. 336-349.
386. Serhan, C.N., S. Krishnamoorthy, A. Recchiuti, and N. Chiang, *Novel anti-inflammatory--pro-resolving mediators and their receptors.* Curr Top Med Chem, 2011. 11(6): p. 629-47.
387. Sessle, B.J., *Recent development in pain research: Central mechanism of orofacial pain and its control.* J. Endodon., 1986. 12: p. 435-444.
388. Sessle, B.J., *Physiology of the trigeminal system,* in *Trigeminal Neuralgia,* G.H. Fromm and B.J. Sessle, Editors. 1991, Butterworth-Heinemann: Boston. p. 71-104.
389. Shelley, B.P. and M.R. Trimble, *The insular lobe of Reil--its anatamico-functional, behavioural and neuropsychiatric attributes in humans--a review.* World J Biol Psychiatry, 2004. 5(4): p. 176-200.
390. Sherman, R.A., C.J. Sherman, and L. Parker, *Chronic phantom and stump pain among American veterans: results of a survey.* Pain, 1984. 18: p. 83-95.
391. Sherrington, C.S., *The Integrative Action of the Nervous System.* 1906, New Haven, CT: Yale Univ. Press.
392. Siddall, P.J., *Pain following spinal cord injury,* in *Wall and Melzak's Textbook of Pain,* S.B. McMahon and M. Koltzenburg, Editors. 2006, Elsevier, Churchill, Livingstone: Amsterdam. p. 1043-1055.
393. Siddall, P.J. and J. McClelland, *Non-painful sensory phenomena after spinal cord injury.* J Neurol Neurosurg Psychiatry. , 1999. 66(5): p. 617-22.
394. Sie, K.C.Y. and E.W. Rubel, *Rapid Changes in Protein Synthesis and Cell Size in the Cochlear Nucleus following Eighth Nerve Activity Blockade and Cochlea Ablation.* J. Comp. Neurol., 1992. 320: p. 501-508.
395. Siegfried, J., *Sensory thalamic neurostimulation for chronic pain.* Pacing & Clin. Electrophysiol., 1987. 10(2): p. 209-210.
396. Simons, D.G. and S. Mense, *Understanding and measurement of muscle tone as related to clinical muscle pain.* Pain, 1998. 75(1): p. 1-17.
397. Simpson, A., K,, J. Cholewicki, and J. Grauer, *Chronic low back pain.* Curr Pain Headache, 2006. 10(6): p. 431-6.
398. Simpson, B.A., *Spinal cord and brain stimulation,* in *Textbook of pain,* P.D. Wall and R. Melzack, Editors. 1999, Churchill Livingstone: Edinburgh. p. 1353-1381.
399. Simpson, B.A., B.A. Meyerson, and B. Linderoth, *Spinal cord and Brain Stimulation,* in *Wall and Melzack's Textbook of Pain,* S.B. Mahon and M. Kolzenburg, Editors. 2006, Elsevier: Amsterdam. p. 563-582.
400. Sindrup, S.H. and T.S. Jensen, *Efficacy of pharmacological treatments of neuropathic pain: an update and effect related to mechanism of drug action.* Pain, 1999. 83: p. 389-400.
401. Singleton, C.K. and P.R. Martin, *Molecular mechanisms of thiamine utilization.* Curr Mol Med., 2001. 1(2): p. 197-207.
402. Sipski, M.L., C.J. Alexander, and R.C. Rosen, *Orgasm in women with spinal cord injuries: a laboratory-based assessment.* Arch. Phys. Med. Rehabil., 1995. 76: p. 1097-1102.
403. Sipski, M.L., C.J. Alexander, and R.R. Rosen, *Sexual arousal and orgasm in women: Effects of spinal cord injury.* Ann. Neurol., 2001. 49(1): p. 35-44.
404. Sivilotti, L. and C.J. Woolf, *The contribution of GABAA and glycine receptors to central sensitization: disinhibition and touch-evoked allodynia in the spinal cord.* J. Neurophysiol., 1994. 72: p. 169–179.
405. Slavin, K.V., *Peripheral nerve stimulation for neuropathic pain.* Neurotherapeutics, 2008. 5(1): p. 100-6.
406. Smith, H.S., *Peripherally-acting opioids.* Pain Physician, 2008. 11, 2 Suppl: p. S121-32.
407. Sola, A.E., *Upper extremity pain,* in *Handbook of Pain,* P.D. Wall and R. Melzack, Editors. 1999, Churchill Livingstone: Edinburgh. p. 559-578.
408. Sola, A.E., M.L. Rodenberg, and B.B. Getty, *Incidence of hypersensitive areas in the neck and shoulder muscles.* Am. J. Phys. Med., 1955. 34: p. 585-90.
409. Sommer, C. and F. Birklein, *Resolvins and inflammatory pain.* F1000 Med Rep. , 2011. 3: p. 19.

410. Sommer, C., M. Marziniak, and R.R. Myers, *The effect of thalidomide treatment on vascular pathology and hyperalgesia caused by chronic constriction injury of rat nerve.* Pain, 1998. 74((1): p. 83-91.
411. Sommera, C. and M. Kressb, *Recent findings on how proinflammatory cytokines cause pain: peripheral mechanisms in inflammatory and neuropathic hyperalgesiaq Claudia Sommera,\*, Michaela Kressb.* Neuroscience Letters, 2004. 361: p. 184–187.
412. Song, P. and Z.-Q. Zhao, *The involvement of glial cells in the development of morphine tolerance.* Neurosci. Res., 2001. 39(3): p. 281-286.
413. Sorensen, J., A. Bengtsson, J. Ahlner, and e. al, *Fibromyalgia - are there different mechanisms in the processing of pain? A double blind crossover comparison of analgesic drugs.* J. Rheumatololgy, 1997. 24: p. 1615-1621.
414. Sorensen, J., A. Bengtsson, E. Backman, K.G. Henrikson, et al., *Pain analysis in patients with fibromyalgia: effects of intravenous morphine, lidocaine and ketamine.* J. Rheumatology, 1995. 24: p. 360-365.
415. Stanton-Hicks, M., *Complex regional pain syndrome.* Anesthesiol Clin North America, 2003 21(4): p. 733-44.
416. Stephani, C., G. Fernandez Baca-Vaca, M. Koubeissi, R. Maciunas, et al. *Stimulation of the insula.* in *Second Congress, International Society of Intraoperative Neurophysiology.* 2009. Dubrovnik.
417. Stephani, C., Fernandez-Baca, G. Vaca, R. Maciunas, et al., *Functional neuroanatomy of the insular lobe.* Brain Struct Funct., 2010
418. Stout, A., *Epidural steroid injections for low back pain.* Phys Med Rehabil Clin N Am., 2010. 21(4): p. 825-34.
419. Straube, S., S. Derry, R.A. Moore, and H.J. McQuay, *Cervico-thoracic or lumbar sympathectomy for neuropathic pain and complex regional pain syndrome.* Cochrane Database Syst Rev, 2010. 7(7).
420. Strong, J., W. Xie, F. Bataille, and J. Zhang, *Preclinical studies of low back pain.* Mol Pain, 2013. 9(17).
421. Sugar, O., *Victor Horsley, John Marshall, nerve stretching, and the nervi nervorum.* Surg. Neurol., 1990. 34(3): p. 184-7.
422. Sullivan, M.J., B. Thorn, J.A. Haythornthwaite, F. Keefe, et al., *Theoretical perspectives on the relation between catastrophizing and pain.* Clin J Pain, 2001. 17(1): p. 52-64.
423. Sun, J., V. Singh, R. Kajino-Sakamoto, and A. Aballay, *Neuronal GPCR controls innate immunity by regulating noncanonical unfolded protein response genes.* Science, 2011. 332: p. 729-32.
424. Sunderland, S., *Microvascular relations and anomalies at the base of the brain.* J. Neurol. Neurosurg. Psychiatry, 1948. 11: p. 243-257.
425. Sweet, W.H., *Deafferentation pain after posterior rhizotomy, trauma to a limb, and herpes zoster.* Neurosurgery, 1984. 15(6): p. 928-32.
426. Sweet, W.H., *The treatment of trigeminal neuralgia (tic douloureux).* N Engl J Med., 1986. 315(3): p. 174-7.
427. Talaei, A., M. Siavash, H. Majidi, and A. Chehrei, *Vitamin B12 may be more effective than nortriptyline in improving painful diabetic neuropathy.* Int J Food Sci Nutr., 2009. 60 Suppl 5: p. 71-6.
428. Tanimoto, T., M. Takeda, and S.S. Matsumoto, *Suppressive effect of vagal afferents on cervical dorsal horn neurons responding to tooth pulp electrical stimulation in the rat.* Experimental Brain Research, 2002. 145(4): p. 468-79.
429. Tawfic, Q., *A review of the use of ketamine in pain management.* Opioid Manag, 2013. 9(5): p. 379-88.
430. Taylor, A., A. Westveld, M. Szkudlinska, P. Guruguri, et al., *The use of metformin is associated with decreased lumbar radiculopathy pain.* J Pain Res., 2013. 6: p. 755-63.
431. Taylor, C., T. Angelotti, and E. Fauman, *Pharmacology and mechanism of action of pregabalin: the calcium channel alpha2-delta (alpha2-delta) subunit as a target for antiepileptic drug discovery.* Epilepsy Res., 2007. 73(2): p. 137-50.

432. Telleria-Diaz, A., M. Schmidt, S. Kreusch, A.K. Neubert, et al., *Spinal antinociceptive effects of cyclooxygenase inhibition during inflammation: Involvement of prostaglandins and endocannabinoids.* Pain., 2010. 148(1): p.:26-35.

433. Thayer, J.F. and E.M. Sternber, *Neural aspects of immunomodulation: Focus on the vagus nerve.* Brain Behav Immun., 2010. 24(8): p. 1223–1228.

434. Thompson, S.W.N., A.E. King, and C.J. Woolf, *Activity-dependent changes in rat ventral horn neurons in vitro: Summation of prolonged afferent evoked post-synaptic depolarization produce a d-APV sensitive wind-up.* Eur. J. Neurosci., 1990. 2: p. 638-649.

435. Tinazzi, M., G. Zanette, D. Volpato, R. Testoni, et al., *Neurophysiological evidence of neuroplasticity at multiple levels of the somatosensory system in patients with carpal tunnel syndrome.* Brain Behav Immun., 1998. 121: p. 1785-94.

436. Todd, A.J., *Neuronal circuitry for pain processing in the dorsal horn.* Nature reviews Neuroscience, 2010. 11: p. 823-36.

437. Tohda, C., T. Yamaguchi, and Y. Kuraishi, *Intracisternal injection of opioids induces itch -associated response through mu-opioid receptors in mice.* Jap. J.Pharmacol., 1997.

438. Tompkins, D.A. and C.M. Campbell, *Opioid-induced hyperalgesia: clinically relevant or extraneous research phenomenon?* Curr Pain Headache Rep., 2011. 15(2): p. 129-36.

439. Torebjoerk, H.E. and J.L. Ochoa, *Pain and itch from C-fiber stimulation.* Society for Neuroscience Abstracts, 1981. 7: p. 228.

440. Towle, V.L., H.A. Yoon, M.C. Castelle, J.C. Edgar, et al., *ECoG Gamma Activity: Differentiating expressive and receptive speech areas.* Brain, 2008. 131: p. 2013-27.

441. Tracey, K., *Physiology and immunology of the cholinergic antiinflammatory pathway.* Journal of Clinical Investigation, 2007. 117(2): p. 289–96.

442. Tracey, K.J., *Reflex control of immunity.* Nat. Rev. Immunol 2009. 9(6): p. 418-28.

443. Tracey, K.J., *Ancient Neurons Regulate Immunity.* Science, 2011. 332: p. 673-4.

444. Travell, J., S. Rinzler, and M. Herman, *Pain and disability of the shoulder and arm, treatment with infiltration with procaine hydrochloride.* JAMA, 1942. 120(6): p. 417-22.

445. Travell, J. and D.G. Simons, *Myofascial pain and dysfunction, the trigger point manual.* 1983, New York: Williams and Wilkins.

446. Tsubokawa, T., Y. Katayama, T. Yamamoto, T. Hirayama, et al., *Chronic motor cortex stimulation for the treatment of central pain.* Acta Neurochir Suppl (Wien), 1991. 52: p. 137-9.

447. Turk, D.C. and R.H. Dworkin, *What should be the core outcomes in chronic pain clinical trials?* Arthritis Research & Therapy, 2004. 6(4): p. 151–154.

448. Turk, D.C. and A. Okifuji, *Pain terms and taxonomies,* in *Bonica's management of pain (3 ed.),* D. Loeser, et al., Editors. 2001, Lippincott Williams & Wilkins. p. 18–25.

449. Turner, J.A., M.P. Jensen, C.A. Warms, and D.D. Cardenas, *Catastrophizing is associated with pain intensity, psychological distress, and pain-related disability among individuals with chronic pain after spinal cord injury.* Pain., 2002. 98(1-2): p. 127-34.

450. Urquhart, D.M., P. Berry, A.E. Wluka, B.J. Strauss, et al., *Increased fat mass is associated with high levels of low back pain intensity and disability.* Spine, 2011.

451. Valat, J.P., S. Genevay, M. Marty, S. Rozenberg, et al., *Sciatica.* Best Pract Res Clin Rheumatol., 2010. 24(2): p.:241-52.

452. van Tulder, M.W., B. Koes, S. Seitsalo, and A. Malmivaara, *Outcome of invasive treatment modalities on back pain and sciatica: an evidence-based review.* Eur Spine J, 2006. Suppl 1: p. S82-92.

453. Veves, A., M. Backonja, and R.A. Malik, *Painful diabetic neuropathy: epidemiology, natural history, early diagnosis, and treatment options.* Pain Med., 2008. 9(6): p. 660-74.

454. Villemure, C. and P. Schweinhardt, *Supraspinal pain processing: distinct roles of emotion and attention.* Neuroscientist., 2010. 16((3): p. 276-84.

455. Vlaeyen, J.W., A.M. Kole-Snijders, R.G. Boeren, and H. van Eek, *Fear of movement/(re)injury in chronic low back pain and its relation to behavioral performance.* Pain, 1995. 62: p. 363-72.
456. Volkmar, F.R. and D. Pauls, *Autism.* The Lancet, 2003. 362: p. 1133-42.
457. Wada, J.A., *Kindling 2.* 1981, New York: Raven Press.
458. Wagner, R. and R.R. Myers, *Endoneurial injection of TNF-alpha produces neuropathic pain behaviors.* Neuroreport., 1996. 7(18): p. 2897-901.
459. Wall, P., *Pain: The Science of suffering.* Maps of the Mind, ed. S. Rose. 2000, New York: Columbia University Press.
460. Wall, P.D., *The presence of ineffective synapses and circumstances which unmask them.* Phil. Trans. Royal Soc. (Lond.), 1977. 278: p. 361-372.
461. Wall, P.D., *The prevention of postoperative pain.* Pain, 1988. 33: p. 289-290.
462. Wall, P.D. and M. Devor, *Sensory afferent impulses originate from dorsal root ganglia as well as from periphery in normal and nerve injured rats.* Pain, 1983. 17: p. 321-339.
463. Wallengren, J., *Neuroanatomy and neurophysiology of itch.* Dermatol Ther., 2005. 18(4): p. 292-303.
464. Walsh, E.G., *Muscles, Masses and Motion: The Physiology of Normality, Hypotonicity, Spasticity and Rigidity.* 1992, Oxford: Blackwell.
465. Walton, K.D. and R.R. Llinás, *Central Pain as a Thalamocortical Dysrhythmia. A Thalamic Efference Disconnection?*, in *Translational Pain Research: From Mouse to Man*, L. Kruger and A.R. Light, Editors. 2010, CRC Press: Boca Raton, FL.
466. Wang, H., M. Yu, M. Ochani, C.A. Amella, et al., *Nicotinic acetylcholine receptor alpha7 subunit is an essential regulator of inflammation.* Nature, 2003. 421(6921): p. 384-8.
467. Wang, J., Q. , L. Mao, and J.S. Han, *Comparison of the antinociceptive effects induced by electroacupuncture and transcutaneous electrical nerve stimulation in the rat.* Int J Neurosci., 1992. 65: p. 117-29.
468. Wang, Z., W. Ma, J.G. Chabot, and R. Quirion, *Morphological evidence for the involvement of microglial p38 activation in CGRP-associated development of morphine antinociceptive tolerance.* Peptides, 2010. 31(12): p. 2179-84.
469. Waters, D., *Is a mechanical or a metabolic approach superior in the treatment of coronary disease? Results of the atorvastatin versus revascularization (AVERT) trial.* Eur Heart J., 2000. 21(13): p. 1029-31.
470. Watson, C.P., M.L. Chipman, and R.C. Monks, *Antidepressants analgesics: a systematic review and comparative study*, in *Wall and Melzack's Textbook of Pain*, S.B. Mahon and M. Kolzenburg, Editors. 2006, Elsevier: Amsterdam. p. 481-497.
471. Weber, H., *The natural history of disc herniation and the influence of intervention.* Spine, 1994. 19: p. 2234-2238.
472. Weiner, D.K., Y.S. Kim, P. Bonino, and T. Wang, *Low back pain in older adults: are we utilizing healthcare resources wisely?* Pain Med, 2006 7(2): p. 101-2.
473. Weltz, C.R., S.M. Klein, J.E. Arbo, and R.A. Greengrass, *Paravertebral block anesthesia for inguinal hernia repair.* World Journal of Surgery, 2003. 27(4): p. 425-9.
474. Wen, Y.R., P.H. Tan, J.K. Cheng, Y.C. Liu, et al., *Microglia: a promising target for treating neuropathic and postoperative pain, and morphine tolerance.* J Formos Med Assoc, 2011. 110(8): p. 487-94.
475. Whipple, B., C.A. Gerdes, and B.R. Komisaruk, *Sexual response to self-stimulation in women with complete spinal cord injury.* J. Sex. Res., 1996. 33: p. 231-240.
476. Whipple, B. and B.R. Komisaruk, *Brain (PET) responses to vaginal-cervical self-stimulation in women with complete spinal cord injury: preliminary findings.* J. Sex & Marital Therapy, 2002. 28(1): p. 79-86.
477. White, J.C. and W.H. Sweet, *Facial and cephalic neuralgias: Trigeminal neuralgia*, in *Pain*. 1955, Charles C. Thomas. p. 433-493.
478. Wieseler-Frank, J., S.F. Maier, and L.R. Watkins, *Glial activation and pathological pain.* Neurochem Int., 2004. 45(2-3): p. 389-95.
479. Willer, J.C., *Relieving effect of TENS on painful muscle contraction produced by an impairment of reciprocal innervation: An electrophysiological analysis.* Pain, 1988. 32: p. 271-274.

480. Willis, W.D., *From nociceptor to cortical activity*, in *Pain and the brain*, B. Bromm and J.E. Desmedt Editors. 1995, Raven Press: New York. p. 1-19.
481. Willis, W.D. and K.N. Westlund, *Neuroanatomy of the pain system and of the pathways that modulate pain.* J Clin Neurophysiol., 1997. 14(1): p. 2-31.
482. Wilsey, B., T. Marcotte, R. Deutsch, B. Gouaux, et al., *Low-dose vaporized cannabis significantly improves neuropathic pain.* J Pain., 2012. 14(2): p. 136-48.
483. Wolf, S., D. Barton, L. Kottschade, A. Grothey, et al., *Chemotherapy-induced peripheral neuropathy: prevention and treatment strategies.* Eur J Cancer., 2008. 44(11): p. 1507-15.
484. Wolfe, F., K. Ross, J. Anderson, and et al, *The prevalence and characteristics of fibromyalgia.* Arthritis and Rheumatism, 1995. 38: p. 18-18.
485. Woolf, C., *What is this thing called pain?.* Journal of Clinical Investigation. J. Clin. Invest., 2010. 120(11): p. 3742–4.
486. Woolf, C.J., *Evidence of a central component of postinjury pain hypersensitivity.* Nature, 1983. 308: p. 686-688.
487. Woolf, C.J., *Central sensitization: Implications for the diagnosis and treatment of pain.* Pain, 2011. 152: p. S1-S15.
488. Woolf, C.J. and R.J. Mannion, *Neuropathic pain: aetiology, symptoms, mechanisms, and managements.* The Lancet, 1999. 353: p. 1959-1964.
489. Woolf, C.J. and M.W. Salter, *Neural plasticity: Increasing the gain in pain.* Science, 2000. 288: p. 1765-1768.
490. Woolf, C.J. and M.W. Salter, *Plasticity and pain: role of the dorsal horn*, in *Wall and Melzak's Textbook of Pain*, S.B. McMahon and M. Koltzenburg, Editors. 2006, Elsevier: Amsterdam. p. 91-105.
491. Woolf, C.J. and S.W.N. Thompson, *The induction and maintenance of central sensitization is dependent on N-methyl-D-aspartic acid receptor activation: Implications for the treatment of post-injury pain hypersensitivity states.* Pain, 1991. 44: p. 293-299.
492. Wu, A., Z. Ying, and F. Gomez-Pinilla, *Dietary omega-3 fatty acids normalize BDNF levels, reduce oxidative damage, and counteract learning disability after traumatic brain injury in rats.* J. Neurotrauma, 2004. 21(10): p. 1457-67.
493. Xiao, W.H. and G.J. Bennett, *Chemotherapy-evoked neuropathic pain: Abnormal spontaneous discharge in A-fiber and C-fiber primary afferent neurons and its suppression by acetyl-L-carnitine.* Pain., 2008. 135(3): p. 262-70.
494. Yakhnitsa, V., B. Linderoth, and B.A. Meyerson, *Spinal cord stimulation attenuates dorsal horn hyperexcitability in a rat model of mononeuropathy.* Pain, 1999. 79: p. 223-233.
495. Yaksh, T.L., *Behavioral and autonomic correlates of the tactile evoked allodynia produced by spinal glycine inhibition: effects of modulatory receptor systems and excitatory amino acid antagonists.* Pain, 1989. 37: p. 111–123.
496. Yosipovitch, G., C. Szolar, X.Y. Hui, and H. Maibach, *Effect of topically applied menthol on thermal, pain and itch sensations and biophysical properties of the skin.* Arch. Arch. Dermatol. Res., 1996. 288: p. 245-8.
497. Young, R.F. and K.M. Perryman, *Pathways for orofacial pain sensation in the trigeminal brain-stem nuclear complex of the Macaque monkey.* J Neurosurg., 1984. 61(3): p. 563-8.
498. Yrjänheikki, J., T. Tikka, R. Keinänen, G. Goldsteins, et al., *A tetracycline derivative, minocycline, reduces inflammation and protects against focal cerebral ischemia with a wide therapeutic window.* Proc Natl Acad Sci U S A., 1999. 96(23): p. 13496-500.
499. Zakrzewska-Pniewska, B. and M. Jedras, *Is pruritus in chronic uremic patients related to peripheral somatic and autonomic neuropathy? Study by R-R interval variation test (RRIV) and by sympathetic skin response (SSR).* Neurophysiol Clinique, 2001. 311(3): p. 181-93.
500. Zhang, Q., L. Peng, and D. Zhang, *Minocycline may attenuate postherpetic neuralgia.* Med Hypotheses., 2009 73(5): p. 744-5.

501. Zhang, S.C., B.D. Goetz, and I.D. Duncan, *Suppression of activated microglia promotes survival and function of transplanted oligodendroglial progenitors.* Glia, 2003. 41(2): p. 191-8.
502. Zhao, Z.Q., *Neural mechanism underlying acupuncture analgesia.* Prog Neurobiol., 2008. 85(4): p. 355-75.
503. Zhou, J. and S. Shore, *Convergence of spinal trigeminal and cochlear nucleus projections in the inferior colliculus of the guinea pig.* J Comp Neurol., 2006. 495(1): p. 100-12.
504. Zhou, L.J., T. Yang, X. Wei, Y. Liu, et al., *Brain-derived neurotrophic factor contributes to spinal long-term potentiation and mechanical hypersensitivity by activation of spinal microglia in rat.* Brain Behav Immun., 2011. 25(2): p. 322-34.
505. Zimmermann, M., *Physiological mechanisms of pain in muscloskeletal system*, in *Muscle spasms and pain*, M. Emre and H. Mathies, Editors. 1988, Parthenon Publishing: Carnforth. p. 7-17.
506. Zin, C.S., L.M. Nissen, M.T. Smith, J.P. O'Callaghan, et al., *An update on the pharmacological management of post-herpetic neuralgia and painful diabetic neuropathy.* CNS Drugs., 2008. 22(5): p. 417-42.
507. Zittermann, A., *The estimated benefits of vitamin D for Germany.* Mol Nutr Food Res., 2010. 54(8): p. 1164-71.
508. Zochodne, D.W., *Epineurial peptides: a role in neuropathic pain?* Canadian. J. Neurol Sci., 1993. 20(1): p. 69-72.

# Subject Index

5-HT, see serotonin, 171

## A

ABL, 95
ACE, 95
acetaminophen, (paracetamol), 170
acetylcholine, 285
   receptors, 309
acetylsalicylic acid, 170
acidity, 158
acute pain, 27
adaptive immune response, 285
addictions, 184, 211
   risk from semisynthetic opioids, 178
   to opioids, 177
adenosine triphosphate (ATP), 281
administration of
   pain medication, 182, 336
   treatments, 335
adrenal medulla, and hyperactivity, 298
adrenocorticotropin, 126
Advil, see ibuprofen, 170
affective disorders, pain and, 60
afferent nerve fibers, in viscera, 114
alcohol, 179
Aleve, see naproxen, 170
allodynia, 151, 203, 215, 289, 351
ALS, 303
altered "self", 206
Alzheimer's disease, 233
AMA, 28
American Food and Drug Administration, 175
American Medical Association, 28
amputation, 227, 346
Amputation pain, 44
amputations, 91
   pain, reducing the incidence of, 362
amygdala, 25, 45, 75, 94, 211, 214, 309
amyotropic lateral sclerosis, 303
analgesics, 168
anesthesia dolorosa, 139, 225, 339
angina, 122
ANS, 298
anterior
   cingulate, 108, 211
      cortex, 75, 352
      gyrus, 309
   insula, 108
   tract, of STT, 80
anti-inflammatory medication, for pain, 289

anti-pyretic effect, 176
apoptosis, and opioids, 290
arthroplasty, 192
Aspirin, 170, 172, 300
astrocytes, 280, 288, 290, 359, 360
astroglia, 290
atopic dermatitis, 104
atypical face pain, 139
Auerbach's plexus, 118
autistic individuals, 44
autoimmune diseases,
   and pain, 290
   disorders, 145
autonomic
   nervous system, 113, 298
      treatment related to, 350
   testing, 316
axoplasmatic flow, 250
A$\beta$ fibers, 73, 76, 77, 97, 115, 154, 162, 191
A$\delta$ fibers, 162, 342

## B

B$_1$, 341
B$_{12}$, 341
back pain, 51
baclofen, 314, 339
basal ganglia, 108, 257
basolateral nucleus, of amygdala, 95
BDNF, 323, 335
Benefit from pain, 38
benzodiazepines, 145
   as pain medications, 180
bicuculine, 236
BMI, 363
body
   image, 346
   mass index, 363
   perception, 206
bottom-up, 47
   communication of pain signals, 75
bradykinin, 157, 281
brain derived neurotrophic factor, 323, 335
brainstem reticular formation, 103
Brodmann's areas, of the cerebral cortex, 373
burn pain, 361
burst firing, 151
bypass operations, 122

## C

C fibers, 76
calcitonin gene-related peptides, 70
cancer pain, 258, 349
capsaicin, 108
    receptor, 114, 120
carbamazepine, 338
cardiac pain, 122
carpal tunnel syndrome, 144, 191, 201, 252, 342, 344, 363
Cartesius, 46
catastrophizing, 23, 34, 205

caudal
    trigeminal nucleus, 89
    ventrolateral medulla, 82
causalgia, 31, 242, 350
cause of pain, 50
    after amputations, 223
    treatment of, 188
CCK, 332
Celebrex, 287
celiac ganglion, 114
central
    action of the sympathetic nervous system, 297
    control of pain, 298
    modulation of physiological pain, anatomical basis for, 96
    neuropathic pain, see chronic neuropathic pain
    nucleus of the amygdala, 95
    pain, CP, 202
    post stroke pain, CPSP, 231
    projections, of pain, 89
    sensitization, 295, 300
C-fibers, 73, 107, 115, 162, 342
    innocuous stimulation of, 74
CGRP, 70
chemokines, 213
chemoreceptors, 281
chickenpox virus, 146, 339
cholecystokinin, 332
chronic
    fatigue syndrome, 275, 367
    neuropathic pain, 26, 27, 28, 30, 39, 47, 146, 196, 199, 201, 214, 366
    pain, 27, 33, 52, 336
    widespread pain, 31, 59, 201, 271
cingulate gyrus, 108, 214
cis-platinum, 145
classification of pain, 25, 28
clonidine, as pain medication, 181
codeine, 178
cognitive-behavioral model, 35
complex regional pain syndrome, 31, 44, 101, 244, 316, 350, 361,
congenital analgesia, 37
coping, 23, 34, 112, 204

cortical representation of the body, 220
cortico-thalamic loop, 225
COX-1 and 2, 157, 170
COX-2, 176, 287
Coxibs, 176
cranial nerve V, 296
critical period, 368
cross-sensitization, 127
CRPS, see complex regional pain syndrome
CTS, 344
CVLM, 82
CWP, 31, 59
cyanocoblamin, 341
cyclooxygenase, see COX 1 and 2
Cymbalta, 338
cytokines, 157, 211, 213, 303
    pro-inflammatory, 303

## D

DBS, see deep brain stimulation
deafferentation pain, 47, 224, 345
deep brain stimulation, 80, 93, 225, 323
deep sensations, 134
definition of pain, 21
degenerative vertebral discs, 148
Dejerine-Roussy syndrome, 231
demyelinating diseases, 152
depression, 211
dermatomes, 129
dermatomyositis, 267
Descartes, 40, 75
descending systems, 97, 305
desimipramin, 338
development, of the nervous system, 369
diabetes, 137, 140
    neuropathies, 51, 145, 181
        painful, 181
    type 2, 364
diagnoses, incorrect, 168, 315
    of pain, 168, 314
Diagnostic and Statistical Manual of Mental Disorders, 185
diagnostic tool, pain as a, 41
diclofenac, 170
Dilantin, 339
disability questionnaires, 341
distorted body image, correcting of, 346
DLPT, 98
DMND, 219
dopamine, 309
dorsal
    and medial thalamus, 75
    cochlear nucleus, 79
    column
        stimulations, 325
        deep pain, 131

dorsal horn
    anatomy of, 75
    changes in, 235
    of the spinal cord, 236
    raphae nucleus, 331
    root ganglia, 75, 114, 224, 248
dorsolateral pontine tegmentum, 98
DQ, 341
DRG, see dorsal root ganglia
DRN, 331
drug
    dependence, 185
    treatments, 320
DSM-IV, see Diagnostic and Statistical Manual of
    Mental Disorders
dualism, 40
duloxetine, 338
Dynorphine, 163, 332
dysfunctional neural networks, 219
dystonia, 31

## E

EA, 332
EAA, 157
electrical
    acupuncture, 332
    stimulation, for neuromodulation, 191
electromyography, 146, 273
EMG, see electromyography, 146
emotional
    brain, 75
    component, 24
    factors, 155
endocannabinoids, 302
endogenous opioids, 37, 163
endomorphine, 163
endorphins, 163
enkephalins, 163, 332
entrapment of spinal nerves, 30
ephaptic transmission, 152
epidemiology of pain, 54
epidural
    corticosteroid injections, 344
    stimulating electrodes, 345
epigenetics, 369
epinephrine, 211
EPSP, see excitatory postsynaptic potential
escapable, 23
evolution
    of pain, 39
    of the immune system, 284
excitatory
    amino acids, 157
    postsynaptic potential, 150
expectation, role of, 188
extralemniscal system, 92

## F

facial pain, 130
FDA, 175
fear, 23
Fentanyl, 178
fibromyalgia, 44, 59, 201, 269, 270, 274, 323, 367
flight and fight reaction, 35, 236, 300
free nerve endings, 262
functional MRI (fMRI), 257
future treatment of physiological pain, 194

## G

$GABA_A$ receptor, 236
gabapentin, 320, 340
gating hypothesis, 45, 191
genetic programs, 369
glia
    activation, in pathological pain, 288
    cells, 194, 304
glossopharyngeal neuralgia, 254, 319, 336, 339
glycinergic transmission, 157
Golgi tendon organs, 264, 349
GPN, 319, 336, 339
Guillain-Barré syndrome, 146

## H

harmful plasticity, 367
heart attacks, 122
Hebb, 370
hemifacial spasm, 138, 255 256, 319
heroin, 178
Herpes
    simplex, 147
    zoster, 147, 192, 339
    zoster oticus, 338
HFS, see hemifacial spasm
high threshold mechanoreceptos, 238
hippocampus, 45, 211
histamine, 105, 157, 281
HPA, 329
HTM see high threshold mechanoreceptos
hydromorphone, 178
hyperactive disorders, 368
hyperalgesia, 186, 235, 281, 289
    developement of, 160
hyperglycemia, 145
hyperpathia, 203, 215, 235, 236, 295
hypertension, 53
hyperthermia, 126
hypnosis, 334
hypothalamus–pituitary–adrenal axis, 126
HZ, see Herpes zoster

## I

ibuprofen, 170, 171
idiopathic pain, 26, 112
IL, see interleukin
illness response, 125
imipramine, 338
immune
    reactions, 125
    reactions and pain, 358
    system, 40, 277
        adaptive, 282
        evolution of, 284
        innate, 282
        role in strokes, 287
        role of in pain, 282
immunoreactivity, involving nerve growth factor, 363
impulse generators, nerves as, 141, 142
incorrect diagnosis, 315
Indocid, see indomethacin, 170
indomethacin, 170, 300
inescapable, 23
inferior mesenteric ganglion, 115
inflammation, 278
    of nerves, 146
    the role of, 157
inflammatory, 196
    cytokines, 125
    disorders, 267
    pain, 197, 277
    processes, 114, 160
reactions, 249
innate (inborn or natural) immune system, 283
innervation, of pain receptors, 73
insula, 309
    anterior, 45, 90, 240, 352
    cortex, 107, 211
    role in visceral pain, 131
interleukin, 125, 211, 289, 359
intermediate zone, of dorsal horn, 83, 97
interpretation of pain, 24
intraoperative neurophysiological monitoring, 192
intrinsic primary afferent neurons, 115
IONM, intraoperative neurophysiological monitoring, 192
ischemia, 114
itch receptor, 105
itching, central representation of, 106

## J

joint replacement surgery, 192

## K

ketamine, 195, 353
kindling, 370
knock-out mice, 301

## L

L-838,417, experimental drug, 354
lateral
    nucleus, of amygdala, 94
    parabrachial area, 82
    spinothalamic tract, 81
    tract, of STT, 80
LC, 331
LEB, 346
leg cramp, 268
leukotrienes, 170
life style,
    change of, 352
    importance of, 363
limbic structures, 71, 214, 240, 309
lipoxins, 180
liver damage, from paracetamol overdosage, 173, 174
local
    effect, of pain stimuli, 70
    twitch response, 273
locus coeruleus, 331
long-term
    depression, 306, 370
    low back pain, 30, 191, 201, 246, 281, 342, 363, 367
        surgical treatment of, 342
    potentiation, 306, 370
low threshold mechanoreceptors (LTM), 238
LPb, 82
LTD, 305, 370
LTP, 305, 370
lumbar epidural blockade, 346
Lyrica, 320

## M

magnetoencephalography, 85
maladaption, 368
manual acupuncture, 331
matters of the mind, 75
mechanoreceptors, 114
    low threshold, 74
MEG, 85
Meissner's plexus, 118
mental activity, and pathological pain, 306
mesencephalic tegmentum, 334
metabolic causes, 51
metformin, 321
methadone, 178
methylcyanobalmin, 341
microglia, 288, 305, 358
    and central sensitization, 302
microvascular decompression, 138, 336, 338
    disorders, 138, 254
    operation, 254
Minnesota Multiphasic Personality Inventory, 33

minocycline, 186, 194, 290, 302, 303, 305, 358, 360
    action of, 304
    and neuroprotection, 303
    and opioid tolerance, 290
    in strokes, 287
mirror box, 348
mirrors, use of, 347
misconceptions, regarding side effects of pain medications, 187
MK 801, 195, 289, 353
MMPI, see Minnesota Multiphasic Personality Inventory
modulation
    of pain, 45
    of pathological pain, 293
    of physiological pain, 153
monoideism, 40
mononeuralgies, 147
mononeuritis, 146
mononeuropathies, 137, 140
mood, 155
morphine, 155, 178
    analgesia, enhancing, 288
    induced respiratory depression, 360
motoneuron, 262
motor cortical areas, 239
Motrin, 170
MRI, 168
muscle
    pain, 234, 261
    spasm, 266
        treatment of pain from, 349
    tone, 263
MVD, 138, 336, 338
myalgia, 265
myocardial infarctions, risk of from NSAID, 172
myofascial pain, 269, 273
myositis, 262

# N

naloxone, 163, 303
naproxen, 170
NA-serotonin pathway, 97, 104, 164
negative
    feedback, 156
    influence, of pain, 24
nerve
    compression, 141
    growth factor, 363
    injuries, cause of, 139, 149
    root compression, 51
    stump, surgical treatment of, 362
nervi nervorum, 51, 140, 144, 148, 213
neural
    pathways, for itch, 106
    plasticity, 52, 138, 193, 366, 367
        activation of, 371

    transmitters, in peripheral sensitization, 157
neuralgia, 137
neuritis, 146
neuroanatomy, of somatic pain, 75
neuroimmune reaction, 358
neurokinase A, 70
neuromas, formation of, 148
neuromodulation, 191, 323
neurontin, 320
neuropathy, 136
    as a side effect of medical treatment, 191
    peripheral nerve, 188
neuroprotection, 303
neurotism, 33
neurotrophic factors, 211
neurotrophines, 213
NG, 115
NGF, 363
niacin, 190
nitric oxide (NO), 281
NKA, 70
NMDA, 194, 332, 353
    receptor, 207, 296, 353
        and sensitization, 186
N-methyl-D-aspartate, see NMDA
nociceptive pain, 196
nociceptors, 29, 45, 72
nodose ganglia, 115
non-active treatment, 352
non-classical pathways, 81, 92
non-steroidal anti-inflammatory drugs, 155, 169, 280, 300, 302, 313, 343, 354
    action of, 170, 175
    antipyretic effect of, 176
noradrenalin, see norepinephine
norepinephrine, 156, 211
nortriptylin, 313
NSAID, see non-steroidal anti-inflammatory drugs,
NST, see nucleus of the solitary tract
nucleus basalis, see nucleus of Meynert
nucleus of Meynert, 89
nucleus of the solitary tract, 82, 88, 123, 125, 328
nucleus tractus solitarii, see nucleus of the solitary tract

# O

obsessive-compulsive disorders, 132
off-cells, 178
omega-3, 170, 180, 313, 352, 355
    substances derived from, 180
omega-6, 355
on-cells, 178
opiates, 177

opioid, 177, 354
   and apoptosis, 290
   action of, 177
   addiction to, 184
   endogenous, 163
   pain relieving effects, and glia cells, 304
   receptors, 177, 290
   tolerance, 290
oxycodone, 178
oxymorphone, 178

# P

PAF, 160
PAG, 23, 97, 178

pain
   after strokes, 231
   and cognition, 32
   and immune reactions, 358
   and stress, 352
   hypersensitivity, 295
   medication, 168
     administration of, 182
   receptors, 72
     throughout muscles, 262
   reducing the risk of, 361
painful diabetic neuropathy, 188, 337, 364
parabrachial nucleus, 331
paracetamol, 170
   and liver damage, 173
   combined with opioids, 175
parallel processing, 214
parasympathetic efferent pathways, 114
paresthesia, 140, 270
Parkinson's disease, 233, 276
pathological pain, 26, 40, 47, 196
   central control of, 295
   modulation of, 293
Pavlovian conditioning, 155
PBN, 331
PDN, 181, 188, 337, 340, 364
Penfield, 220
pentoxifylline, 186
penumbra, 287
perception of
perception of
   pain, 24
   self, 227, 228, 347
periaqueductal gray, 23, 97, 178, 258, 306, 352
peripheral
   control of central pain, 295
   nerve neuropathy, 188
     as side effect of therapy, 191
   nerve stimulation, 324
   nerves, 135, 282
   sensitization, 72, 155, 157
peroneal nerve, 145
personality profiles, 33

PET scans, 36 298
phantom limb
   limb syndrome, 196, 206, 222
     neurophysiological basis for, 349
   pain, 44
     reducing risk of, 193
   perceptions, 24, 44
phantom sensations, 206
pharmacogenetic testing, 309
phenytoin, 339
PHN, 192, 303, 337, 340, 360
physical exercise, 335
physiological pain, 26, 47, 367
   central modulation of, 96
pins and needles, 140
pituitary-adrenal axis, 329
placebo effect, 155, 187, 298, 352
plastic changes, 152, 223
plasticity diseases, 366
platelet activating factor, 160
pleasant touch, stimulation of C-fibers, 74
pleasure, from scratching, 107
PLP, 44
PMA, 326
polyneuropathies, 137, 145
positive feedback, 156, 241
positron emission tomography, 298
post herpetic neuralgia, 192, 303, 337, 360
post traumatic stress disorders, 132
posterior cingulate, 108
postoperative pain, 192
prefrontal cortex, 211, 352
pregabalin, 320, 340
premotor area, 108, 234, 326, 345
pressure hyperalgesia, 295
prevalence of pain, 55
primary
   motor cortex, 345
   somatosensory cortex, 82, 345
pro-inflammatory cytokines, 289, 359
pro-resolving lipid mediators, 180
prostacyclines, 170
prostaglandins, 170, 356
   and central sensitization, 300
   sensitizing effect of, 176
prostaglandin D, 301
prostaglandin $E_2$, 7, 15, 170, 281, 297
prostaglandin $E_3$, 356
prostanoids
   and central sensitization, 300
proteins
   misfolded, 283
   synthesis of, 369
PTSD, 132
punishment, pain as a, 45
puritus, 104
purposefulness of pain, 38

## Q

quality of life, 25

## R

RA, see rheumatoid arthritis
Ramsay-Hunt syndrome, 146, 147
randomized controlled trials, 345
raphe nucleus, 89, 97
RCT, 345
RDA, 190

receptors
    of visceral pain, 113
    opioid, 177
    pain, 29, 72
        innervation of, 73
recommended daily allowance, 190
reducing risk
    of pain, 192
    of postoperative pain, 192
referred pain, 112, 127
reflex sympathetic dystrophy, 31, 242, 350
reorganization of central pain pathways, 216
repetitive transcranial magnetic stimulation, 327
resolvins, 180
respiratory suppression, from opioids, 179
resting muscle tone, 264
restless legs syndrome, 267
reward system, 211, 309
Reye's syndrome, and Aspirin, 172
rhabdomyolysis, 267
rheumatoid arthritis, 44, 279, 282, 290
rostral ventromedial medulla, 98, 178, 305
RSD, 31, 350
rTMS, 327
RVM, 98, 178, 305

## S

schizophrenia, 132
sciatic nerve, 145
sciatica, 143, 248, 344
secondary somatosensory cortex, 82, 108
secosteroid, 341
secretion of noradrenalin, by C-fibers, 157
selective serotonin re-uptake inhibitors, 179, 340
self,
    perception of, 347
    experience, 22
    inflicted pain, 44
semi-synthetic opioids, 155

sensitization
    central, 300
    of receptors, 156
    peripheral, 72
serotonin, 105, 157, 171, 281
    noradrenalin reuptake inhibitors, 340
severed nerves, 148
sexual functions, 329
shingles, 146, 147, 339
SII, 82, 108
slightly injured nerves, 149
SMA, 326
SMP, 47, 350
SNRI, 340
somatic pain, 26, 29, 68
    neuroanatomy of, 75
somatosensory cortices, 45
somatotopic organization, of the insula, 90
spasm, 145, 367
spasmodic torticollis, 268
spasticity, 367
spinal cord injuries, 231
spinal stenosis, 252
spinoreticular tracts, 86
spinothalamic tracts, 75, 80, 162, 299
    anterior part, 83
    lateral part of, 81
SPM, 180
spondylitis, 281
sprouting, of axons, 148
SSRI, 179, 340
stents, 122
stomach bleeding, risk of, 171
stretch receptors, 114
strokes, ischemic, 287
STT, 75, 80, 162, 299
substance abuse, 185
substance P, 70
substantia gelantinosa, 76
suffering, 23, 24
supplemental areas, SMA, 234, 326
surgical
    operations, severed nerves, 148
    treatment of pain, 191, 336
    treatment, of low back pain, 342
sympathectomy, 351
sympathetic nervous system, 52, 130, 156, 224, 241, 291, 297
    central action of, 297
sympathetically maintained pain, 47, 350
sympatholytica, 351
synaptic efficacy, 369
synthesis of proteins, 369
synthetic opioids, 155

## T

tapentadol, 179
Taxol, 140, 145, 191
Tegretol, 338
telescoping, 349
temporal
    integration, 253
    summation, 295
temporo-mandibular joint disorders, 271, 334
tenderness, 273
tendinitis, 267
TENS, see transderm electrical nerve stimulation,
tension headaches, 265
TGN, 138, 225, 319, 336, 337, 338
thalamic
    pain, 30
    syndrome, 196
thalamo-cortical dysrythmia, 226
Thalidomide, 354
The International Association for the Study of Pain (IASP), 21
thiamine, 341
Thromboxane, 170, 301, 356
tic douleroux, see trigeminal neuralgia, 138
Tinel sign, 142
tinnitus, 79, 204
    retraining therapy, 25
tissue damage, 71
TMD, 334
TMS, 308, 345
TNF-α, 211, 249, 289, 306
tolerance, 184
    opioid, 290
top-down, 47
    communication of pain signals, 75
torture, 45
tramadol, 179
transcranial magnetic stimulation, 229, 308, 345
transderm electrical nerve stimulation, 155, 162, 191, 295, 321, 324, 335
trauma, to peripheral nerves, 148
treatment of
    pain, 48, 191
        methods for, 319
        surgical, 336
    pathological pain, 311
    physiological pain, 165
    specific pain disorders, 337
treatments
    administration of, 335
    non-drug, 321
    related to autonomic nervous system, 350
tricyclic antidepressants, 340
trigeminal neuralgia, 79, 137, 254, 319, 336, 337, 338
    treatment of, 338
trigeminal nucleus, 75, 78, 236
    caudal part, 78
trigeminothalamic tract, 80, 81
trigger point, 269
trismus, 268
TRPV1, 114, 120, 133, 158
TRT, 25
TTT, 80, 81
tumor necrosis factor-alpha, 211, 289, 306
TX, 301
Tylenol, see paracetamol, 170

## U

Ulnar nerve entrapment, 145, 319
uremia, 104

## V

vaculities, 146
vagus nerve, 115, 122, 125, 323
    and immune reactions, 125
    and visceral pain, 123
    stimulation, 124, 285, 329
valporate, 195
vanilliod receptors, 158
varicella zoster virus, 146, 147
VAS, 341
ventral
    posterior inferior thalamus, 82
    posterior lateral thalamus , 82
    thalamus, 75
    ventromedial posterior thalamus, 93
vicious circle, 156
vincristine, 145
Vviral infections, 51, 147, 192
visceral
    pain, 26, 29
    sensations, 89
viscero-sensory cortex, 132
visual analog scales, 341
vitamins, 140, 145, 313, 352
    $B_1$ and $B_{12}$, 140, 340, 354
        as pain medications, 181
    $B_3$, 190
    D (D3) , 190, 314, 341, 354
    deficiencies, 137
VMpo, 93, 107
VNS, 124, 323, 329
Voltaren, see diclofenac, 170
VZV, 146, 147

## W

Wallerian degeneration, 158
WHO, see World Health Organization
wide dynamic range neurons, 237, 297
withdrawal reflex, 40, 71, 75
World Health Organization, 185

Made in the USA
San Bernardino, CA
06 August 2014